AN ATLAS OF
DIAGNOSTIC RADIOLOGY
IN GASTROENTEROLOGY

An Atlas of Diagnostic Radiology in Gastroenterology

RAMSAY VALLANCE

MB, ChB, FRCS (Glasg), FRCR, DMRD
Consultant Radiologist
West Glasgow Hospitals University NHS Trust
Honorary Clinical Senior Lecturer in Radiology
University of Glasgow

With contributions by

RICHARD D. EDWARDS
MRCP, FRCR

J. GRAEME HOUSTON
MA, MRCP, FRCR

ALISON McLEAN
FRCP, FRCR

b

Blackwell
Science

This book is dedicated with love to
Norma, Laura, Gillian and Elizabeth

© 1999 by
Blackwell Science Ltd
Editorial Offices:
Osney Mead, Oxford OX2 0EL
25 John Street, London WC1N 2BL
23 Ainslie Place, Edinburgh EH3 6AJ
350 Main Street, Malden
  MA 02148 5018, USA
54 University Street, Carlton
  Victoria 3053, Australia
10, rue Casimir Delavigne
  75006 Paris, France

Other Editorial Offices:
Blackwell Wissenschafts-Verlag GmbH
Kurfürstendamm 57
10707 Berlin, Germany

Blackwell Science KK
MG Kodenmacho Building
7–10 Kodenmacho Nihombashi
Chuo-ku, Tokyo 104, Japan

First published 1999

Set by Excel Typesetters Co., Hong Kong
Printed and bound in Great Britain
at the University Press, Cambridge

A catalogue record for this title is available
from the British Library

ISBN 0-632-05022-5

Library of Congress
Cataloging-in-publication Data

Vallance, Ramsay.
    An atlas of diagnostic radiology in
gastroenterology/Ramsay Vallance;
with contributions by Richard D. Edwards,
Graeme Houston, Alison McLean.
        p.   cm.
    Includes bibliographical references.
    ISBN 0-632-05022-5
    1. Digestive organs—Radiography
—Atlases.   I. Title.
    [DNLM: 1. Digestive System Diseases
—diagnosis atlases.
    WI 17 V177a   1998]
RC804.R6V34   1998
616.3'0754—dc21
DNLM/DLC
for Library of Congress   98-15826
                                CIP

DISTRIBUTORS

Marston Book Services Ltd
PO Box 269
Abingdon, Oxon OX14 4YN
(*Orders*: Tel: 01235 465500
            Fax: 01235 465555)

USA
Blackwell Science, Inc.
Commerce Place
350 Main Street
Malden, MA 02148 5018
(*Orders*: Tel: 800 759 6102
                781 388 8250
            Fax: 781 388 8255)

Canada
Login Brothers Book Company
324 Saulteaux Crescent
Winnipeg, Manitoba R3J 3T2
(*Orders*: Tel: 204 837-2987)

Australia
Blackwell Science Pty Ltd
54 University Street
Carlton, Victoria 3053
(*Orders*: Tel: 3 9347 0300
            Fax: 3 9347 5001)

For further information on
Blackwell Science, visit our website:
www.blackwell-science.com

Contents

Foreword

In my days as one of three junior house officers in the University Department of Surgery at the Western Infirmary in Glasgow, headed by the late Sir Charles Illingworth, we were beholden to have the previous days radiographs available for the morning ward round, and woe betide us if we failed to retrieve these from the Department of Radiology. Woe betide us also if we did not ensure that the plates were returned to the Department of Radiology immediately after the ward round so that they could, as we were reminded, 'be properly examined and correctly reported'. In those days the range of radiological examinations, in respect of the gastrointestinal tract, comprised straight films, barium studies, cholecystograms and, occasionally, angiographic studies.

To us, as junior house officers, these plates were often of an unconvincing grey appearance, impossible to decipher. However, double contrast barium enemas were being introduced at about this time and even we could appreciate the greater detail which they showed (not that our opinion was ever sought). We were often initially impressed by the apparent interpretative skills of the senior surgeons using the windows as viewing boxes, but we realized the greater skills which the radiologist required in producing the definitive report, a report which was as avidly sought by the surgeon prior to operative intervention as the plates had been on a preliminary ward round.

I contrast these early experiences with the illustrations which are presented in this atlas, illustrations which are of superb artistic merit but, in addition, show in much greater detail a wide range of pathology in the alimentary tract. This indeed is an atlas of macroscopic pathology (together with some normal anatomy) produced by virtue of the increased sophistication introduced by improved imaging techniques such as spiral CT, magnetic resonance and digital-subtraction angiography. Interventional radiology has not been included but I am aware of the still further sophistication which this has introduced into radiology. Thus, over the past 15–20 years there has been a blossoming of radiology such that in the investigation of the gastrointestinal tract and liver, indeed of all body organs, the radiologist plays a key role in establishing many clinical diagnoses. The definitive tissue diagnosis may be with the histopathologists but in many instances this simply serves to confirm the radiological diagnosis. Radiologists and histopathologists thus frequently operate together to establish the clinical diagnosis which determines patient management. Our two specialities work closely together and in each the use of pattern recognition establishes our key roles in the provision of the clinical services.

It has been a great pleasure for me to study this atlas and to more fully appreciate the advances which have taken place in gastrointestinal radiology. I welcome the emphasis Dr Vallance and his colleagues have placed on the role of diagnostic radiology in the investigation of gastrointestinal disease. The aims which he has set out in his preface have been abundantly met. This volume brings credit to radiology as a discipline.

Roddy MacSween
Glasgow, August 1998

Preface

The practice of gastrointestinal radiology is at the present time undergoing an exciting process of rapid change. Partly in response to demands to reduce the dose of ionizing radiation, the traditional methods of plain film radiography and barium studies have to a considerable extent given way to alternative imaging methods and endoscopy. At the same time, a much greater emphasis on subspecialization in diagnostic radiology is emerging, actively promoted by the Royal College of Radiologists. These parallel developments call for a much more focused, systematic approach to training in gastrointestinal radiology.

The purpose of this completely new publication, consisting very largely of previously unpublished material, is to illustrate in the form of an atlas, a wide range of pathology in the alimentary tract and its accessory organs in a systematic fashion, integrating the principal imaging modalities currently in use. A cursory glance will show that it is not a textbook and it therefore needs to be used in conjunction with a standard text. Carefully selected references have been included to encourage further reading. A comprehensive mix of ultrasound, spiral CT, magnetic resonance and digital-subtraction angiography is combined with a wide range of conventional plain films and barium studies to highlight all of the important radiological signs of disease in the alimentary tract. Of necessity, in a compact volume of this kind, I have had to be selective, so that topics in paediatric radiology and nuclear medicine have not been included, and interventional radiology is outside the scope of this title.

The highest possible technical standards, with a distinct emphasis on image quality, have been employed to display normal structures, as well as morbid anatomy, in a format that is not currently available. This work is intended to meet some of the needs of the radiologist in training, the practising gastrointestinal radiologist, physicians and surgeons in gastroenterology and also radiographers whose task it is to provide high-quality images in the alimentary tract and its accessory organs. I hope, therefore, that it will make a modest contribution to education in the rapidly expanding field of alimentary tract diagnostic imaging. In addition, I hope very much that it might encourage and stimulate those who strive to improve patient care in the field of clinical radiology.

Ramsay Vallance

Acknowledgements

So many have contributed to the publication of this atlas. I am very glad of this opportunity to express my thanks to each and all of them. When Professor R.N.M. MacSween kindly agreed to write the foreword, I was tremendously encouraged and greatly honoured. The readiness of Dr Alison McLean, Dr Richard Edwards and Dr Graeme Houston to contribute their widely acclaimed expertise from the fields of endoscopic ultrasound, angiography and magnetic resonance is very much appreciated. I am also indebted to Dr Marie Callaghan and Dr Alasdair Taylor who have so generously provided additional material in CT cholangiography and MR respectively, and to Dr Peter Mills and Mr Grant Fullarton for ERCP cases. Individual cases have also been contributed by colleagues, for which I am most grateful, and I have endeavoured to acknowledge all of these in the text. It is a great pleasure for me to thank the numerous radiographers, particularly at Gartnavel General Hospital, whose technical contributions have made this work possible.

Typing the manuscript has been a monumental task and Ms Linda Chambers has fulfilled this role with great expertise, patience and remarkable cheerfulness. Thanks are due also to Ms Kathy McFall for assistance with medical illustration. I am greatly indebted to Dr Stuart Taylor, senior editor at Blackwell Science, for his encouragement and guidance, without whose initial enthusiasm this atlas would not have been written. I am also grateful to Ms Jane Andrew, production editor at Blackwell Science, for her professional skills in fashioning the raw material into the finished work, and to Ms Caroline Sheard for her expertise in compiling the index.

Finally, my wife and family have been very patient and a source of great encouragement during these months of preparation. Thank you!

Ramsay Vallance

1: The Salivary Glands and Pharynx

Introduction

The principal salivary glands consist of the paired parotid, submandibular and sublingual glands. The parotid is irregularly shaped like an inverted pyramid lying in the prestyloid portion of the parapharyngeal space (PPS), between the mastoid process posteriorly and the ramus of mandible anteriorly [1]. Its anterior process extends over the masseter muscle and it has two posterior processes, one of which lies between the mastoid process and the sternomastoid muscle and the other anterior to the styloid process in the retropharyngeal space (RPS). Its large, single (Stenson's) duct opens on to a papilla in the mouth opposite the second upper molar tooth. The submandibular gland lies below the mandible, is approximately 50% of the size of the parotid, is triangular in shape and is drained by Wharton's duct on to a papilla in the floor of the mouth adjacent to the frenulum of the tongue.

The salivary glands are usually investigated by conventional radiography [2]. Plain films are of use in showing calculi and soft-tissue swelling. Further information can be obtained by means of sialography, in which the appropriate duct orifice is intubated by means of a metal cannula or fine polythene catheter, approximately 0.5–1.5 ml of contrast medium — for example, Lipiodol ultrafluid — is injected and appropriate films are obtained.

Ultrasound (US) is able to image all three major salivary glands and to detect most pathology [3]. In many cases, it is the first imaging procedure [4]. Success depends upon combining multiple scanning planes and high-resolution, real-time transducers, varying between 5 and 10 MHz. On US, the parotid gland has a homogeneous texture, but marginal definition is indistinct and the deep portion of the gland cannot be evaluated [1, 3]. The parotid duct may be visualized and in expert hands, with high-resolution transducers, the facial nerve may be recognized in one-third of subjects [3]. The submandibular gland has a homogeneous texture on US, similar to the parotid.

On computerized tomography (CT), the parotid and submandibular glands are visible without contrast enhancement, but the assessment of disease normally requires intravenous (IV) contrast and dynamic scanning [5].

Magnetic resonance imaging (MRI), by virtue of its exquisite soft-tissue contrast, is able to depict the three main salivary glands with great clarity. On T_1-weighted and T_2-weighted images, the parotid gives a higher signal than the others because of its increased fat content [6]. The facial nerve can be clearly delineated by modern MR techniques. A major limitation of MR is its inability to detect calcification, which can be readily depicted on CT with a high degree of sensitivity. However, CT images may be severely degraded by the presence of dental amalgam.

According to Rubesin and Yousem [7], the pharynx is the crossroads of speech, swallowing and respiration. Consequently, disorders of the pharynx may present in a variety of ways to a variety of clinics and it is not unusual for lesions of the pharynx to manifest themselves by recurrent pneumonia. The pharynx is a funnel-shaped musculomembranous tube and extends for approximately 12 cm from the base of the skull to the lower margin of the cricoid cartilage. It is bounded posteriorly by the cervical spine, the prevertebral muscles and the loose areolar tissue of the RPS. Laterally, the pharynx is bounded by the muscles of the neck, the lateral portions of the hyoid bone and thyroid cartilage and the carotid sheath. Arbitrarily, it is subdivided into three zones, namely: (i) the nasopharynx, which is primarily a respiratory tract structure; (ii) the oropharynx, which is limited superiorly by the soft palate and inferiorly by the hyoid bone; (iii) the hypopharynx, which includes the piriform fossae, lies posterior and lateral to the larynx and extends from the hyoid bone level to the lower margin of the cricopharyngeus muscle at the level of the inferior border of the cricoid cartilage, where it is continuous with the oesophagus. The pharynx forms a propulsive conduit, conducting the food bolus from the mouth to the oesophagus and functioning in conjunction with the laryngeal muscles to protect the upper airway [8]. The nerve supply of the pharynx is vital. Sensory stimuli that initiate swallowing are transmitted centrally via the superior laryngeal nerves. The pharyngeal muscles required for swallowing are controlled by the cranial nerves V, VII, IX, X, XI and XII. The upper oesophageal sphincter, formed by the cricopharyngeus muscle, is closed at rest and relaxes when the pharynx contracts [9]. Laxity of the mucosa over the submucosal venous plexus behind the cricoid frequently produces a variable filling defect on the anterior wall of the pharynx during swallowing. This postcricoid impression is commonly seen in the fully distended hypopharynx on barium studies. It is of no pathological significance and is seen in 80% of normal adults [10].

The RPS is located between the visceral compartment anteriorly and the prevertebral space (PVS) posteriorly and extends from the base of skull to the level of T3. Retropharyngeal lymph nodes are present only in the suprahyoid portion of the RPS, whereas the infrahyoid portion contains only fat [11]. Lymphoma and lymph-node metastases are common in the RPS. Abscesses and primary tumours occur rarely in this compartment, but these conditions may extend from a neighbouring fascial space into the RPS much more commonly. The PVS is separated from the RPS by the deep (prevertebral) layer of the deep cervical fascia. This compartment is continuous posterolaterally with the paraspinal space and contains the vertebral artery and vein, phrenic nerve and brachial plexus. Lesions in the PVS originate commonly in the cervical spine and include spondylosis, metastases and infective spondylitis. The PVS is completely enclosed by the deep cervical fascia. The PPS, consisting of prestyloid and poststyloid compartments, has no mucosa, muscle, bone, lymph-node or salivary-gland tissue, except for the parotid gland in its superficial portion. Disease uncommonly originates in the PPS. Instead, this largely fatty, tubular compartment, extending from the base of skull to the superior margin of the hyoid, acts as an 'elevator shaft', through which infection and neoplasm originating in adjacent spaces may travel [11].

Plain film radiography

Plain film radiography is particularly valuable in the assessment of trauma and the impaction of foreign bodies, and the hyoid bone can be clearly seen. The thickness of the prevertebral muscle layer may be determined, together with pathology in the vertebral bodies—for example, Forestier's disease [8, 12, 13].

Barium and other contrast studies

Barium and other contrast studies are valuable in providing both morphological and functional information, in the form of high-resolution, real-time images. The double-contrast technique enables the mucosa to be examined in detail. This method is greatly enhanced by fluoroscopy, with or without video or cine recording.

Cross-sectional imaging

The extramucosal anatomy is depicted in unparalleled detail by cross-sectional imaging, namely CT, MR and US. Both MR and CT are particularly valuable for tumour staging and the demonstration of central nervous system (CNS) and peripheral nerve lesions responsible for pharyngeal disorders. Magnetic resonance has become the modality of choice for the detailed demonstration of adjacent structures and CNS lesions [8]. In addition, MR and, to a lesser extent, US provide unrestricted slice orientation and they share the advantage of producing no ionizing radiation. Magnetic resonance is not degraded by dental amalgam and bone. It is more expensive, is relatively poor in imaging bone structure and is contraindicated in patients with cardiac pacemakers and ferromagnetic implants—for example, aneurysm clips. Also, MR is degraded by motion artefact and, because of the relatively long acquisition time compared with CT and US, it is less appropriate for small children, the very elderly and severely sick and injured patients.

Selective angiography

Selective angiography has a limited role in pharyngeal disease, but is of value in assessment of vascular lesions and injuries—for example, in gunshot wounds and blunt trauma [14].

References

1 Candiani F. & Martinoli C. (1995) Salivary glands. In: Solbiati L. & Rizzatto G. (eds) *Ultrasound of Superficial Structures*. Edinburgh: Churchill Livingstone, 125–139.
2 Simpkins K.C. (1993) The salivary glands, pharynx and oesophagus. In: Sutton D. (ed.) *A Textbook of Radiology and Imaging*, 5th edn. Edinburgh: Churchill Livingstone, 755–787.
3 Derchi L.E. & Solbiati L. (1993) The salivary glands. In: Cosgrove D.O., Meire H. & Dewbury K. (eds) *Abdominal and General Ultrasound*, Vol. 2. Edinburgh: Churchill Livingstone, 677–681.
4 Gritzmann N. (1989) Sonography of the salivary glands. *American Journal of Roentgenology* **153**, 163–166.
5 Isherwood I. & Forbes W.StC. (1993) CT of salivary glands. In: Sutton D. (ed.) *A Textbook of Radiology and Imaging*, 5th edn. Edinburgh: Churchill Livingstone, 757–758.
6 Isherwood I. & Jenkins J.P.R. (1993) MRI of salivary glands. In: Sutton D. (ed.) *A Textbook of Radiology and Imaging*, 5th edn. Edinburgh: Churchill Livingstone, 758–759.
7 Rubesin S.E. & Yousem D.M. (1994) Pharynx: normal anatomy and techniques. In: Gore R.M., Levine M.S. & Laufer I. (eds) *A Textbook of Gastrointestinal Radiology*. Philadelphia: W.B. Saunders, 202–225.
8 Cunningham E.T., Jones B. & Donner M.W. (1994) Normal anatomy and techniques of examination of the pharynx. In: Freeny P.C. & Stevenson G.W. (eds) *Margulis and Burhenne's Alimentary Tract Radiology*, 5th edn. St Louis: Mosby, 94–113.
9 Bartram C.I. & Kumar P. (1981) *Clinical Radiology in Gastroenterology*. Oxford: Blackwell Scientific Publications, 1–49.
10 Dahnert W. (1996) *Radiology Review Manual*, 3rd edn. Baltimore: Williams & Wilkins, 621.
11 Burgener F.A. & Kormano M. (1996) *Differential Diagnosis in Computed Tomography*. Stuttgart: Thieme Medical Publishers.

12 Zerhouni E.A., Bosma G.F. & Donner M.W. (1987) Relationship of cervical spine disorders to dysphagia. *Dysphagia* **1**, 129–134.

13 Ekberg O. (1994) Benign structural diseases of the pharynx. In: Freeny P.C. & Stevenson G.W. (eds) *Margulis and Burhenne's Alimentary Tract Radiology*, 5th edn. St Louis: Mosby, 114–126.

14 Cross D.T., Kido D.K. & Moran C.J. (1997) Abnormalities of cerebral vessels. In: Baum S. (ed.) *Abrams' Angiography*, 4th edn. Boston: Little, Brown, 342–355.

Suggested further reading

Chapman A.H. (1998) The salivary glands, pharynx and oesophagus. In: Sutton D. (ed.) *Textbook of Radiology and Imaging*, 6th edn. Edinburgh: Churchill Livingstone, 789–827.

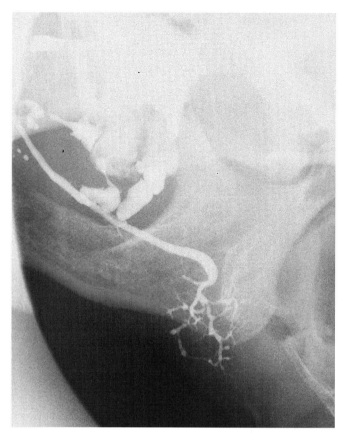

Fig. 1.1 Submandibular sialectasis. There was a history of intermittent swelling and pain in the right submandibular region. The submandibular sialogram shows normal filling of the main submandibular duct, but there is distortion of the tributaries, which have a stretched and tapered appearance, together with relatively slight punctate dilatation (grade 2/3) [2].

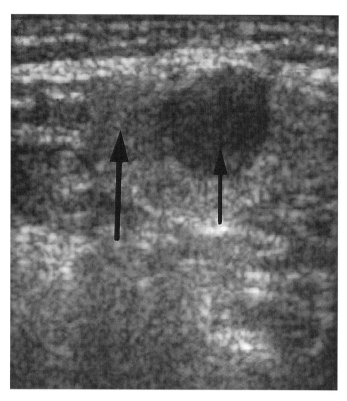

Fig. 1.2 Submandibular pleomorphic adenoma. A middle-aged female patient presented with several weeks' history of painless swelling in the left submandibular region. A 7 MHz US scan shows a solid low attenuation 11 mm mass lesion (small arrow) within the submandibular gland (large arrow). Surgical confirmation.

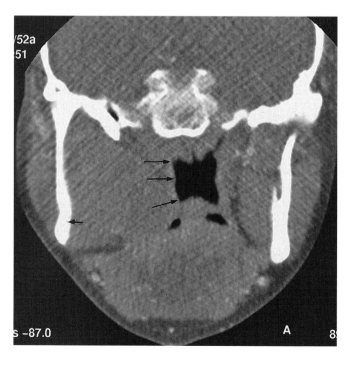

Fig. 1.3 Parotid pleomorphic adenoma. A 24-year-old female patient with increasing swelling in the oropharynx for several months. Coronal CT scan with 3 mm collimation shows marked soft-tissue swelling affecting the oropharynx on the left side, the medial margin of the lesion causing considerable encroachment on the airspace (large arrows). (Patient was scanned prone with neck extended.) The radiological appearance is non-specific. Provisional diagnosis was lymphoma; histological diagnosis was pleomorphic salivary adenoma. Small arrow, mandible.

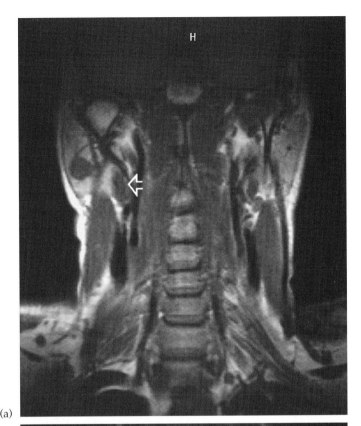

(a)

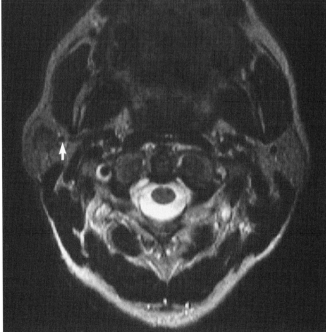

(b)

Fig. 1.4 Mucoepidermoid carcinoma of the parotid gland. (a) A 45-year-old female patient with 4 months' history of enlarging mass in the right side of neck. A coronal T_1 spin echo (SE) MRI scan of the neck shows a well circumscribed 1.5 cm low-signal mass in the superficial portion of the right parotid gland. A deep cervical lymph node (2 cm) is also visible (open arrow). (b) Axial T_2 fast spin echo (FSE) confirms a low-signal mass lateral to the retromandibular vein (small arrow). Surgical confirmation. (Courtesy of Dr J. Graeme Houston.)

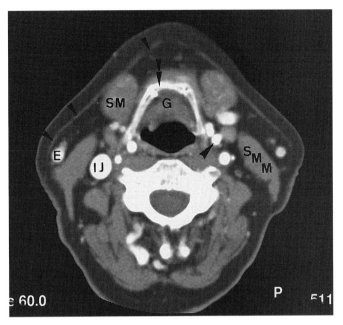

Fig. 1.5 Normal pharynx. Spiral contrast-enhanced CT (CECT) at the level of the hyoid bone (double arrowheads). The platysma is clearly shown (small arrowheads) as well as the right submandibular gland (SM) and left sternomastoid muscle (SMM). The pharyngeal airspace is limited anteriorly by the epiglottis and glossoepiglottic fold (G). E, external jugular vein; IJ, internal jugular vein; large arrowhead, left internal carotid artery.

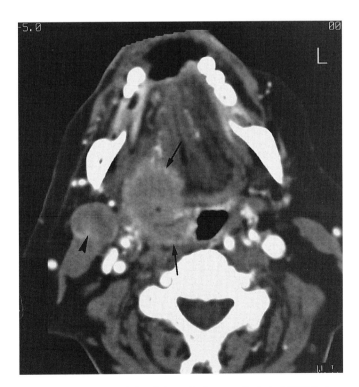

Fig. 1.6 Carcinoma of the right palatine tonsil. Spiral CECT at the level of the hard palate shows an irregular soft-tissue mass lesion (arrows) involving the posterolateral wall of the pharynx on the right side as well as the palate and partly obstructing the airspace. An enlarged lymph node is shown (arrowhead). Histological confirmation.

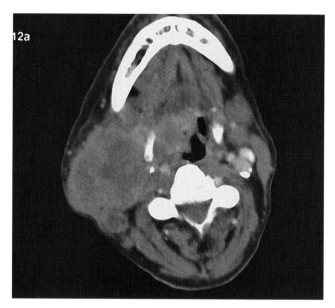

Fig. 1.7 Carcinoma of the tongue with massive lymphadenopathy. A 56-year-old male patient presented with right-sided neck swelling and increasing difficulty in swallowing. A spiral CECT shows massive soft-tissue swelling in the right side of the neck at the level of the upper border of the hyoid bone. This is in continuity with an infiltrative process, the medial extent of which seriously compromises the airspace of the pharynx.

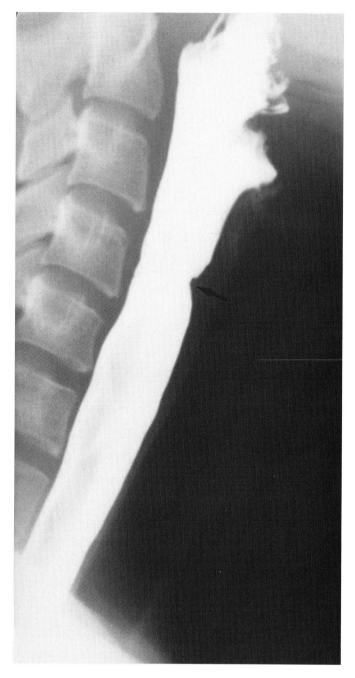

Fig. 1.8 Normal pharynx, barium swallow. A lateral projection of the pharynx and upper oesophagus filled with barium shows a normal anterior indentation (arrow) at C4 level. This is due to laxity of the mucosa over the submucosal venous plexus behind the cricoid cartilage. It is of no pathological significance [10]. the normal retropharyngeal space and prevertebral space together measure only a few millimetres.

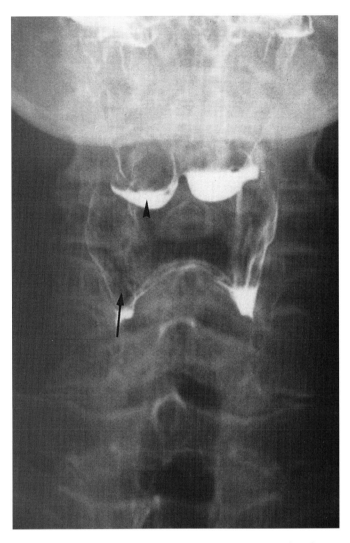

Fig. 1.9 Normal pharynx, barium swallow, AP view. After the passage of the bolus of barium, a small quantity is retained in the valleculae (arrowhead) and piriform fossae (arrow).

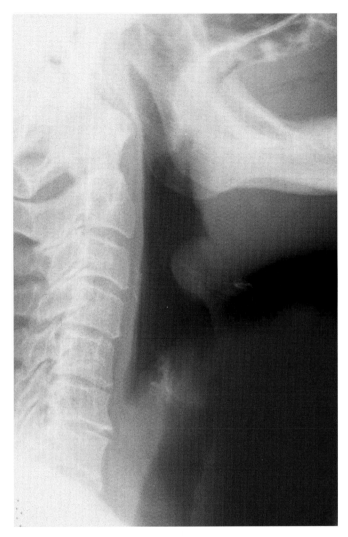

Fig. 1.10 Simple cyst of the epiglottis. Most patients who present with a feeling of something in the throat have no visible structural abnormality. This patient has a smooth mass lesion of soft-tissue density arising from the epiglottis on this soft-tissue lateral view of neck. Biopsy revealed a simple cyst. The differential diagnosis includes epiglottitis and carcinoma.

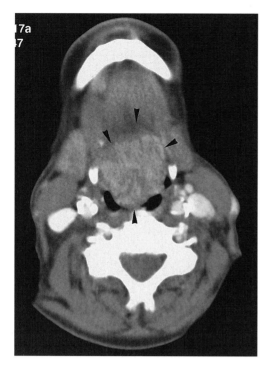

Fig. 1.11 Carcinoma of the epiglottis. Spiral CECT in a 67-year-old patient with increasing dysphagia. A solid mass lesion (arrowheads) almost completely obstructs the pharyngeal airspace immediately superior to the hyoid bone.

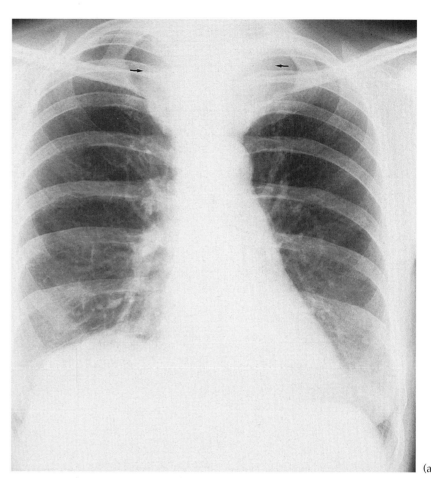

(a)

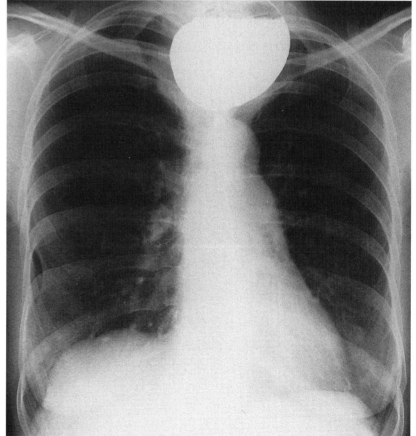

(b)

Fig. 1.12 Posterior pharyngeal pouch (Zenker's diverticulum). (a) This posteroanterior chest X-ray in a female patient with a long history of dysphagia, shows a marked, fairly symmetrical, soft-tissue swelling at the thoracic inlet (arrows). (b) Ten minutes following a barium-swallow examination, the soft-tissue swelling is represented by a large barium-filled Zenker's diverticulum.

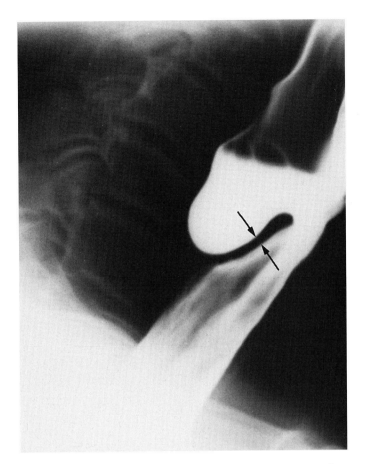

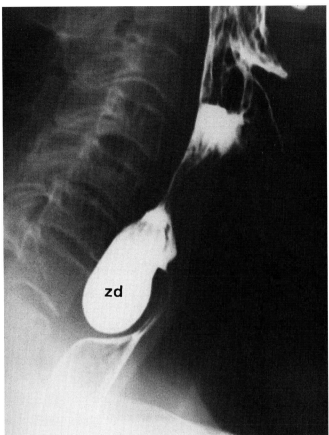

Fig. 1.13 Pharyngeal pouch (Zenker's diverticulum). A second patient with moderate dysphagia. The lateral filled view of the pharynx and upper oesophagus shows the characteristic posterior location of the pouch, the anterior wall of which, together with the posterior wall of the oesophagus, form a prominent spur (arrows). One method of treatment consists of division of the spur by diathermy between forceps introduced orally (Dohlmann's procedure).

Fig. 1.14 Posterior pharyngeal pouch. A larger diverticulum is seen to displace the upper oesophagus anteriorly and partly obstruct it. zd, Zenker's diverticulum.

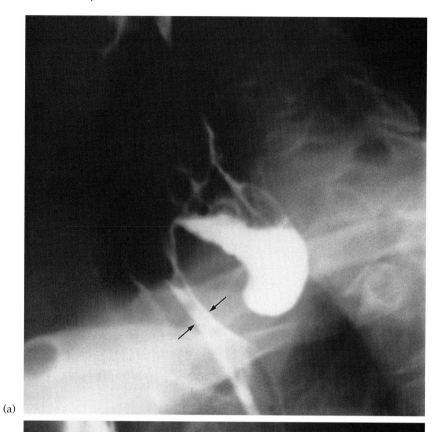

(a)

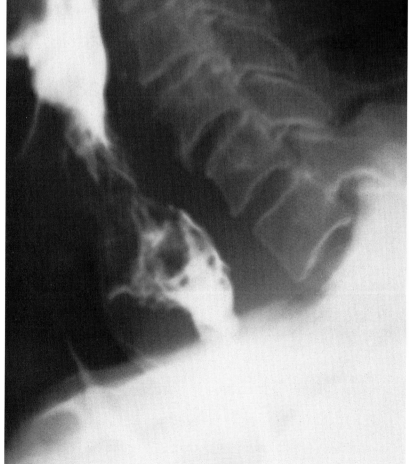

(b)

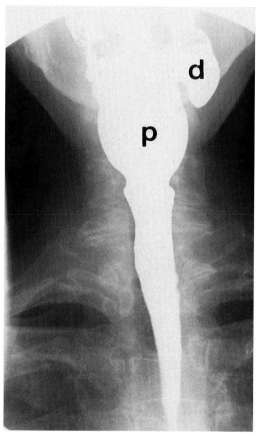

Fig. 1.16 Lateral pharyngeal diverticulum. An AP barium swallow shows transient filling of a lateral diverticulum ('pharyngeal ear'). This is likely to be the result of impaired tonicity of the pharyngeal constrictors. The condition may be bilateral. d, diverticulum; p, hypopharynx.

Fig. 1.15 Carcinoma arising within a Zenker's diverticulum. (a) A moderately large posterior pharyngeal pouch is shown in a patient with increasing dysphagia. The compressed oesophageal lumen is indicated by the arrows. The filling defects within the pouch were misinterpreted as a food residue. (b) Five months later, there is a more obvious irregular filling defect involving the lumen of the pouch, which also shows considerable loss of distensibility and an increase in the prevertebral space, in keeping with tumour infiltration of its wall. Histological confirmation.

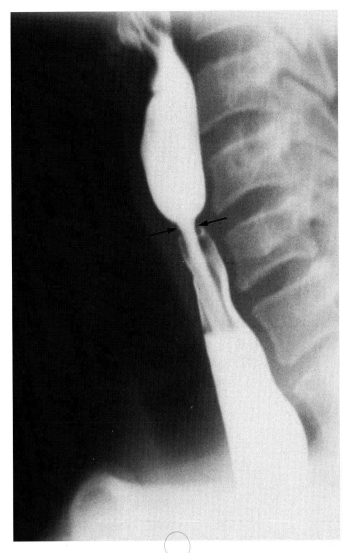

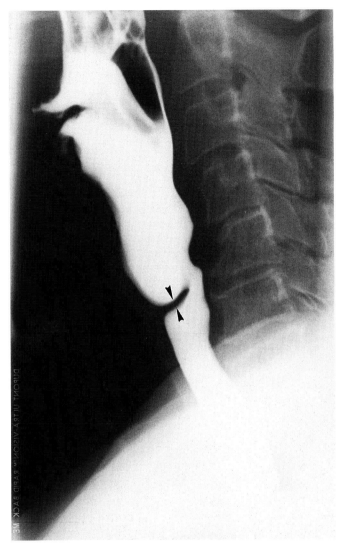

Fig. 1.17 Pharyngeal web. A lateral-projection barium swallow shows a clearly defined circumferential membrane with a central orifice (arrows) through which the barium is projected as a jet. This condition predisposes to malignancy.

Fig. 1.18 Pharyngeal web. A lateral barium swallow in a 60-year-old female patient with dysphagia shows a constant shelf-like anterior diaphragm arising from the wall of the pharynx 3 mm in thickness (arrowheads) at the level of the C5/6 disc space. This is the commonest site for cervical webs. In this patient, extrinsic impressions on the posterior wall of the pharynx are caused by marked changes of cervical spondylosis.

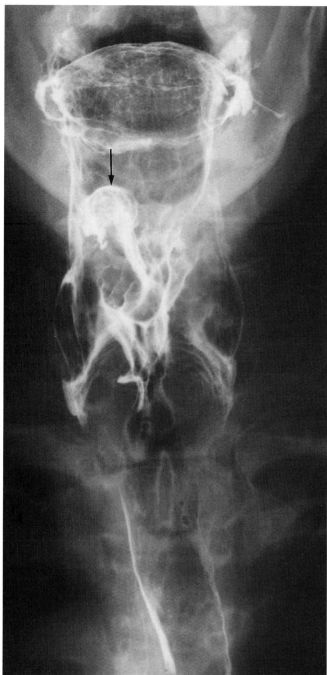

(a)

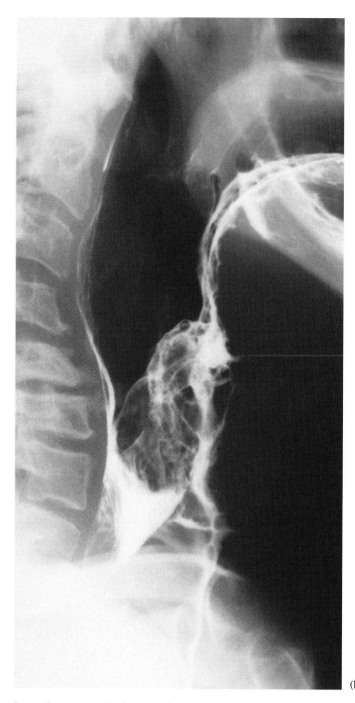

(b)

Fig. 1.19 Carcinoma of the hypopharynx. (a) Anteroposterior and (b) lateral projections of the pharynx during a barium swallow show a large, lobulated filling defect in the airspace of the hypopharynx, particularly on the right side (arrow). A small amount of contrast has been aspirated into the trachea.

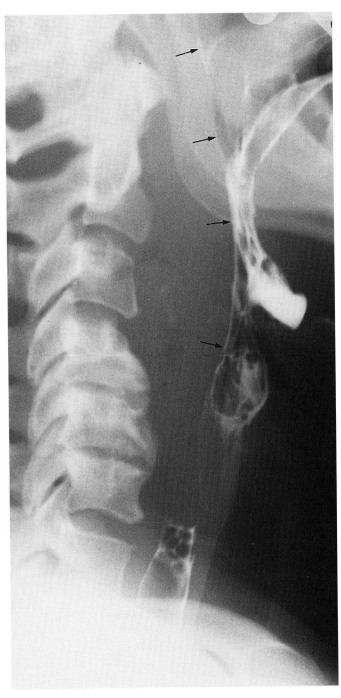

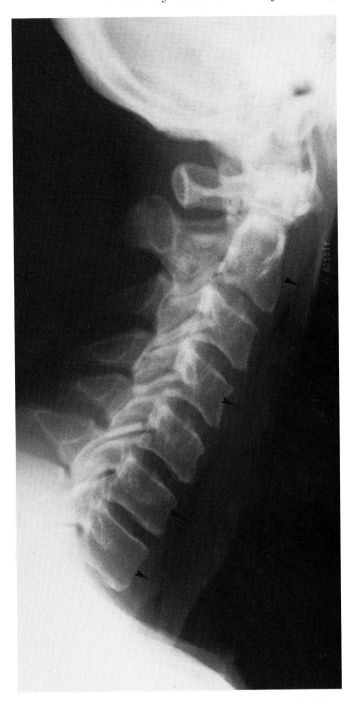

Fig. 1.20 Perforation of the pharynx. A 40-year-old female patient was stabbed in the side of the neck with a pair of scissors. A water-soluble contrast study at 72 h shows marked anterior displacement of the posterior wall of the pharynx right up to the base of the skull (arrows). No perforation site has been demonstrated at this stage, but pockets of air are shown in the soft tissues within a retropharyngeal haematoma. The patient was apyrexial and with a normal white-cell count. A retropharyngeal abscess could produce a similar appearance. Marked degenerative changes are shown in the lower cervical spine as an incidental finding.

Fig. 1.21 Pharyngeal perforation. This patient developed neck and throat pain after swallowing a chicken bone. This lateral soft-tissue neck view shows no foreign body, but a retropharyngeal track of air is shown in the soft tissues (arrowheads).

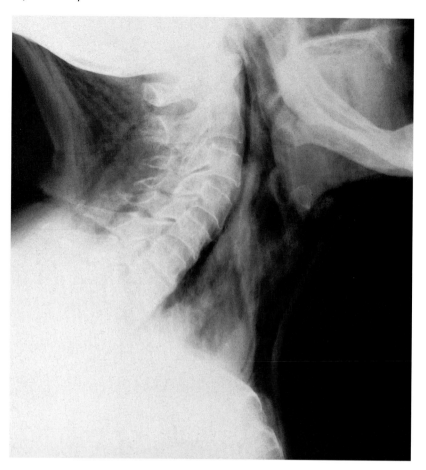

Fig. 1.22 Soft-tissue emphysema in the neck associated with perforation of the thoracic oesophagus. Spontaneous thoracic oesophageal perforation resulted in massive thoracic soft-tissue emphysema and a tension pneumothorax. The soft-tissue emphysema is seen to extend into the soft tissues of the neck.

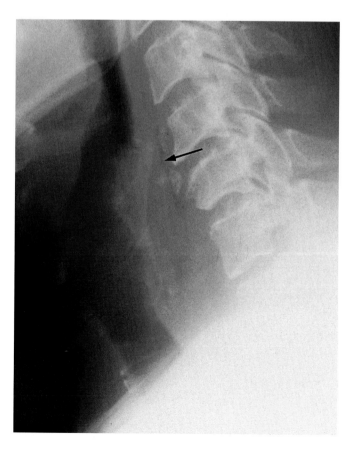

Fig. 1.23 Soft-tissue emphysema following sclerotherapy of oesophageal varices. Lateral view of the neck 2 h following injection of the oesophageal varices shows a small amount of air in the retropharyngeal space (arrow). More obvious soft-tissue emphysema was apparent in the mediastinum.

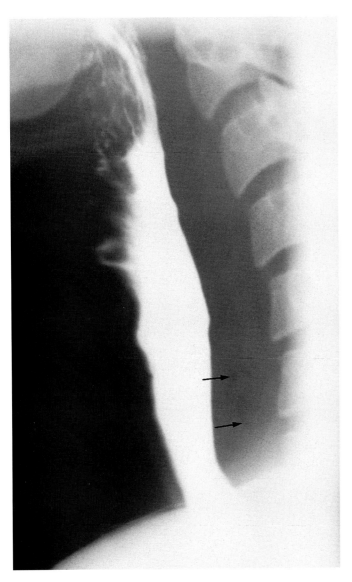

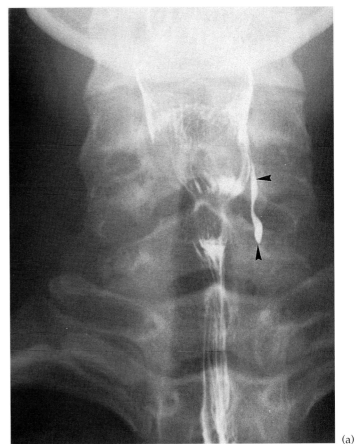

(a)

Fig. 1.24 Retropharyngeal abscess. A patient had severe throat pain with a high temperature and elevated white-cell count. The lateral barium swallow shows marked diffuse, retropharyngeal, soft-tissue swelling, with multiple bubbles of gas within the soft tissues (arrows).

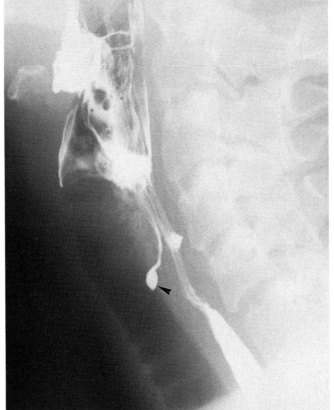

Fig. 1.25 Persistent fourth branchial arch sinus. A 20-year-old student nurse had multiple recurrences of a discharging abscess on the left side of her neck. (a) Anteroposterior and (b) lateral views of the barium swallow show a persistent track of barium extending downwards and anterolaterally from the left piriform sinus, with no communication with the skin surface at the time of the examination. The track is indicated by arrowheads.

(b)

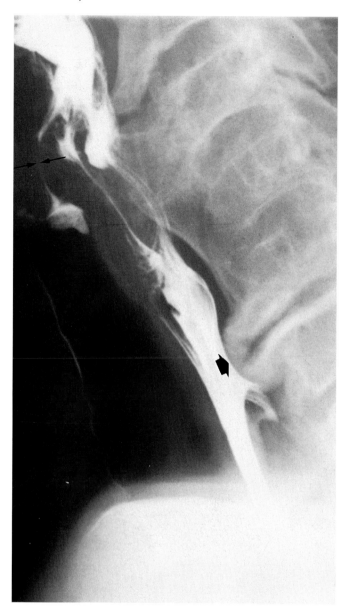

Fig. 1.26 Extrinsic compression of the pharynx by diffuse idiopathic skeletal hyperostosis (Forestier's disease). A lateral barium swallow in an elderly male patient with persistent dysphagia shows gross hypertrophic ankylosis in the cervical spine, producing marked deformity of the posterior wall of the pharynx (arrowhead) at multiple levels. If these changes are sufficiently severe, the normal closure of the airway by backward flexion of the epiglottis during swallowing may be prevented and aspiration may occur (arrows).

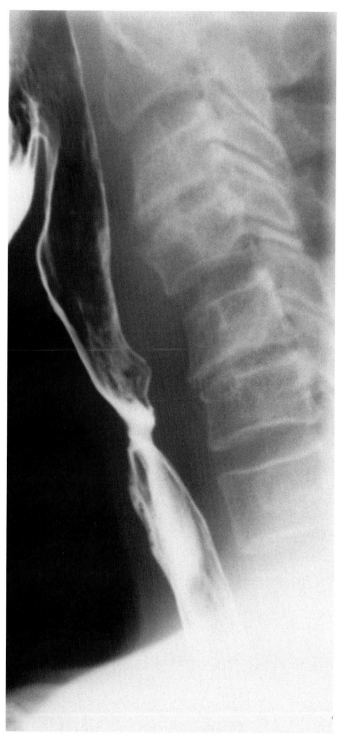

Fig. 1.27 Pharyngeal stricture following radiotherapy. A 69-year-old male patient had a total laryngectomy for carcinoma 3 years previously, followed by radiotherapy; he has had increasing dysphagia in recent weeks. The lateral barium swallow shows a persistent relatively smooth stricture of the pharynx at C5/6 level. The larynx has, of course, been removed. The differential diagnosis includes a circumferential web, pharyngeal carcinoma, peptic stricture, corrosive stricture and post-traumatic stricture.

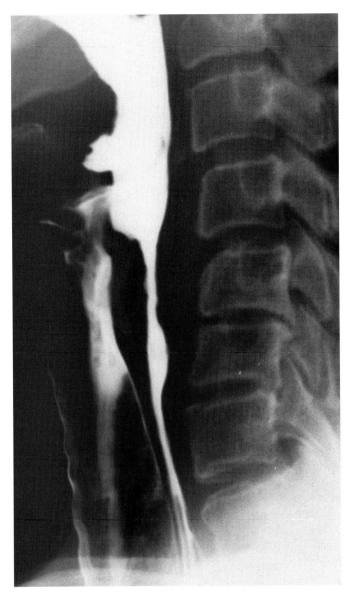

Fig. 1.28 Radiation-induced pharyngeal stricture. The lateral barium swallow shows a relatively smooth, tight postcricoid stricture in a patient with a previous history of radiotherapy. Aspiration of contrast into the airway is apparent. Recurrent chest infection is a common presentation of a variety of pharyngeal lesions.

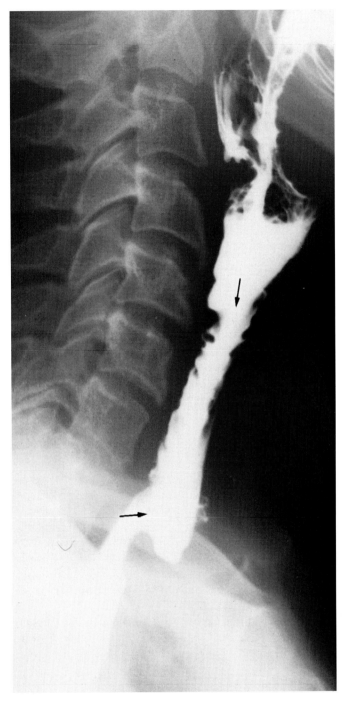

Fig. 1.29 Jejunal interposition following pharyngectomy and laryngectomy for carcinoma. A lateral barium swallow shows the typical mucosal pattern of jejunum in a patient in whom a segment of small bowel has been used to replace the hypopharynx. The proximal and distal anastomoses are indicated by the arrows.

2: The Oesophagus

Introduction

The morphology of the gullet is well adapted to its primary function in actively conveying food and liquids from the pharynx to the stomach. It has virtually no secretory or absorptive function. Lying mainly in the posterior mediastinum and measuring 20–24 cm in length, the oesophagus is lined by non-keratinizing squamous epithelium covering a lamina propria, which contains nerves and lymphatics, as well as blood vessels. The outer half of the oesophageal wall consists of a prominent muscularis arranged in an outer longitudinal and inner circular muscle layer. In the proximal third of the oesophagus, striated muscle predominates, reflecting the initial voluntary phase of swallowing. The striated muscle of the pharynx and upper third of the oesophagus has a motor nerve supply delivered via cranial nerves IX and X. In the distal half to two-thirds of the gullet, with a variable intermediate zone, the muscular wall consists of smooth muscle under control of the autonomic nervous system. This is responsible for the peristaltic activity of the more distal oesophagus, including relaxation of the cardia. Its parasympathetic nerve supply is mediated via the vagus nerves. Sympathetic nerves have a minimal role in the regulation of oesophageal motor function.

The oesophagus commences at the level of C5/6, where the upper oesophageal sphincter [1] is formed by the horizontal fibres of the inferior constrictor (cricopharyngeus), which is responsible for a zone of high pressure approximately 2.5 cm in length and which separates the pharynx from the oesophagus. The lower oesophageal sphincter is not a discrete anatomical structure, but denotes the lowest 2–3 cm of the oesophagus, where there is a second high-pressure zone [2, 3] extending upwards from the oesophagogastric junction. This corresponds to the slightly more distensible portion, known as the vestibule or phrenic ampulla. At the proximal end of the high-pressure zone, a ring of muscle spasm is occasionally visible on barium studies and this is known as the A-ring, to distinguish it from the B-ring or Schatski ring [4]. This is sometimes visible at the distal end of the sphincter at the oesophagogastric junction. The junction is also demarcated by the oblique muscle fibres of the stomach, which loop over the junction before passing downwards on the anterior and posterior aspects of the body of the stomach. The acute angle between the stomach and the oesophagus is probably dependent on these fibres. The oesophagus has no serosal covering, except in a small distal section, and the general lack of this layer contributes to the rapid spread of primary oesophageal carcinoma [5]. The lymphatic drainage of the oesophagus is in three directions. The upper oesophagus drains to cervical supraclavicular nodes, while tracheobronchial nodes drain the middle third. The lymphatic drainage of the distal third is to coeliac and adjacent gastric nodes. In normal barium studies, there are normal extrinsic impressions in the wall of the oesophagus, caused by the aortic arch, the left main-stem bronchus and the diaphragmatic hiatus. Important venous anastamoses occur in the distal oesophagus between tributaries of the azygos and hemiazygos systemic veins and oesophagogastric tributaries of the hepatic portal system. These may distend in the presence of portal hypertension and are an important and serious cause of oesophagogastric haemorrhage (uphill varices). Less commonly, varicose collaterals may occur more proximally in the oesophagus in the presence of obstruction of the superior vena cava (SVC), principally resulting from extension of bronchial carcinoma. In this situation, the azygos system is used to bypass the obstructed SVC, and oesophageal collaterals may be a manifestation of this collateral circulation (downhill varices) [5].

An important part of the radiological examination of the oesophagus is an assessment of its motility. This is probably best done in the recumbent position without the influence of gravity. Peristalsis refers to the normal coordinated propulsive contraction of the oesophagus. Three kinds of motor activity are recognized. Primary peristalsis is the orderly, coordinated, propulsive sequence of contraction resulting in progressive stripping waves crossing the whole length of the oesophagus, with complete emptying of the barium column. This centrally mediated swallow reflex via the glossopharyngeal nerve is initiated by active swallowing. Secondary peristalsis is a local wave but elicited through oesophageal distension. Tertiary contractions are non-propulsive oesophageal contractions, characterized by disorderly 'to and fro' movements of the bolus without clearing of the gullet. This may be observed in the absence of disease in older subjects.

Plain film radiography

As a rule, plain films are of very limited value in the oesophagus, but will occasionally show fluid levels or gaseous distension of the gullet—for example, in achalasia [2, 5]. Air in the lumen of the oesophagus is a normal feature on CT scans. Opaque foreign bodies may also be seen.

Barium studies

A complete examination of the oesophagus assesses both its structure and its function. Frequent clinical indications are resistant heartburn, dysphagia, pain on swallowing, atypical chest pain, globus (a feeling of a lump in the throat) and treatment planning. It may also be the initial part of an overall evaluation of the upper gastrointestinal tract. For patients with globus, chest pain or dysphagia, barium radiology is likely to be a more useful initial test than endoscopy.

Computerized tomography scanning

This technique has proved useful for staging oesophageal malignancy [6], particularly in advanced disease. It may also be used to assess the extent of invasion of bronchial carcinoma producing oesophageal symptoms. It is also an indispensable tool in the planning of radiotherapy. Modern spiral scanners very rapidly produce useful information regarding the primary lesion, including the presence or absence of direct spread to neighbouring structures (for example, the aorta), enlarged lymph nodes and the presence or absence of distant metastases (for example, in the liver or lungs). The main disadvantages of CT, apart from the radiation dose, are its inability to distinguish the individual layers of the wall of the oesophagus and its inability to detect tumour pathology in normal-sized glands. On CT, the thickness of the oesophageal wall should be no greater than 0.5 cm and it is demarcated internally by air or contrast in the lumen and externally by the presence of perioesophageal fat and the airways. There is often no fat plane between the posterior wall of the trachea and the oesophagus. At the distal end of the oesophagus, there is apparent thickening or pseudo-tumour effect, stemming from a combination of incomplete distension of the fundus of the stomach and the oblique course of the oesophagogastric junction in relation to the transverse plane of the CT section [2].

Magnetic resonance imaging

The normal oesophagus produces a signal intensity similar to that of muscle in the chest wall on both T_1- and T_2-weighted images. Mostly, the perioesophageal fat is hyperintense, but, as with CT, between the oesophagus and trachea there is no visible fat plane and, in most subjects, there is at least partial effacement of the hyperintense fat plane between the oesophagus and aorta [2]. At the present time, there are no essential indications for magnetic resonance imaging (MRI) in the gullet and its clinical superiority over CT has not yet been shown. Its potential advantage lies in the variety of projections and exquisite contrast resolution, as well as the lack of ionizing radiation. In the preoperative staging of oesophageal cancer, MRI is potentially superior to CT in the detection of mediastinal invasion, by virtue of the easy differentiation of fat from other soft-tissue structures. Nevertheless, motion artefacts due to long acquisition times may limit its use.

Endoscopic ultrasound

This exciting technique represents the successful integration of gastrointestinal endoscopy and ultrasound, utilizing a miniaturized high-frequency transducer [7]. The oesophagus and other hollow gastrointestinal viscera can be accessed by ultrasound with the aid of a latex balloon placed over the transducer tip and filled with water. In this way, acoustic contact can be established between the wall of the oesophagus and the transducer and valuable information obtained. Because the area under scrutiny is so close to the transducer, relatively high-frequency probes—for example, 5–12 MHz—can be used. These permit evaluation of individual layers of the oesophageal wall and can detect pathology not seen with other modalities. Smaller probes are currently being evaluated from 12 to 20 MHz, which can be passed down the biopsy channel of a standard endoscope [7]. Major current applications include the staging of tumour invasion in the oesophagus [8–10]. Endoscopic ultrasound, particularly if combined with biopsy, may help to differentiate benign from malignant lymph nodes in the mediastinum [6]. Despite its obvious advantages, endoscopic ultrasound is a difficult technique and extremely operator-dependent.

References

1 Ott D.G. (1994) Motility disorders. In: Gore R.M., Levine M.S. & Laufer I. (eds) *A Textbook of Gastro-intestinal Radiology.* Philadelphia: W.B. Saunders, 346–359.
2 Ekberg O. (1994) Normal anatomy and techniques of examination of the oesophagus. In: Freeny P.C. & Stevenson G.W. (eds) *Margulis and Burhenne's Alimentary Tract Radiology*, 5th edn. St Louis: Mosby, 168–185.
3 Stewart E.T. & Dodds W.J. (1994) Radiology of the oesophagus. In: Freeny P.C. & Stevenson G.W. (eds) *Margulis and Burhenne's Alimentary Tract Radiology*, 5th edn. St Louis: Mosby, 192–263.
4 Dahnert W. (1996) *Radiology Review Manual*, 3rd edn. Baltimore: Williams & Wilkins, 571.
5 Harrell G.S. (1997) The oesophagus. In: Grainger R.G &

Allison D.J. (eds) *Diagnostic Radiology*, 3rd edn. New York: Churchill Livingstone, 909–939.

6 Levine M.S. & Halvorsen R.A. (1994) Oesophageal carcinoma. In: Gore R.M., Levine M.S. & Laufer I. (eds) *A Textbook of Gastro-intestinal Radiology*. Philidelphia: W.B. Saunders, 446–478.

7 McLean A. & Fairclough P. (1996) Endoscopic ultrasound—current applications. *Clinical Radiology* **51**, 83–98.

8 Botet J.F. & Lightdale C.J. (1994) Normal anatomy and techniques of examination of the oesophagus—endosonography. In: Freeny P.C. & Stevenson G.W. (eds) *Margulis and Burhenne's Alimentary Tract Radiology*, 5th edn. St Louis: Mosby, 186–191.

9 Botet J.F., Lightdale C.J., Zauber A.G. *et al.* (1991) Pre-operative staging of oesophageal cancer: comparison of endsocopic ultrasound and dynamic CT. *Radiology* **181**, 419–425.

10 Ziegler K., Sanft C., Zeitz M. *et al.* (1991) Evaluation of endosonography in T.N.: staging of oesophageal cancer. *Gut* **32**, 10–16.

11 Sheiner N.M. & La Chance C. (1980) Congenital oesophago-bronchial fistula in the adult. *Canadian Journal of Surgery* **23**, 483–491.

12 Rubesin S.E. & Rosato E.F. (1994) The post-operative oesophagus. In: Gore R.M., Levine M.S. & Laufer I. (eds) *A Textbook of Gastro intestinal Radiology*. Philadelphia: W.B. Saunders, 542–556.

13 MacSween R.N.M. & Whaley K. (eds) *Muir's Textbook of Pathology*, 13th edn. London: Arnold, 689.

14 Beauchamp J.M., Nice C.M., Belanger M.A. & Neitzschman H.R. (1974) Oesophageal intramural pseudodiverticulosis. *Radiology* **113**, 273–276.

15 Lupovitch A. & Tippins R. (1974) Oesophageal intramural pseudodiverticulosis: disease of adnexal glands. *Radiology* **113**, 271–272.

16 Bruhlmann W.F., Zollikofer C.L., Maranta E. *et al.* (1981) Intramural pseudodiverticulosis of the oesophagus. *Gastrointestinal Radiology* **6**, 199–208.

17 Levine M.S. (1994) Infectious oesophagitis. In: Gore R.M., Levine M.S. & Laufer I. (eds) *A Textbook of Gastro-intestinal Radiology*. Philadelphia: W.B. Saunders, 385–402.

18 Simpkins K.C. (1993) The salivary glands, pharynx and oesophagus. In: Sutton D. (ed.) *A Textbook of Radiology and Imaging*, 5th edn. Edinburgh: Churchill Livingstone, 755–787.

19 Tio T.L., Tytgat G.N.J. & den Hartog Jaeger F.C.A. (1990) Endoscopic ultrasonography for the evaluation of smooth muscle tumours in the upper gastro-intestinal tract. *Gastro-intestinal Endoscopy* **36**, 342.

20 Burkitt H.G., Quick C.R.G. & Gatt D. (1990) *Essential Surgery*. Edinburgh: Churchill Livingstone, 255–263.

21 Rankin S.C. (1996) CT in the staging of gastro-intestinal malignancy. In: *Proceedings of the London CT/MRI Course*. Gleneagles, Scotland, 64–68.

22 Quint L.E., Francis I.R., Glazer G.M. *et al.* (1994) CT and MR staging of tumours of the oesophagus. In: Freeny P.C. & Stevenson G.W. (eds) *Margulis and Burhenne's Alimentary Tract Radiology*, 5th edn. St Louis: Mosby, 272–281.

23 Picus D., Balfe D.M., Koehler R.E., Roper C.L. & Owen J.W. (1983) Computed tomography in the staging of oesophageal carcinoma. *Radiology* **146**, 433–438.

24 Takashima S., Takeuchi N., Shiozaki H. *et al.* (1991) Carcinoma of the oesophagus: CT versus MR imaging in determining resectability. *American Journal of Roentgenology* **156**, 297–302.

25 Bartram C.I. & Kumar P. (1981) *Clinical Radiology in Gastroenterology*. Oxford: Blackwell Scientific Publications, 56.

26 Enterline H. & Thompson J. (1984) *Pathology of the Oesophagus*. New York: Springer Verlag, 55–71.

27 Wyschulis A.R., Woolam G.L., Andersen H.A. *et al.* (1971) Achalasia and carcinoma of the oesophagus. *Journal of the American Medical Association* **215**, 1638–1641.

28 Buschman D.L. (1991) Barium sulphate bronchography: report of a complication. *Chest* **99**, 747–749.

29 Beckly D.E. (1994) Gastro-intestinal bleeding: endoscopy and diagnostic approach. In: Freeny P.C. & Stevenson G.W. (eds) *Margulis and Burhenne's Alimentary Tract Radiology*, 5th edn. St Louis: Mosby, 967–982.

Suggested further reading

Saunders H.S., Wolfman N.T. & Ott D.J. (1997) Oesophageal cancer radiologic staging. In: Gore R.M. (ed.) *Staging Gastrointestinal Malignancy*. Radiologic Clinics of North America, Vol. 35(2). Philadelphia: W.B. Saunders, 281–294.

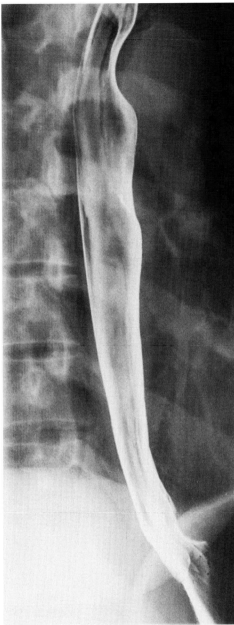

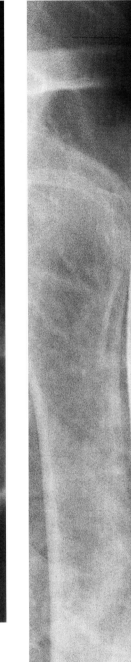

Fig. 2.1 Normal oesophagus.
The gullet has been distended
with gas and coated with
barium. In this RAO position,
normal extrinsic impressions on
the wall of the oesophagus are
produced by the aortic arch and,
to a slight extent, by the left
main-stem bronchus. The fundus
of the stomach is distended
with gas.

Fig. 2.2 Normal oesophagus, feline cross-striation. This transient transverse ridging
in the double-contrast swallow is said to be due to contraction of the muscularis
mucosa [11]. This is said to be a constant feature of the cat oesophagus.

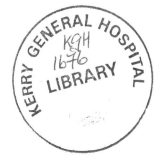

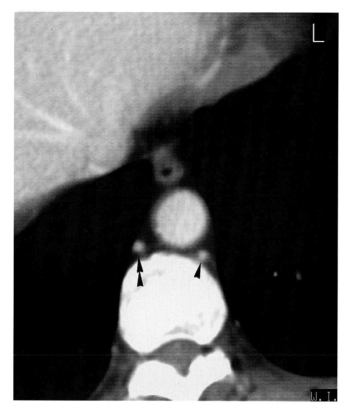

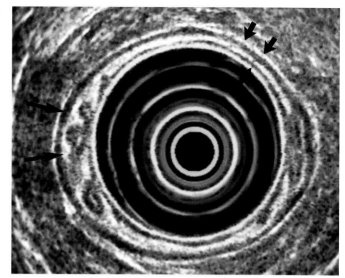

Fig. 2.5 Normal oesophagus, endoscopic ultrasound. The normal oesophageal wall is shown at the proximal margin of a hiatus hernia. The normal-layered structure of the oesophageal wall is visible (short arrows). The gastric-fold pattern can be seen within the hiatus hernia (longer arrows). (Courtesy of Dr Alison McLean.)

Fig. 2.3 Normal oesophagus, spiral CECT scan. The oesophagus in transverse section is clearly visible anterior to the contrast-filled descending thoracic aorta. The right and left pleural reflections, azygos (double arrowhead) and hemiazygos (single arrowhead) veins are visible.

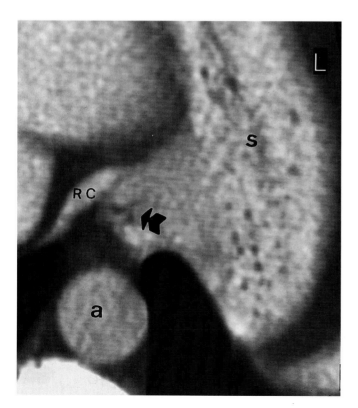

Fig. 2.4 Normal oesophagogastric junction. A spiral CT scan through the oesophagogastric junction. The stellate collapsed lumen is just visible (arrow). The oesophageal hiatus is marked by the right crus of the diaphragm (RC). The undistended stomach (S) and aorta (a) are also shown.

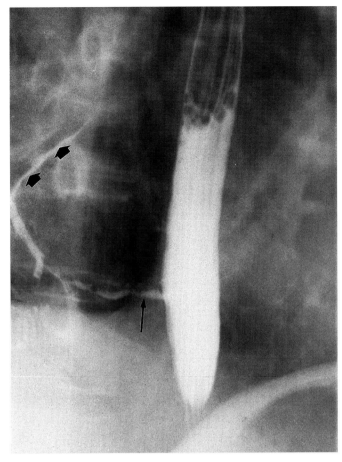

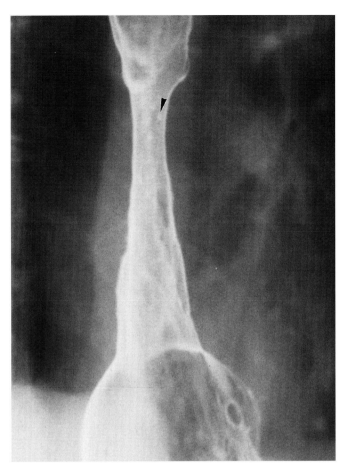

Fig. 2.6 Congenital broncho-oesophageal fistula. It is unusual for congenital oesophageal lesions to present in adult life. Oesophageal lesions of various kinds are an important cause of recurrent chest infections. This barium swallow shows contrast escaping from the distal oesophagus into a narrow fistulous track (arrow), which is seen to communicate with the bronchial tree (arrowheads) [11].

Fig. 2.7 Reflux oesophagitis. The double-contrast barium swallow (DCBS) shows a moderate-sized hiatus hernia associated with a moderate stricture of the distal oesophagus 6 cm in length. Multiple tiny erosions are seen, one of which is indicated by the arrowhead, in keeping with peptic oesophagitis.

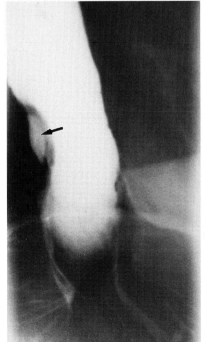

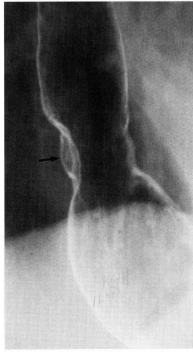

Fig. 2.8 Oesophageal peptic ulcer. (a) Single contrast and (b) double contrast views indicate a large, discrete, penetrating ulcer crater (arrows) in the wall of the distal oesophagus at the level of the oesophagogastric junction immediately above a hiatus hernia, resulting from gastro-oesophageal reflux disease.

(a)

(b)

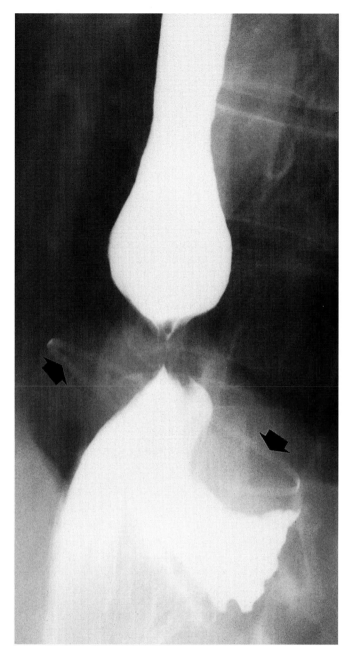

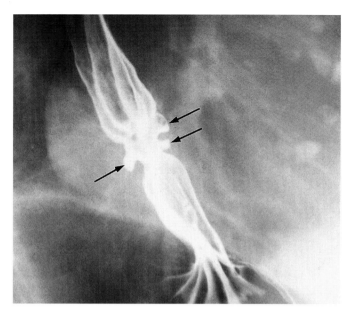

Fig. 2.10 Reflux oesophagitis, postinflammatory sacculations. In this female patient with long-standing symptoms of reflux oesophagitis, there is considerable deformity at the oesophagogastric junction produced by postinflammatory sacculations resulting from a gross degree of cicatrization (arrows).

Fig. 2.9 Gastro-oesophageal reflux. This barium study shows gross gastro-oesophageal reflux of barium from the stomach to the oesophagus in the recumbent position, despite the presence of an Angelchik antireflux prosthesis (arrowheads) [12].

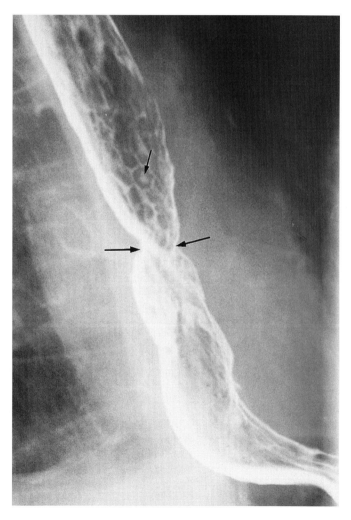

Fig. 2.11 Reflux oesophagitis with stricture. This male patient, with symptoms of severe gastro-oesophageal reflux, recent weight loss, small haematemesis and dysphagia, had an endoscopy which demonstrated oesophagitis, but the endoscope could not be advanced beyond a distal oesophageal stricture. The DCBS shows multiple discrete erosions (small arrow), with a stricture at or near the gastro-oesophageal junction (large arrows). There was also evidence of a sliding hiatus hernia. The patient was treated with a proton-pump inhibitor and 4 months later his oesophagus was completely normal at endoscopy.

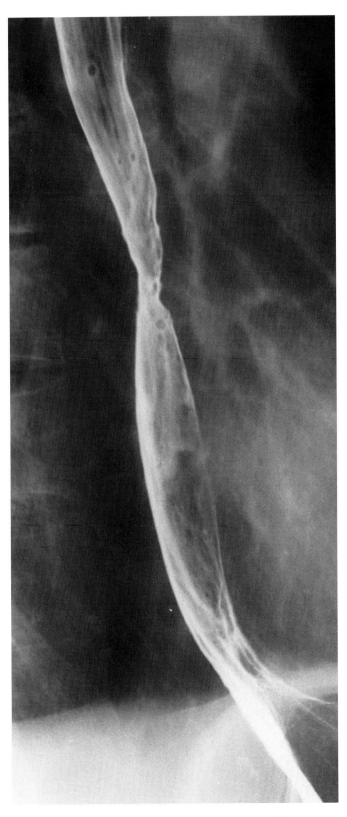

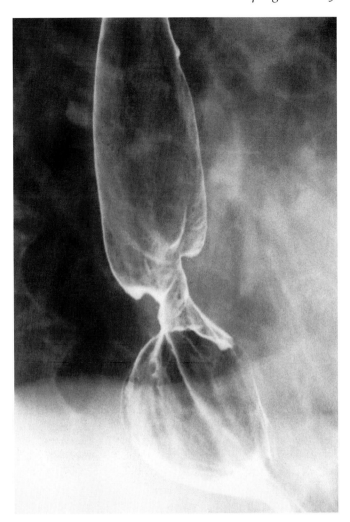

Fig. 2.13 Barrett's oesophagus. A 72-year-old male patient with a long history of reflux symptoms and a recent history of dysphagia. The DCBS shows a 2.5 cm long stricture of the distal oesophagus with a slightly shouldered margin. A sliding hiatus hernia is also present. Oesophagoscopy confirmed the presence of a stricture, and the histology indicated dysplastic changes within Barrett's oesophagus [5]. There was no evidence of malignancy. The patient lived for a further 10 years until he developed a bronchial carcinoma.

Fig. 2.12 Barrett's oesophagus. The DCBS shows a slightly irregular stricture of the middle third of the oesophagus in a male patient with dysphagia. Later in the examination, marked gastro-oesophageal reflux of barium was apparent. Endoscopy confirmed a peptic stricture, and mucosal biopsy indicated columnar lined epithelium (Barrett's oesophagus) [13].

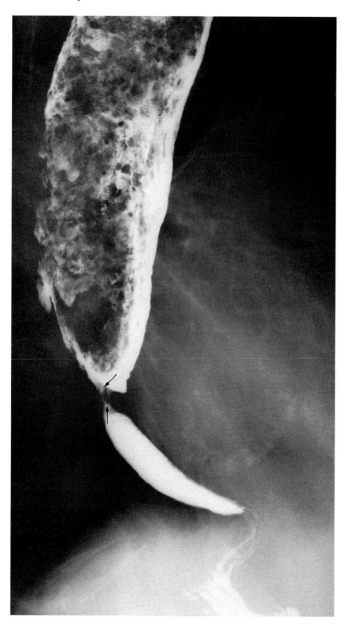

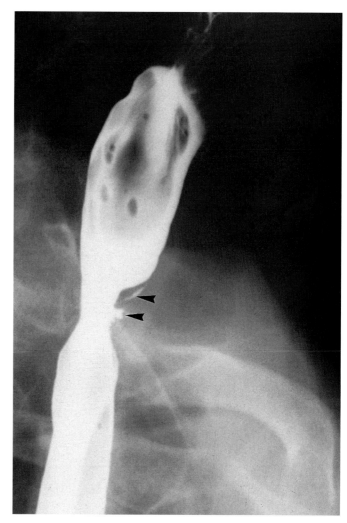

Fig. 2.15 Barrett's oesophagus. Barium swallow in this patient with dysphagia shows moderate constriction of the oesophagus at the level of the thoracic inlet. Two discrete ulcers are shown filling with contrast (arrowheads) at the level of the stricture.

Fig. 2.14 Barrett's oesophagus. An elderly female patient with increasing dysphagia over several months. Barium swallow shows quite marked dilatation of the gullet, which contains a very large fasting residue above a short, tight stricture (arrows) 7 cm above the oesophagogastric junction. A benign stricture was confirmed by endoscopy at 30 cm. Histology revealed no evidence of malignancy.

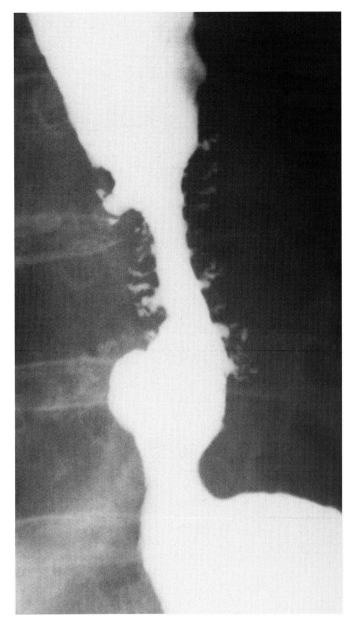

Fig. 2.16 Intramural pseudodiverticulosis. Flask-like collections of contrast are seen to fill dilated mucous glands associated with gross reflux oesophagitis and a sliding hiatus hernia. This is a rare complication of chronic reflux oesophagitis [3].

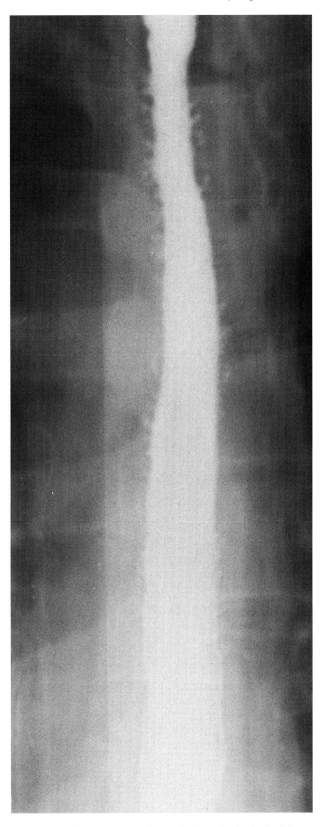

Fig. 2.17 Diffuse intramural pseudodiverticulosis. In this single-contrast barium swallow, numerous flask-like collections of barium are seen to extend from the lumen of the oesophagus [14–16].

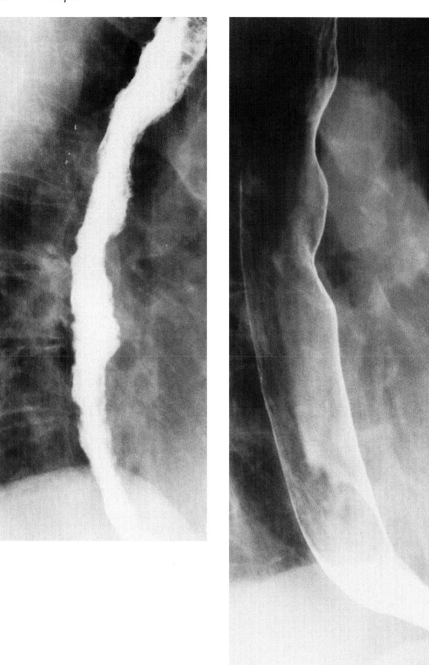

(a)

(b)

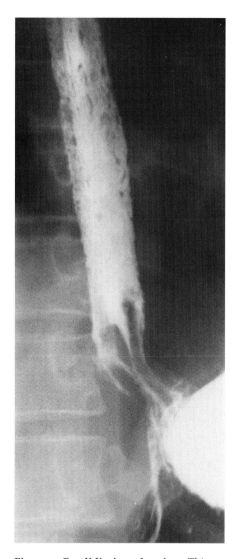

Fig. 2.19 Candidiasis and varices. This 32-year-old female patient with alcoholic liver disease, hepatic failure, ascites and portal hypertension has diffuse mucosal irregularity on barium swallow and, in addition, there are serpiginous filling defects in the distal oesophagus, characteristic of varices. Both diagnoses were confirmed endoscopically.

Fig. 2.18 Candidiasis (moniliasis). (a) Before treatment, the barium swallow shows a grossly abnormal oesophageal wall, with a diffuse shaggy appearance, which is typical of candidiasis. (b) Five weeks later, following treatment with nystatin, the DCBS shows a completely normal oesophageal mucosa [17].

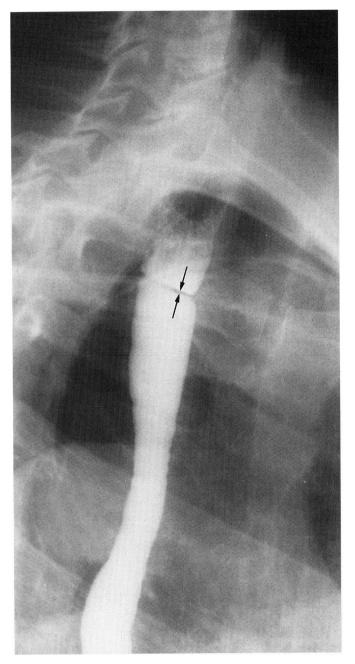

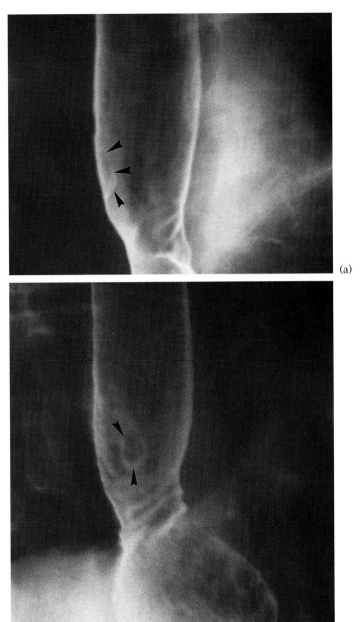

(a)

(b)

Fig. 2.20 Oesophageal web [18]. This middle-aged male patient complained of a sensation of food sticking. Single-contrast barium swallow shows a very fine membranous diaphragm, 2 mm thick, in the oesophagus at the level of the thoracic inlet (arrows).

Fig. 2.21 Leiomyoma. This 56-year-old male patient had a history of dyspeptic symptoms but no dysphagia. The DCBS shows a well-circumscribed ovoid filling defect 1 cm in diameter (arrowheads), shown in (a) profile and (b) *en face* in opposite oblique projections of the distal oesophagus. At endoscopy, a smooth polypoid lesion was confirmed and mucosal biopsy was normal [19].

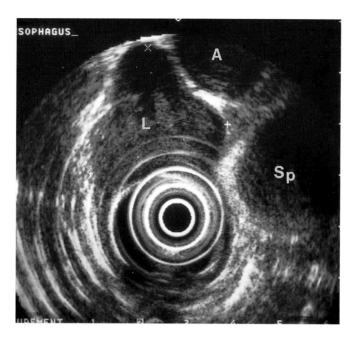

Fig. 2.22 **Leiomyoma.** Endoscopic US reveals a clearly defined hypoechoic mass arising from the deep hypoechoic area of the oesophageal wall, with preservation of the mucosal layer over the surface of the lesion (L). The mass is of the same reflectivity as the muscular layer from which it arises. A, aorta; Sp, spine. (Courtesy of Dr Alison McLean.)

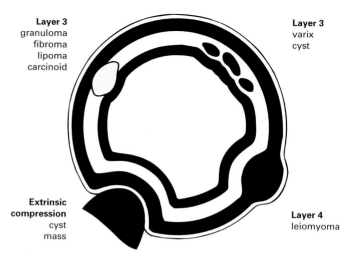

Fig. 2.23 **Submucosal disease on endoscopic US.** The nature of a submucosal mass demonstrated endoscopically can be clarified on endoscopic US. Intrinsic and extrinsic lesions may be differentiated and the histological nature of a mass may be suggested by its echo characteristics and layer of origin. Leiomyomata are typically hypoechoic, arising from the muscularis propria. Varices and cysts are seen as anechoic structures within the third hyperechoic submucosal layer. Other benign submucosal lesions may have variable echogenicity. Lipomata are characteristically hyperechoic. (Courtesy of Dr Alison McLean.)

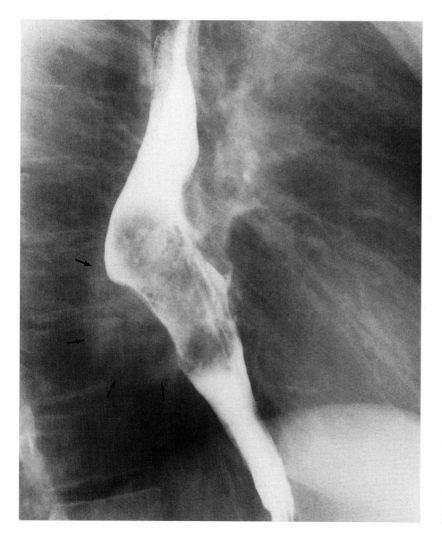

Fig. 2.24 **Leiomyoma.** A barium swallow in this 52-year-old male patient who had dysphagia for several months shows extensive deformity caused by filling defects in the wall of the middle third of the oesophagus. The posterior margin of the soft-tissue mass (arrows) is seen to extend backwards for approximately 3.5 cm from the mucosal surface. The appearance is typical of leiomyoma. Mucosal biopsy was normal.

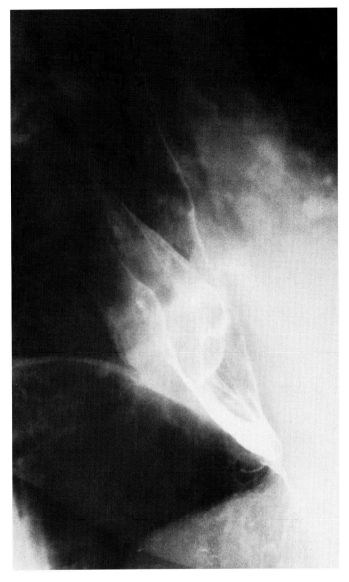

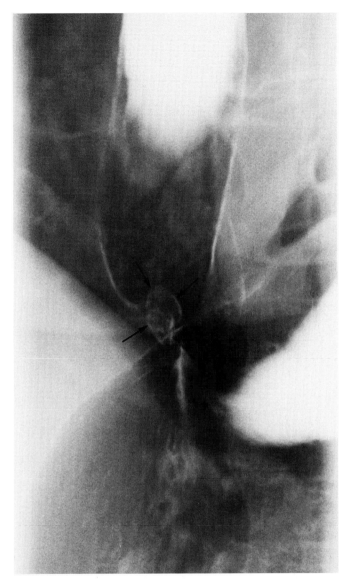

Fig. 2.25 Leiomyoma. This DCBS shows a large, smooth, extramucosal filling defect in the distal oesophagus in a 68-year-old female patient with a 12-month history of dysphagia for solids. Mucosal biopsy was normal and the lesion showed no change in appearance over a 4-year period.

Fig. 2.26 Inflammatory polyp. The DCBS of this 70-year-old patient with a long history of heartburn shows a constant, smooth, 1 cm filling defect (arrows) at the distal end of the oesophagus. The patient was also shown to have gastro-oesophageal reflux. Endoscopy indicated a 1 cm polyp at the squamocolumnar junction. Biopsy of this lesion showed papillary folds of inflamed gastric mucosa, with no evidence of malignancy.

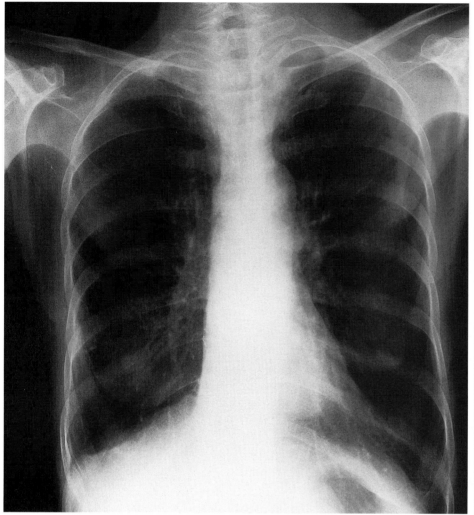

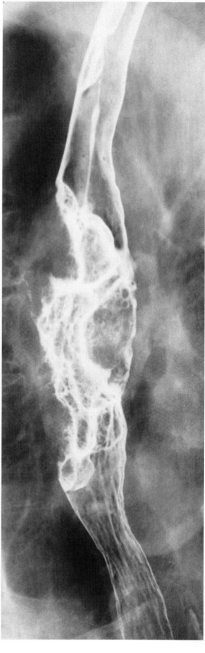

Fig. 2.27 Oesophageal carcinoma with lymph-node metastases. (a) A posteroanterior chest X-ray shows no abnormality in the mediastinum or lung fields, but there is a soft-tissue mass in the left supraclavicular fossa. (b) The DCBS shows a very extensive exophytic mass lesion occupying the middle third of the oesophagus. The appearance is characteristic of carcinoma [20].

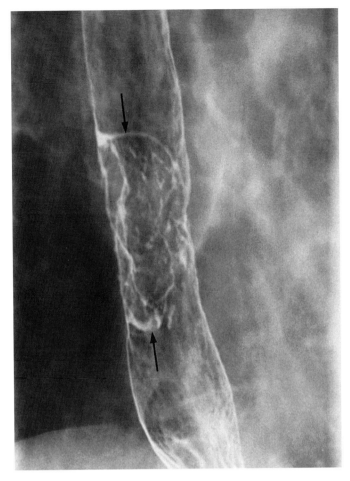

Fig. 2.28 Oesophageal carcinoma. The DCBS in this 66-year-old male patient with recent dysphagia shows a 6 cm long, relatively well-defined, but irregular, eccentric filling defect (arrows) in the distal third of the oesophagus. Endoscopic biopsy confirmed carcinoma.

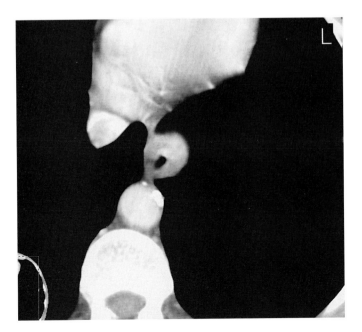

Fig. 2.29 Oesophageal carcinoma. A spiral CT scan shows eccentric circumferential wall thickening with no evidence of local spread.

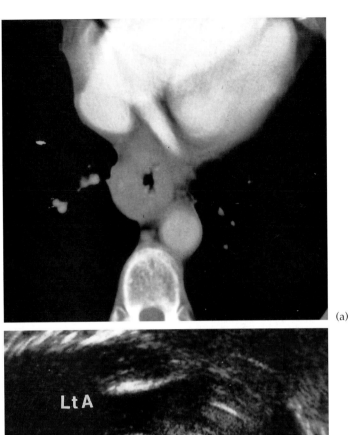

(a)

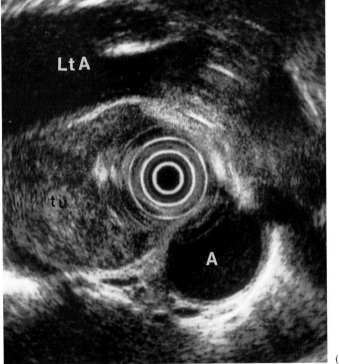

(b)

Fig. 2.30 Oesophageal carcinoma, endoscopic ultrasound. Circumferential thickening of the distal oesophagus seen on (a) CT and (b) endoscopic ultrasound. Tumour stenosis may prevent the passage of the echoendoscope in about one-third of cases. However, high accuracy of T staging (between 80 and 100%) is possible even when assessment is limited to the proximal end of a stricture. In tumour stenosis, miniprobes, which can be introduced down the operating channel of a normal endoscope, may facilitate T staging, although the limited depth of penetration with these high-frequency probes prevents adequate nodal assessment. A, descending aorta; LtA, left atrium; tu, tumour. (Courtesy of Dr Alison McLean.)

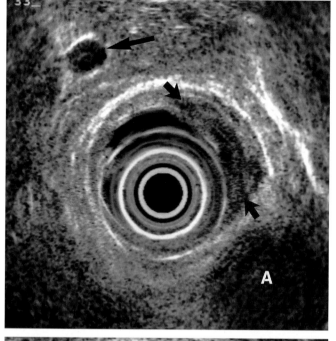

(a)

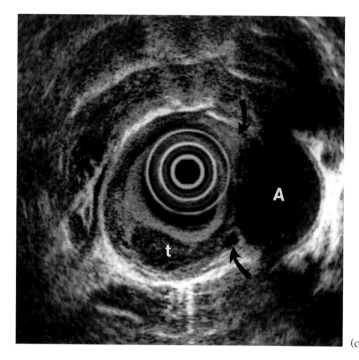

(c)

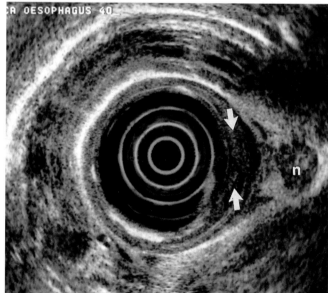

(b)

Fig. 2.31 T staging of oesophageal carcinoma by endosonography. (a) T2. Hypoechoic tumour mass (short arrows) expands and destroys the layers of the oesophageal wall, but does not extend beyond the wall. A rounded hypoechoic paraoesophageal lymph node is demonstrated (long arrow). A, aorta. (b) T3. Hypoechoic tumour destroyed the layered structure of the wall with tumour pseudopodia (small arrows) extending into the adventitia. The lack of a clearly defined serosa in the oesophagus allows for early spread into the paraoesophageal tissues, with longitudinal extension of disease. An enlarged, irregular paraoesophageal node (n) is also demonstrated. (c) T4. There is circumferential thickening of the oesophageal wall with displacement of the layers. Hypoechoic tumour is extending beyond the wall and encasing the aorta (A; curved arrows). t, tumour. (Reprinted from [7] with permission; courtesy of Dr Alison McLean.)

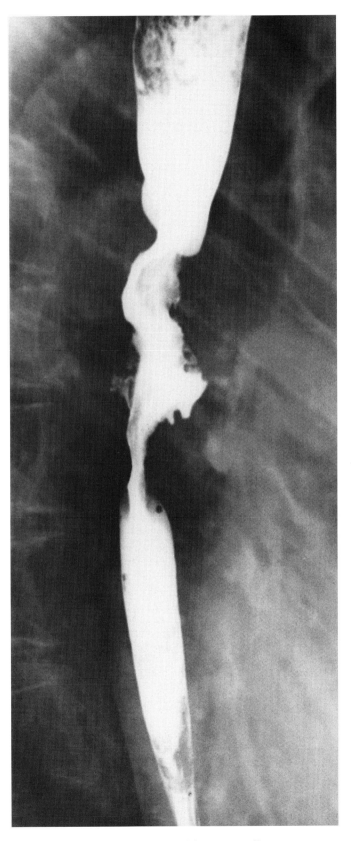

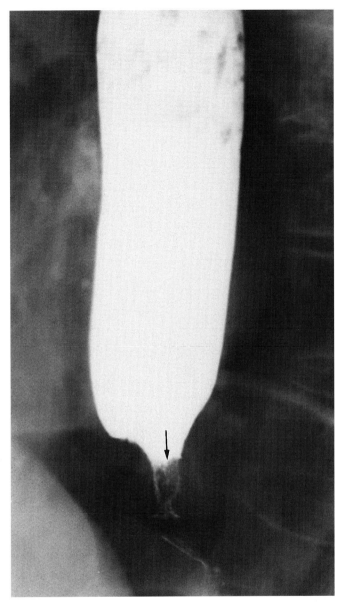

Fig. 2.33 Oesophageal carcinoma. A barium swallow demonstrates a short, tight stricture in the distal end of the oesophagus (arrow), less than 2 cm in length, with an irregular filling defect within the stricture. Endoscopy confirmed a tight malignant stricture at 38 cm. Histology revealed poorly differentiated mucin-secreting adenocarcinoma.

Fig. 2.32 Oesophageal carcinoma. A barium swallow demonstrates a very extensive, 9 cm long stricture and exophytic mass involving the middle third of the oesophagus. The relative lack of proximal oesophageal dilatation is typical of carcinoma. Although this method clearly detects the primary lesion, it is of no value in staging the disease.

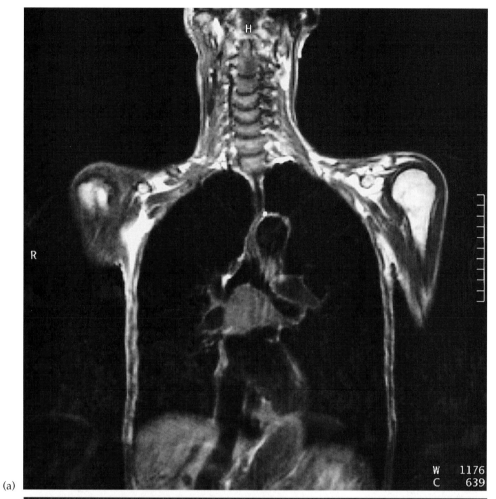

(a)

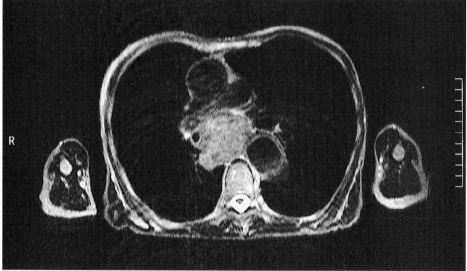

(b)

Fig. 2.34 Oesophageal carcinoma. A 65-year-old female patient with a 4-month history of increasing dysphagia. MRI scans: (a) coronal T_1 FSE mediastinum (TR 570 ms, TE 15 ms) shows a subcarinal, 5 cm long signal homogeneous mass, displacing the bronchi and left atrium; (b) axial T_2 FSE (TR 5500 ms, TE 115 ms) shows an intermediate signal mass in the azygo-oesophageal recess, with less than 90° contact with the mildly dilated thoracic aorta. These changes were due to biopsy-proved oesophageal carcinoma producing a middle mediastinal mass, including lymphadenopathy. (Courtesy of Dr J. Graeme Houston.)

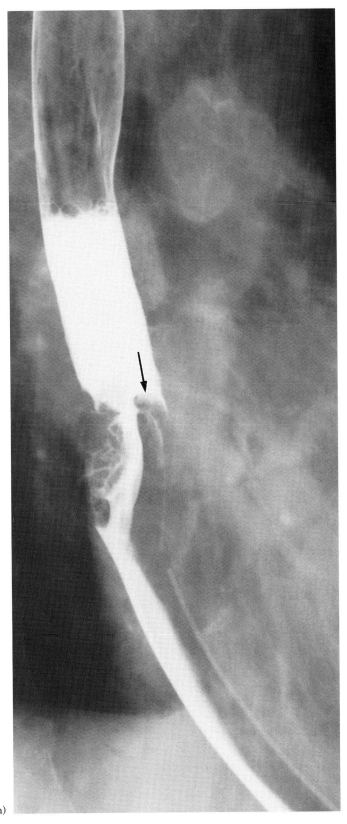

(a)

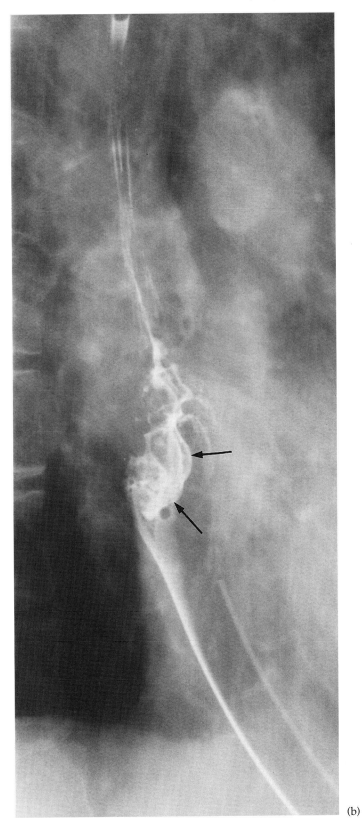

(b)

Fig. 2.35 Progression of oesophageal carcinoma following intubation. Carcinoma of the distal third of the oesophagus had been treated palliatively by the insertion of a Celestin tube. A good initial symptomatic result was followed by a recurrence of dysphagia after 8 weeks. A repeat barium swallow shows tumour extending over the upper margin of the tube and into the lumen of the tube (arrows) [12]. (a) Early and (b) late phases of the same barium study.

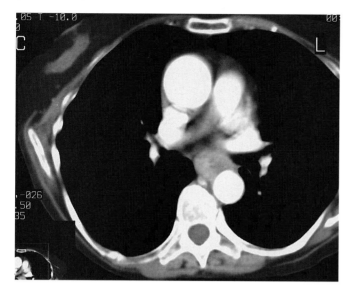

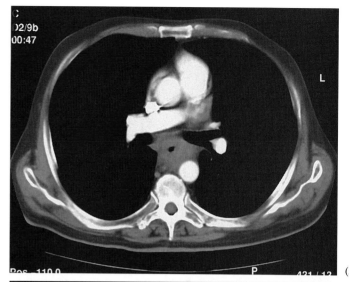

(a)

Fig. 2.36 Oesophageal carcinoma with mediastinal spread. A spiral contrast-enhanced CT (CECT) shows circumferential thickening of the wall of the oesophagus 2 cm below the level of the carina. The tumour is seen to extend backwards, making contact with the circumference of the aorta through an arc of about 150°, making aortic invasion likely [21].

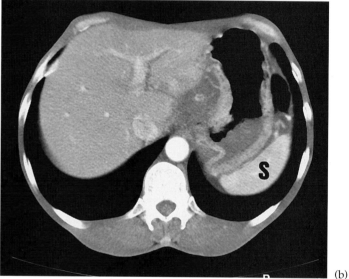

(b)

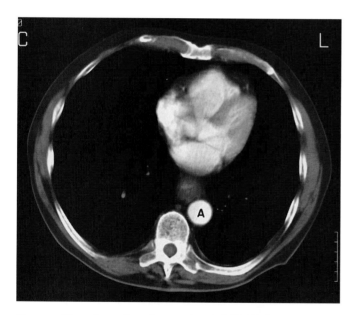

Fig. 2.37 Oesophageal carcinoma. A spiral CECT shows circumferential thickening of the wall of the gullet at the level of the left atrium. There is evidence of extramural soft-tissue stranding, suggestive of mediastinal fat invasion, but there is still a fat plane between the lesion and the aorta (A) [22]. Liver metastases were visible on lower slices.

Fig. 2.38 Oesophageal and oesophagogastric carcinoma. (a) A spiral CECT scan in histologically proved adenocarcinoma of the oesophagus revealed a very long lesion extending from the level of the aortic arch to the proximal stomach. This section shows widespread extension of tumour into the subcarinal area and also posteriorly as far as the dorsal spine and encases a 180° arc of the aorta [23, 24]. (b) Spiral CECT with oral CO_2 and IV hyoscine showing an extensive lesion of the distal oesophagus and stomach, which shows a marked loss of distensibility proximally and thickening of the lesser and greater curves. S, spleen.

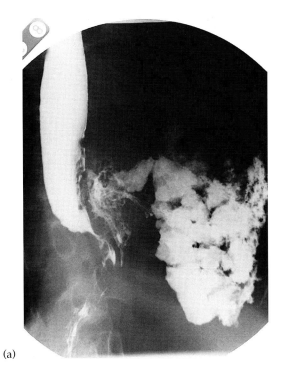

(a)

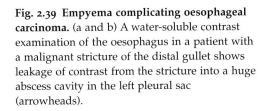

**Fig. 2.39 Empyema complicating oesophageal
carcinoma.** (a and b) A water-soluble contrast
examination of the oesophagus in a patient with
a malignant stricture of the distal gullet shows
leakage of contrast from the stricture into a huge
abscess cavity in the left pleural sac
(arrowheads).

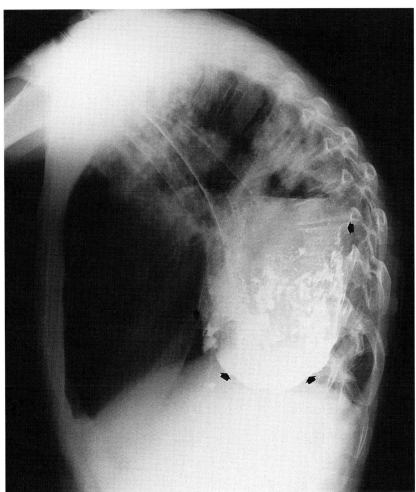

(b)

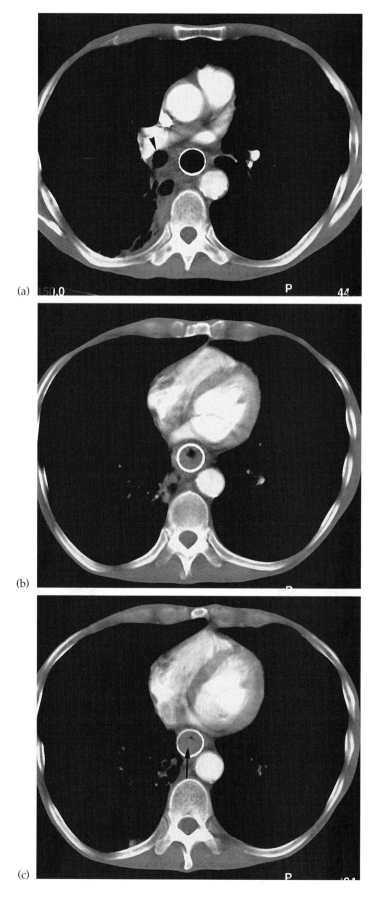

(a)

(b)

(c)

Fig. 2.40 Progression of oesophageal carcinoma after stenting.
A 59-year-old male patient with a carcinoma of the distal half of
the oesophagus was treated by an uncovered metal stent. After
several weeks, dysphagia recurred and this spiral CECT shows:
(a) mediastinal extension of tumour, but the stent is widely patent
proximally (right main bronchus (arrowhead)); (b) 5 cm more
distally, there is obvious extension of the tumour through the
stent, with a small residual lumen; (c) 2 cm distal to (b) the stent
is virtually completely occluded with tumour (arrow).

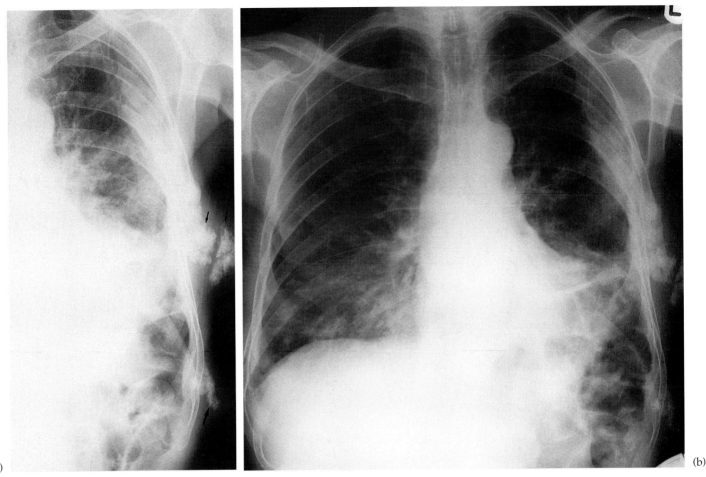

(a)

(b)

Fig. 2.41 Recurrent oesophageal carcinoma. A 55-year-old male patient, who had had an oesophagectomy for a mucin-secreting adenocarcinoma 1 year previously, recently noticed two tender swellings on his left lateral chest wall and also became increasingly breathless. (a) There is a conglomeration of calcification (small arrows) in the soft tissues of the left lateral chest wall, which clinically was related to the thoracotomy scar. A similar but smaller lesion is apparent at the scar of a previous chest-drainage site (large arrow). These lesions represent local recurrence of the patient's mucin-secreting adenocarcinoma in the chest wall. (b) The chest X-ray also shows extensive bilateral perihilar shadowing, in keeping with lymphangitis carcinomatosis. There is also evidence of superadded infection at the right base.

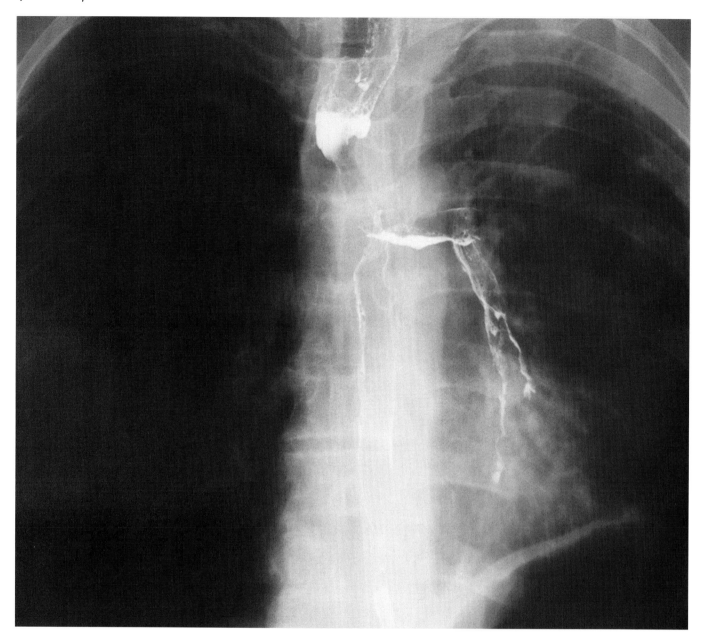

Fig. 2.42 Bronchial carcinoma with an oesophageal fistula.
A 60-year-old male patient with known bronchial carcinoma developed increasing dysphagia and recurrent chest infections. A water-soluble swallow examination shows obstruction of the oesophagus by a stricture at the level of the aortic arch, with some of the contrast entering the left bronchial tree via a fistula. The mechanism needs to be distinguished from aspiration of contrast into the airway. The patient also has a left phrenic nerve palsy.

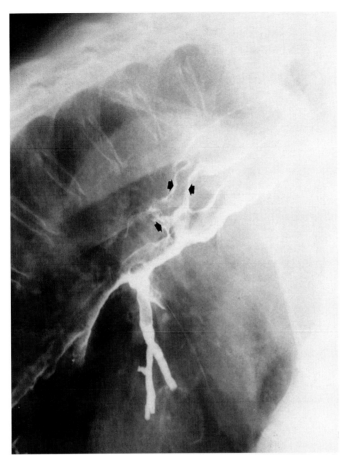

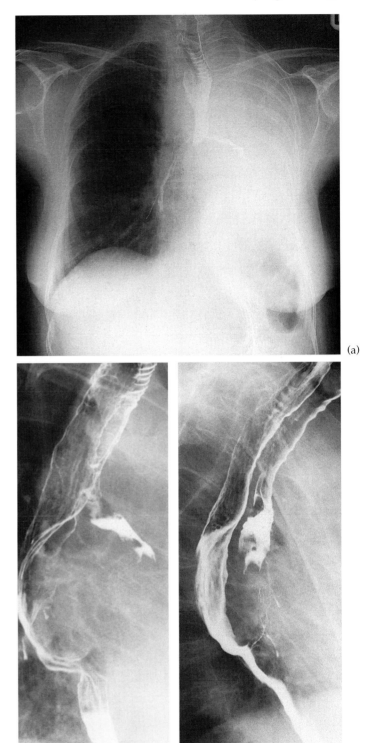

Fig. 2.43 Bronchial carcinoma with an oesophageal fistula. A lateral view of a contrast study of the oesophagus shows a large fistula (arrowheads) between the middle third of the oesophagus and a main-stem bronchus.

Fig. 2.44 Oesophageal obstruction caused by bronchial carcinoma. (a) A chest X-ray immediately after a barium swallow shows total collapse of the left lung and complete obstruction of the oesophagus immediately below the level of the carina; barium is seen in the tracheobronchial tree. (b) The barium swallow shows massive deformity of the lower oesophagus, the appearance being consistent with a large extrinsic mass compressing or invading the wall, but apparently not involving the mucosa. Barium is also shown in the tracheobronchial tree, resulting from aspiration, there being no evidence of a fistula. The primary bronchial lesion is apparent in the left main-stem bronchus.

(a)

(b)

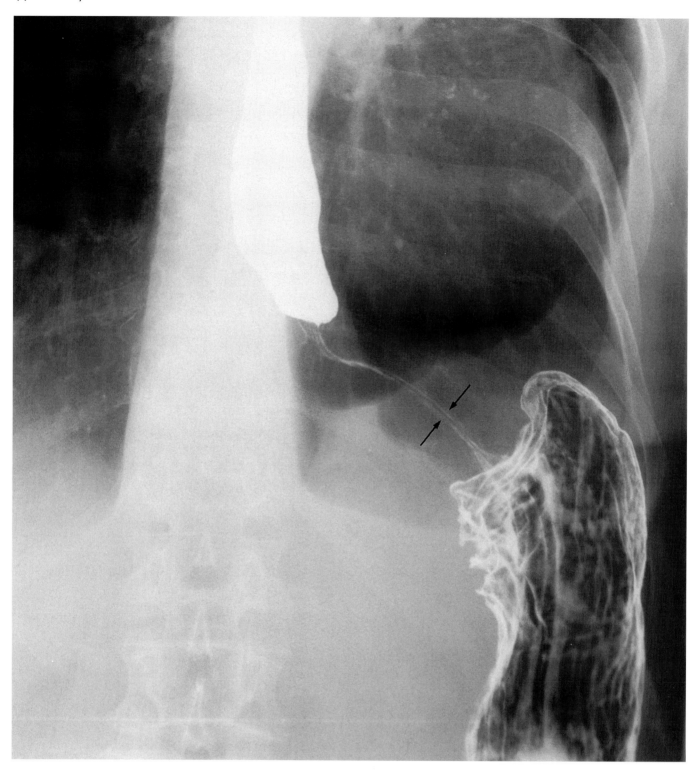

Fig. 2.45 Pancreatic carcinoma invading the oesophagus. Barium swallow in a 76-year-old female patient with 2 months' history of progressive dysphagia and weight loss. Endoscopic biopsy revealed normal mucosa. There is a smooth tight stricture, 8 cm in length, of the distal oesophagus (arrows) associated with an irregular filling defect involving the cardia and fundus of the stomach. The final diagnosis was established at laparotomy. The route of tumour spread is via the superior recess of the lesser sac [18].

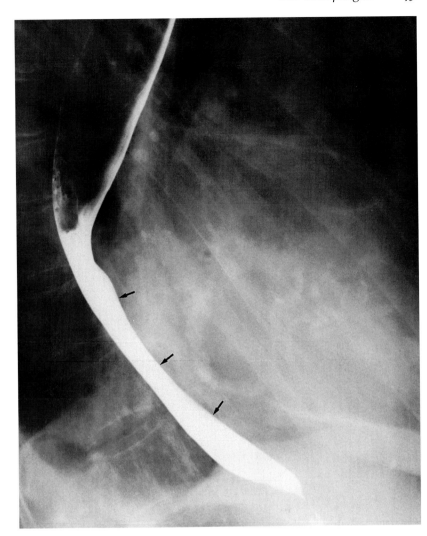

Fig. 2.46 Extrinsic displacement and compression of the oesophagus by an enlarged left atrium. This barium swallow in a patient with rheumatic heart disease shows posterior displacement and smooth extrinsic compression of the distal third of the oesophagus (arrows) by an enlarged left atrium. This method used to be employed to assess left atrial size, but has been completely replaced by more accurate methods, e.g. ultrasound. The oesophagus, however, may still be used to provide access for cardiac ultrasound delivered via a transoesophageal transducer, made possible by the intimate relationship between the left atrium and the gullet.

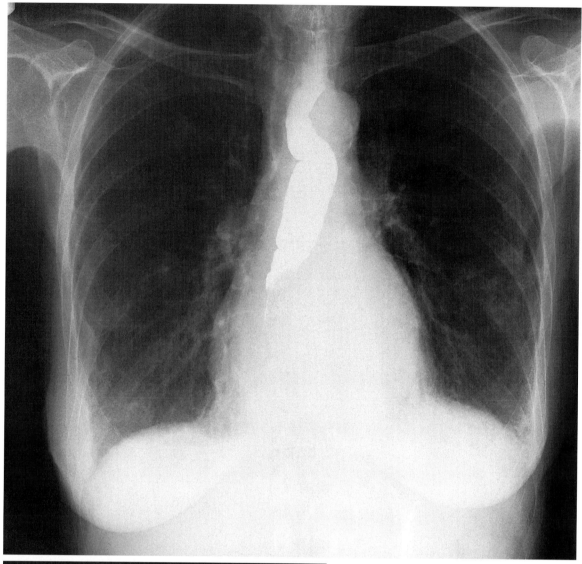

(a)

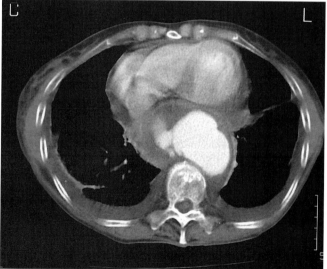

(b)

Fig. 2.47 Oesophageal obstruction caused by an aneurysm of the descending thoracic aorta. This 75-year-old female patient presented with progressive dysphagia over several weeks. (a) The chest X-ray taken immediately after the barium swallow shows almost complete obstruction of the distal third of the oesophagus. (b) A spiral CECT shows a huge, very tortuous aneurysm of the descending thoracic aorta, which completely obstructed the lumen of the gullet (not visible on this section). The aneurysm was treated surgically, but the patient did not survive. (Courtesy of Dr M.D. Cowan.)

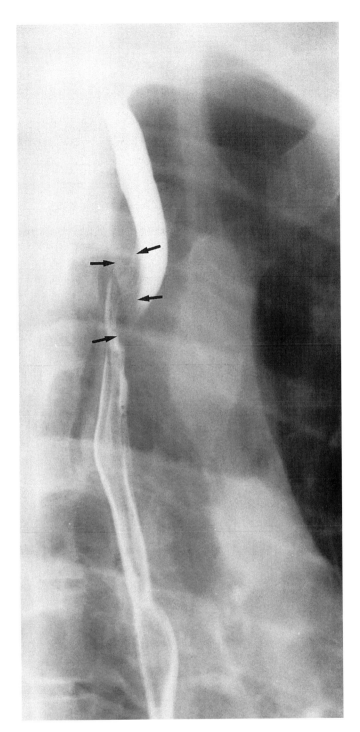

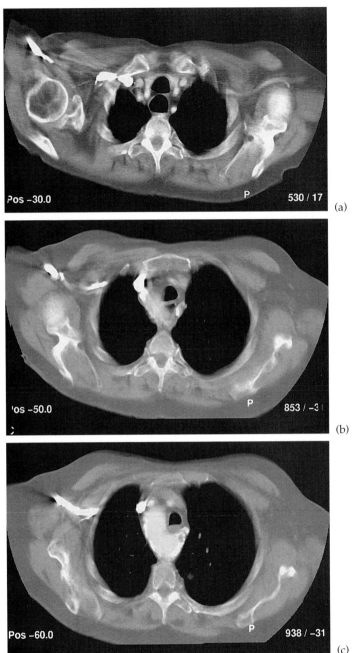

(a)

(b)

(c)

Fig. 2.48 Oesophageal extrinsic compression by an aberrant right subclavian artery [5, 25]. This young adult male patient complained of mild dysphagia. The barium swallow shows an oblique, smooth, extrinsic compression in the upper third of the oesophagus (arrows), resulting from compression by an aberrant right subclavian artery, which arises as the last branch of the aortic arch and which obliquely compresses the gullet as it traverses the mediastinum from left to right. The incidence is one in 200 [5].

Fig. 2.49 Extrinsic compression of the upper oesophagus by a right-sided aortic arch. A spiral CT scan shows (a) a moderately dilated, gas-filled oesophagus above the level of the aortic arch and, at (b), through the superior aspect of the aortic arch, the gas-filled lumen is small but still visible. (c) No gas is seen in the lumen at the level of the right-sided aortic arch. The patient was an 82-year-old female with mild dysphagia in whom no other cause was demonstrated.

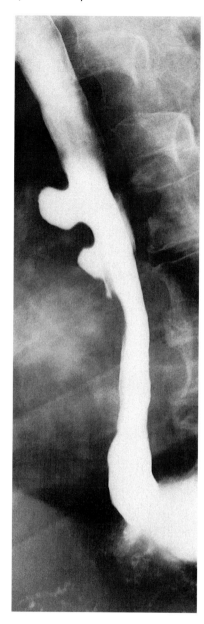

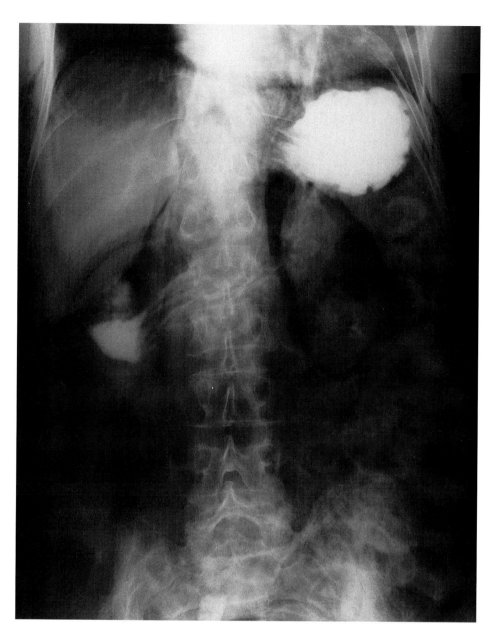

Fig. 2.50 Traction diverticula of the oesophagus. Single-contrast barium swallow in a patient with symptoms of gastro-oesophageal reflux. Two wide-necked diverticula in the middle third of the oesophagus are shown. These are generally asymptomatic and said to be the result of adherent mediastinal lymph nodes.

Fig. 2.51 Oesophageal perforation. An elderly patient experienced chest pain immediately after endoscopy. This supine abdominal X-ray after oral gastrografin shows extraluminal contrast within the mediastinum. There is also evidence of mediastinal air and there is extensive retroperitoneal air surrounding both kidneys and separating the bare area of the liver from the diaphragm. These changes were caused by a perforation of the distal end of the oesophagus.

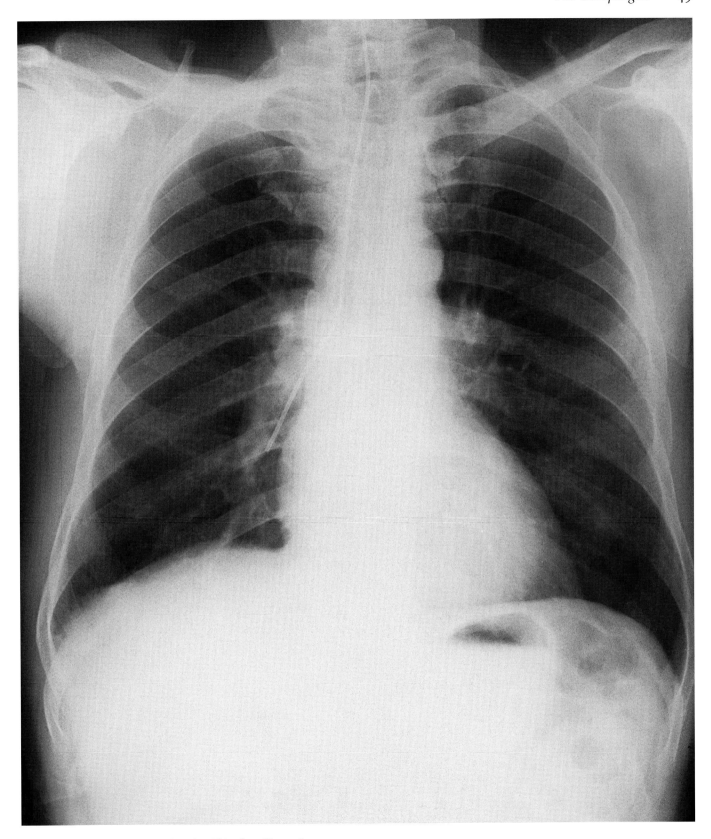

Fig. 2.52 Misplaced nasogastric tube. This chest X-ray shows
that the nasogastric feeding tube has been inadvertently placed in
the tracheobronchial tree on the right side, rather than in the
oesophagus and stomach.

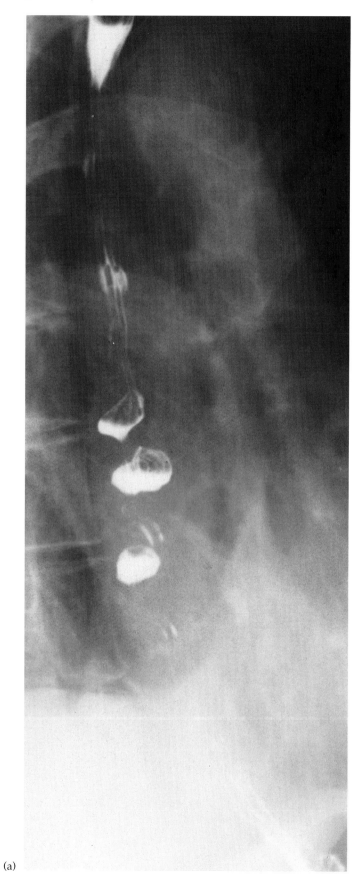

(a)

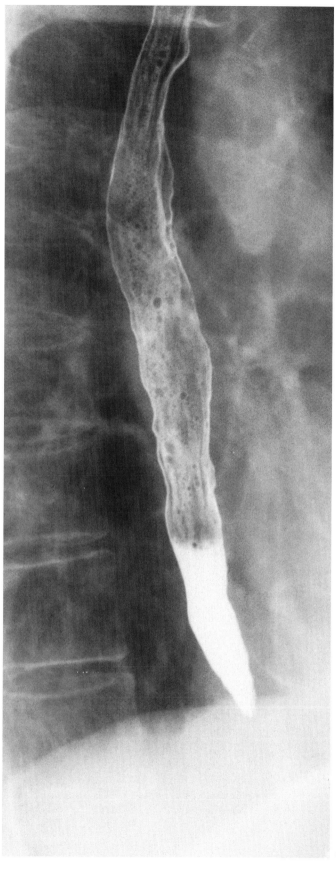

(b)

Fig. 2.53 Oesophageal motility disorder, tertiary contractions.
(a) Transient segmental non-propulsive contractions are seen in
this barium swallow. (b) A few seconds later, the oesophagus
filled normally.

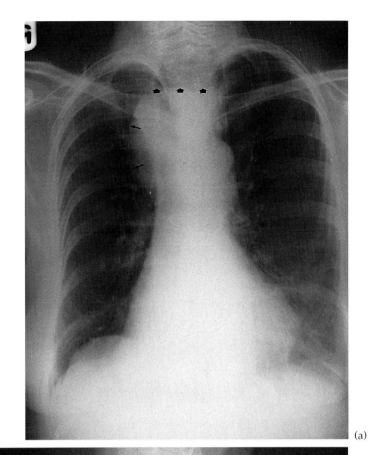

(a)

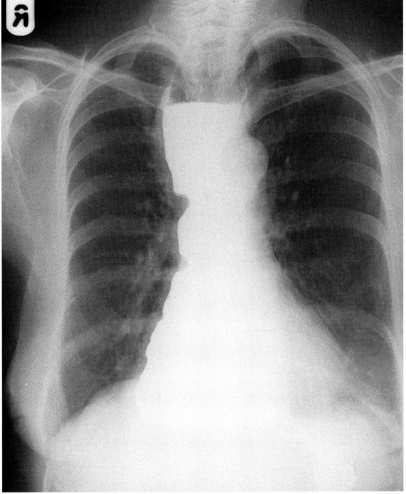

Fig. 2.54 Achalasia of the cardia. (a) This chest X-ray in a 61-year-old female patient with several years' history of progressive dysphagia shows widening of the mediastinal shadow, particularly superiorly on the right side (arrows). There is also a gas–fluid level at the level of the thoracic inlet (arrowheads). (b) A chest X-ray after barium swallow confirms the presence of gross dilatation of the oesophagus with a long fluid level, consistent with long-standing achalasia [26].

(b)

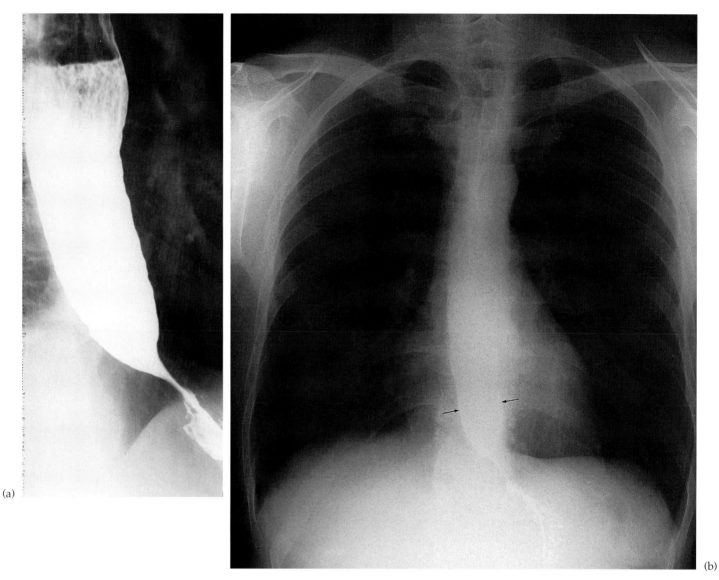

(a)

(b)

Fig. 2.55 Achalasia of the cardia. A 47-year-old male patient presented with difficulty in swallowing for approximately 2 years. (a) The barium swallow shows marked dilatation of the oesophagus, which on fluoroscopy shows virtually no peristalsis and a failure of the distal end of the oesophagus to relax, except infrequently and incompletely. (b) The chest X-ray 45 min after the barium swallow shows a persistent residue of barium in the oesophagus (arrows). No gas is visible in the fundus of the stomach.

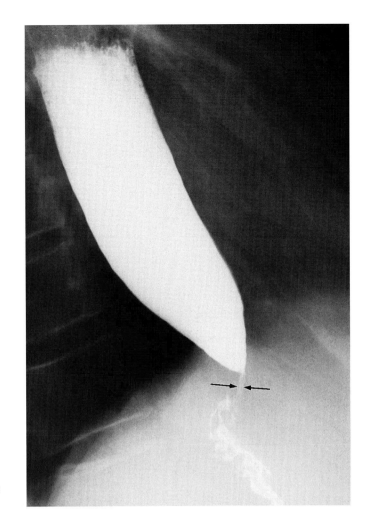

Fig. 2.56 Achalasia of the cardia. A 49-year-old male patient had an 18-month history of dysphagia and weight loss. Endoscopy revealed a large fasting residue, but the mucosa was normal and there was no actual stricture. The barium swallow in this patient also shows oesophageal dilatation and a smooth, tapering constriction of the distal end (arrows), with a very small intermittent trickle of contrast into the stomach and virtually no visible peristalsis on fluoroscopy. Balloon dilatation of the distal end unfortunately resulted in perforation of the oesophagus, requiring surgical repair. The patient made a satisfactory outcome and was alive and well 4 years later.

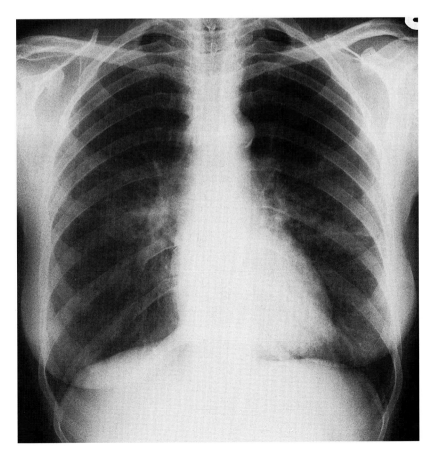

Fig. 2.57 Chronic aspiration resulting from achalasia. A chest X-ray in this patient with known achalasia shows bilateral mid-zone pulmonary shadowing resulting from repeated aspiration.

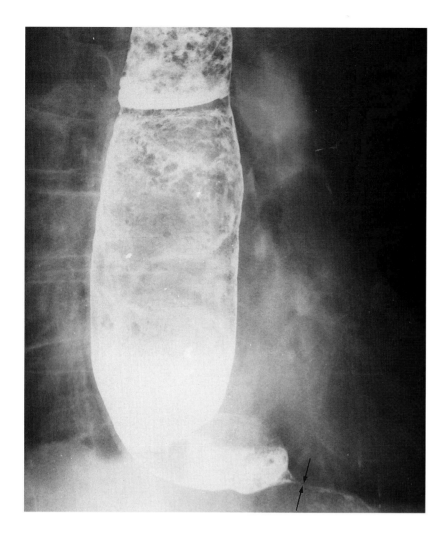

Fig. 2.58 Achalasia with large residue. The barium swallow shows gross oesophageal dilatation, a very large food residue, no peristalsis on fluoroscopy and a distal end which relaxes only very slightly (arrows).

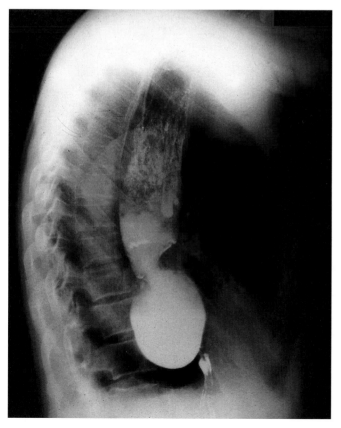

Fig. 2.59 Achalasia complicated by carcinoma. The barium swallow in this case shows generalized oesophageal dilatation, loss of peristalsis and a cigar-shaped distal end, in keeping with achalasia. In addition, however, there is an annular stricture of the oesophagus several centimetres above the distal end. Endoscopic biopsy confirmed carcinoma. The association between achalasia and cancer varies, but, in one study of 1318 patients, the risk of carcinoma was found to be 2.7–14 times greater than that in the general population [27].

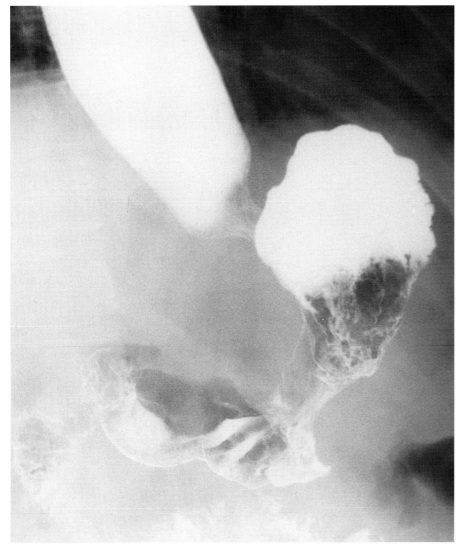

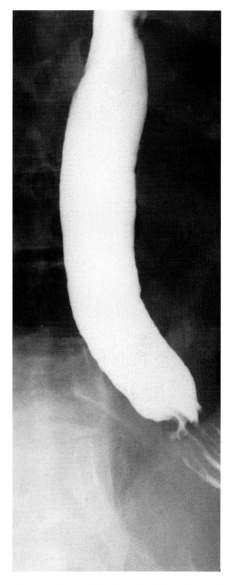

Fig. 2.60 Pseudoachalasia in carcinoma of the stomach. A barium study in this patient with proved diffuse, infiltrating gastric carcinoma shows marked oesophageal dilatation in the absence of a stricture [1].

Fig. 2.61 Systemic sclerosis (scleroderma) [13]. In this patient with known systemic sclerosis, the barium swallow shows moderate oesophageal dilatation; there is almost complete loss of peristalsis, but, unlike achalasia, the oesophagogastric junction is seen to be wide open and, in the recumbent position, there is marked gastro-oesophageal reflux. In patients in whom gastro-oesophageal reflux results in a peptic stricture, the radiological findings may resemble achalasia.

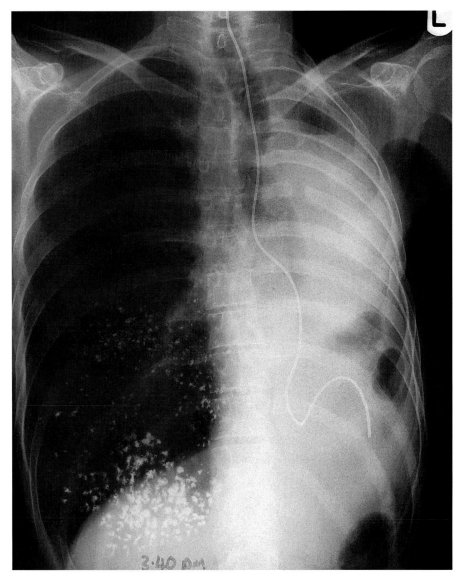

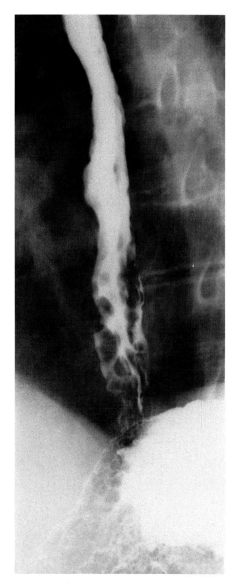

Fig. 2.62 Aspiration of barium. This 70-year-old male patient had had a left pneumonectomy for lung cancer 6 weeks previously. A barium study was performed because of some difficulty in swallowing, but no obstructing lesion was demonstrated. This chest X-ray, however, shows the result of extensive aspiration of barium, which forms numerous clumps in the right mid and lower zones. A nasogastric tube is shown in the stomach. If the aspirated barium reaches the alveoli, prolonged retention can result [28].

Fig. 2.63 Oesophageal varices. Widespread serpiginous filling defects are shown on this barium swallow in a patient with portal hypertension. These varicose collaterals, involving the proximal stomach and oesophagus, connect the left gastric vein with the azygos and hemiazygos systemic veins.

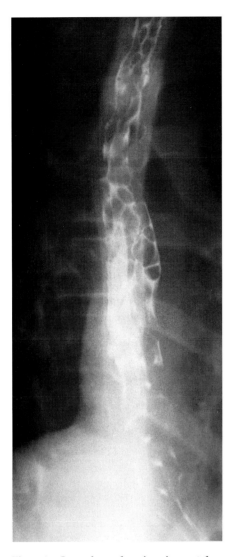

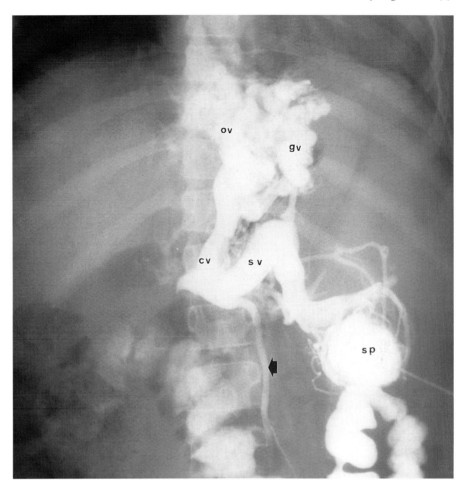

Fig. 2.64 Oesophageal varices in portal hypertension. This is a barium swallow in a 17-year-old male who had presented with variceal bleeding at the age of 3 resulting from portal vein thrombosis in infancy. In his childhood, he had had numerous haematemeses. The barium swallow shows gross filling defects throughout the oesophagus, typical of varices.

Fig. 2.65 Oesophageal varices, portal vein thrombosis. This splenoportogram produced by direct puncture and injection of contrast into the splenic pulp (sp) is seen to fill a massively distended splenic vein (sv), and most of the contrast is diverted into a markedly distended left gastric vein (coronary vein, cv), which is seen to fill huge oesophageal varices (ov) and gastric varices (gv). No portal vein filling has been demonstrated. There is retrograde filling of the inferior mesenteric vein (arrowhead). Some barium is incidentally present in the transverse colon. This direct technique has been replaced by indirect splenoportography using digital-subtraction angiography.

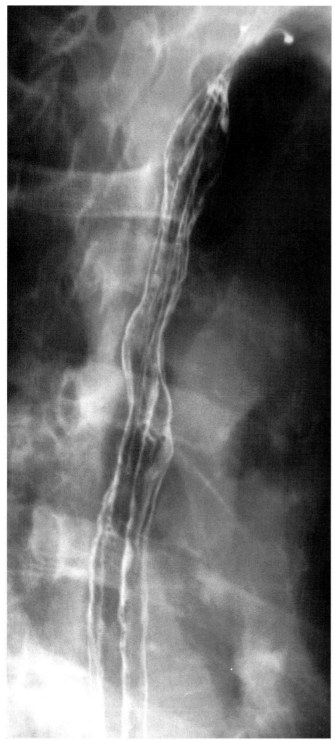

(a)

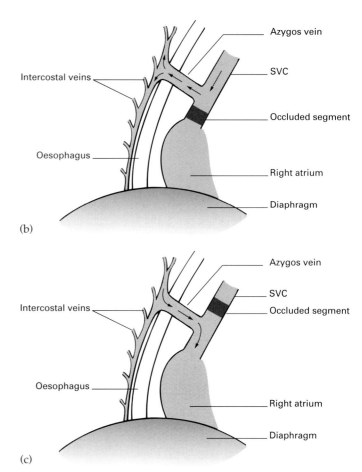

(b)

(c)

Fig. 2.66 Oesophageal varices associated with SVC obstruction. This 71-year-old male patient was found to have a widened mediastinum on chest X-ray. Adenocarcinoma was diagnosed by bronchoscopic biopsy and he subsequently developed obstruction of his superior vena cava (SVC) as well as some difficulty in swallowing. (a) The DCBS shows serpiginous filling defects in the proximal half of the oesophagus, consistent with varices. There was no clinical evidence of portal hypertension. These are sometimes called *downhill* varices, while varices related to portal hypertension are referred to as *uphill* varices [5]. (b) When the SVC is occluded below the junction of the SVC and azygos vein, the venous drainage from the SVC is diverted into the azygos vein and oesophageal collaterals, proximally and distally. (c) When the SVC is occluded above the termination of the azygos vein, blood is diverted round the obstruction via the proximal portion which, together with adjacent oesophageal veins, becomes engorged. Blood enters the SVC distal to the occlusion. In this type of case varices are likely to be confined to the proximal gullet.

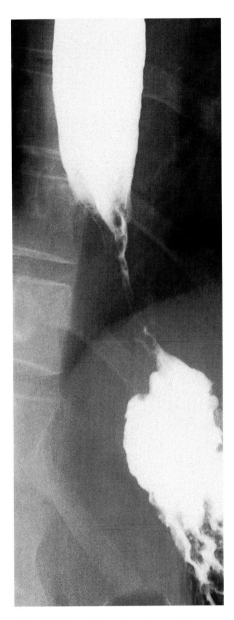

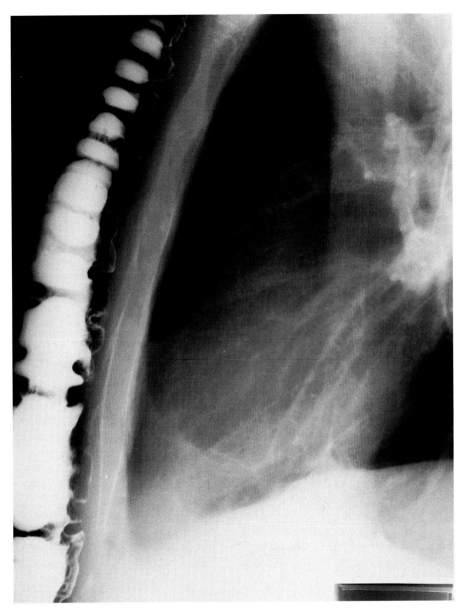

Fig. 2.67 Oesophageal varices and stricture following repeated injection sclerotherapy. A 45-year-old female patient with a history of alcoholic liver disease, portal hypertension and proved oesophageal varices, treated by repeated injection sclerotherapy, developed dysphagia. The barium swallow shows longitudinal filling defects, in keeping with varices. In addition, there is a stricture of the distal oesophagus, without shouldering and with no evidence of reflux. Gastric varices are also visible [29]. The stricture was successfully treated by the insertion of a metal stent.

Fig. 2.68 Oesophagectomy with colonic subcutaneous bypass. A barium swallow in a patient who had had an oesophagectomy for carcinoma, bypassed with a colonic conduit from the pharynx to the stomach, shows normal colonic filling in a subcutaneous presternal tunnel on this lateral view of the anterior chest.

3: The Stomach

Anatomy

Anatomically, the stomach is divided into several parts. The fundus, which is the highest part seen on erect projections, lies above the level of the oesophagogastric junction. However, in the supine position, the fundus of the stomach is the most dependent part and a circular pool of fluid occupying the normal fundus, sometimes seen on a supine plain X-ray, should not be mistaken for pathology in the fundus, the left adrenal gland or the upper pole of the left kidney. The cardia is the area surrounding the oesophagogastric junction and lacks precise marginal definition. The main part of the stomach, or body, extends from the fundus to the antrum. The proximal limit of the antrum is defined by a line that transects the stomach at the incisura. The antrum extends distally to the pyloric canal, which is surrounded by a prominent circular sphincter of smooth muscle; this regulates the process of gastric emptying, in conjunction with peristaltic waves, which course through the stomach under the influence of the vagus nerves. The shape of the stomach is variable. In slim subjects, it tends to have a vertical J-shaped orientation, but, in muscular or obese individuals, its long axis tends to lie transversely.

The stomach lies within the peritoneal cavity and has important peritoneal attachments or ligaments. The lesser omentum (gastrohepatic ligament) attaches the lesser curve of the stomach to the liver. The greater omentum is attached to the convexity of the greater curve of the stomach. The posterior wall of the stomach forms part of the anterior wall of the lesser sac and is therefore closely related to the anterior surface of the pancreas.

The mucosal lining of the stomach has a distinct appearance on account of long parallel folds, known as rugae, which are 3–5 mm in thickness. In addition, the mucosal surface has a fine mosaic pattern, which is readily demonstrated on double-contrast examinations and consists of tiny nodular elevations, known as areae gastricae. Unlike the rugae, the areae gastricae are visible in both the distended and non-distended state. The quality of the mucosal coating on a double-contrast barium meal can be assessed by the presence or absence of areae gastricae [1].

The blood supply of the stomach is provided by two major vascular arcades, one of which is related to the lesser curve and formed by the right and left gastric arteries, while the other lies in close proximity to the greater curve and is formed by the right and left gastroepiploic arteries. The left gastric artery normally originates as one of the three major branches of the coeliac axis, the artery of the primitive foregut. The territory of the left gastric artery accounts for about 85% of gastric haemorrhages [2]. The right gastric artery is small and it almost always arises in the region of the common hepatic artery bifurcation. The terminal branch of the gastroduodenal artery is the right gastroepiploic artery, which anastamoses with the left gastroepiploic artery. This vessel usually arises from the main splenic artery. The most important of the gastric veins is the left gastric vein, or coronary vein, which is closely related to the lesser curve of the stomach. The point at which it joints the confluence of the superior mesenteric vein and splenic vein is variable. In portal hypertension, the left gastric vein is frequently an important collateral for spontaneous portosystemic shunting and, in splenic vein occlusion, it may provide spleno-portal collateral flow.

Plain film radiography

Plain films are of limited value, but may provide diagnostic information in specific situations—for example, hiatus hernia, gastric volvulus, gastric ulcer perforation or gastric outlet obstruction—or in the detection of ingested opaque foreign bodies.

Barium studies

The original and simplest form of barium study consisted of observing, by means of fluoroscopy and appropriate films, the stomach filled with barium in search of contour defects, a loss of distensibility or rigidity of the wall. While this may detect gross pathology, such as linitis plastica, it provides no information about the gastric mucosa. For this purpose, the double-contrast technique has been used very successfully during the past 25 years. This modification involves distending the fasted stomach with a gas-producing agent, normally carbon dioxide (CO_2) [3]. This product consists of sodium bicarbonate, together with a weak acid and antifoaming agent. Approximately 300–500 ml CO_2 may be generated by a single dose. This is followed by a relatively small volume, typically 100–150 ml, of a high-density, low-viscosity barium sulphate suspension up to 250% w/v. An essential feature of the method is to coat or paint the mucosa of the gas-distended stomach with this low-viscosity barium suspension. This can be achieved by turning the patient several times. In this way, quite small mucosal lesions may be detected. The examination may be significantly enhanced by the use of hyoscine-*N*-butyl bromide (Buscopan) 20 mg IV or glucagon 0.1 mg IV. The stomach is examined in a variety of projections, using a combination of fluoroscopy and appropriate films. The advent of digital technology has significantly improved the overall performance of the method. The thoroughness of the technique, however, is limited in severely ill or immobile patients.

Water-soluble contrast studies

In the specific circumstances in which perforation of a gastric ulcer is suspected or in the postoperative period to confirm or exclude anastamotic leaks, a water-soluble contrast medium—for example, meglumine diatrizoate (Gastrografin)—should be used instead of barium suspension, since the latter is a cause of peritoneal fibrosis [4].

Computerized tomography scanning

Cross-sectional imaging using CT can provide an accurate assessment of the thickness of the stomach wall, provided there is adequate gastric distension. Normally, the wall of the suitably distended stomach measures approximately 3 mm and should not exceed 5 mm. A suitable regime would be 500 ml of 10–15% water-soluble contrast—for example, Gastrografin—or 1–2% barium suspension 30 min prior to the examination and a further 200 ml immediately before the scan. The patient is fasted beforehand. Excellent demonstration of the stomach can be achieved, particularly with modern rapid scanners employing a spiral (helical) method of data acquisition. The normal oesophagogastric junction may produce an intraluminal bulge at the cardia and should not be confused with pathology. A suspected mass lesion on CT should be confirmed by the administration of additional contrast (CO_2) and IV hyoscine 20 mg or glucagon 0.1 mg. Lateral and prone positioning may also be required [5]. Diagnostic criteria include normal distensibility, a lack of rigidity, the thickness of the gastric wall and focal mural lesions. Lymphadenopathy should also be confirmed or excluded. The CT diagnosis of lymph node spread (like MRI) is based on node size only and these methods cannot identify malignant disease in normal-sized nodes [6]. The lesser omentum is usually visible on CT [7]. Non-enhancing nodules are likely to represent significant lymphadenopathy if they exceed 8 mm in diameter in this region [8].

Magnetic resonance imaging

This technique, which has been so valuable in many clinical situations, has so far failed to make a major impact on the assessment of gastric pathology. Several factors are responsible, including the limitation of anatomical resolution caused by cardiovascular, peristaltic and respiratory motion artefacts.

Angiography

The widespread use of more effective medical treatment—for example, proton-pump inhibitors and H_2-receptor antagonists—has led to a reduced incidence of gastrointestinal haemorrhage. In addition, endoscopic equipment has undergone refinement, in terms of both diagnosis and treatment, and improvements in cross-sectional imaging have resulted in fewer indications for diagnostic and therapeutic procedures. Intra-arterial digital-subtraction angiography (DSA) is now an essential component of a properly equipped gastrointestinal vascular unit [9]. Much smaller volumes of contrast may be used, unwanted background detail is eliminated from the images and intra-arterial DSA facilitates imaging of the portal, splenic and mesenteric veins, as well as the arterial circulation. Intravenous DSA is of no value in this vascular territory [9].

Endoscopic ultrasound

The ease with which the stomach may be distended with water renders it remarkably suitable for acoustic access. This allows close evaluation of the gastric wall with a directable endoscope [10]. Five layers of the stomach wall can be identified, namely the mucosa, deep mucosa, submucosa, muscularis propria and the serosa. Endoscopic ultrasound can also evaluate the perigastric nodes, and nodes as small as 5 mm may be visible. The technique has therefore become a valuable tool in tumour staging [11].

References

1 Laufer I. (1994) Barium studies. In: Gore R.M., Levine M.S. & Laufer I. (eds) *A Textbook of Gastro-intestinal Radiology*. Philadelphia: W.B. Saunders, 292–303.
2 Kelemouridis V., Athanasoulis C.A. & Waltman A.C. (1983) Gastric bleeding sites: an angiographic study. *Radiology* **149**, 643–648.
3 Gelfand D.W. & Haschiya J. (1969) The double contrast examination of the stomach using gas producing granules and tablets. *Radiology* **93**, 1381–1382.
4 Westfall R.H., Nelson R.H. & Musselman M.M. (1966) Barium peritonitis. *American Journal of Surgery* **112**, 760–764.

5 Burgener F.A. & Kormano M. (1996) *Differential Diagnosis in Computed Tomography.* Stuttgart: Thieme Medical Publishers, 293–308.

6 Tio T.L. & Tytgat G.N.J. (1986) Endoscopic ultrasonography in analysing peri-intestinal lymph node abnormality: preliminary results of studies *in vitro* and *in vivo. Scandinavian Journal of Gastro-enterology* **21**, 158–163.

7 Balfe D.M., Mauro M.A., Koehler R.E. *et al.* (1984) Gastro-hepatic ligament: normal and pathological CT anatomy. *Radiology* **150**, 485–490.

8 Harris K.M., Roberts G.M. & Laurie B.W. (1994) Normal anatomy and techniques of examination of the stomach and duodenum. In: Freeny P.C. & Stevenson G.W. (eds) *Margulis and Burhenne's Alimentary Tract Radiology,* 5th edn. St Louis: Mosby, 282–310.

9 Allison D.J. (1997) Gastro-intestinal angiography. In: Grainger R.G. & Allison D.J. (eds) *Diagnostic Radiology,* 3rd edn. New York: Churchill Livingstone, 1091–1108.

10 Botet J.F. & Lightdale C.J. (1994) Endosonography: normal anatomy and techniques of examination of the stomach and duodenum. In: Freeny P.C. & Stevenson G.W. (eds) *Margulis and Burhenne's Alimentary Tract Radiology,* 5th edn. St Louis: Mosby, 311–317.

11 McLean A. & Fairclough P. (1996) Endoscopic ultrasound — current applications. *Clinical Radiology* **51**, 83–98.

12 Bruneton J.N., Caramella E., Cazenave P. *et al.* (1987) Gastric leiomyosarcoma: comparative value of barium examinations, ultrasonography and CT scans. *European Journal of Radiology* **7**, 160–162.

13 Simpkins K.C. (1993) The stomach and duodenum. In: Sutton D. (ed.) *A Textbook of Radiology and Imaging,* 5th edn. Edinburgh: Churchill Livingstone, 789–829.

14 Thoeni R.F. & Moss A.A. (1979) The radiographic appearance of complications following Nissen fundoplication. *Radiology* **131**, 17–21.

15 Gelfand D.W. (1997) The stomach. In: Grainger R.G. & Allison D.J. (eds) *Diagnostic Radiology,* 3rd edn. New York: Churchill Livingstone, 941–972.

16 Aleman S. (1948) Jejunogastric intussusception: a rare complication of the operated stomach. *Acta Radiologica* **29**, 383–395.

17 Dahnert W. (1996) *Radiology Review Manual,* 3rd edn. Baltimore: Williams & Wilkins, 554 and 602.

18 Eisenberg R.L. (1994) Miscellaneous gastric and duodenal abnormalities. In: Gore R.M., Levine M.S. & Laufer I. (eds) *A Textbook of Gastro-intestinal Radiology.* Philadelphia: W.B. Saunders, 717–741.

Suggested further reading

Bragg D.J., Thompson W.M. & Humphrey E.W. (1994) Applications and limitations of imaging in staging and follow-up of gastro-intestinal neoplasms. In: Freeny P.C. & Stevenson G.W. (eds) *Margulis and Burhenne's Alimentary Tract Radiology,* 5th edn. St Louis: Mosby, 881–887.

Burkett H.G., Quick C.R.G. & Gatt D. (1990) *Essential Surgery.* Edinburgh: Churchill Livingstone, 219–242.

Davies J., Chalmers A.G., Sue-Ling H.M. *et al.* (1997) Spiral CT and operative staging of gastric carcinoma: a comparison with histopathological staging. *Gut* **41**, 314–319.

Fischbach W., Kestel W., Kirschner T. *et al.* (1992) Malignant lymphomas of the upper gastro-intestinal tract. *Cancer* **70**, 1075–1080.

Goldberg H.I. (1994) Malignant tumours of the stomach. In: Freeny P.C. & Stevenson G.W. (eds) *Margulis and Burhenne's Alimentary Tract Radiology,* 5th edn. St Louis: Mosby, 429–436.

Gore R.M., Levine M.S., Ghahremani G.C. & Miller F.H. (1997) Gastric cancer radiologic diagnosis. In: Gore R.M. (ed.) *Staging Gastrointestinal Malignancy.* Radiologic Clinics of North America, Vol. 35(2). Philadelphia: W.B. Saunders, 311–329.

Levine M.S. & Megibow A.J. (1994) Carcinoma (stomach). In: Gore R.M., Levine M.S. & Laufer I. (eds) *A Textbook of Gastro-intestinal Radiology.* Philadelphia: W.B. Saunders, 660–683.

MacSween R.N.M. & Whaley K. (1993) In: *Muir's Textbook of Pathology,* 13th edn. London: Arnold, 695–699.

Megibow A.J. (1994) The gastro-intestinal tract. In: Haaga J.R., Lanzieri C.F., Sartoris D.J. & Zerhouni E.A. (eds) *Computed Tomography and Magnetic Resonance Imaging of the Whole Body,* 3rd edn. St Louis: Mosby, 855–895.

Miller F.H., Kochman M.L., Talamonti M.S., Ghahremani G.C. & Gore R.M. (1997) Gastric cancer radiologic staging. In: Gore R.M. (ed.) *Staging Gastrointestinal Malignancy.* Radiologic Clinics of North America, Vol. 35(2). Philadelphia: W.B. Saunders, 311–349.

Ng C.S., Husband J.E.S., MacVicar A.D.L., Ross P. & Cunningham D.C. (1998) Correlation of CT with histopathological findings in patients with gastric and gastro-oesophageal carcinomas following neoadjuvant chemotherapy. *Clinical Radiology* **53**(6), 422–427.

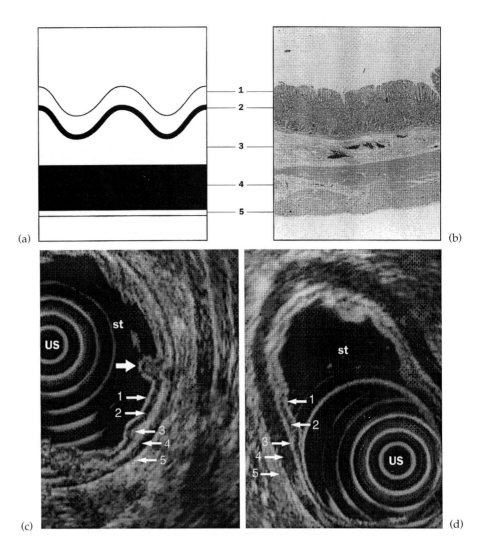

Fig. 3.1 Endoscopic ultrasound. Standard endoscopic ultrasound transducers operate at frequencies of 7.5–12 MHz. At these frequencies, the structure of the bowel wall can be resolved into five distinct alternative hyper- and hypoechoic bands, which correspond to the histological structure of the bowel wall. The thickness of individual layers varies throughout the gut and may be influenced by technical scanning factors. High-resolution probes (up to 20 MHz) can resolve more detailed wall structure and demonstrate between seven and nine distinct layers. (a) Diagramatic presentation of the five-layered structure of the bowel. (b) Histological section through the gastric wall. (c) Water-filled stomach with a section through the body. Bold arrow, gastric fold. (d) Antrum of the stomach demonstrating the five-layered structure. 1, mucosa (echogenic); 2, deep mucosa (hypochoic); 3, submucosa (echogenic); 4, muscularis propria (hypoechoic); 5, serosa/adventia (echogenic). st, stomach; US, ultrasound source. (Reprinted from [11] with permission; courtesy of Dr Alison McLean.)

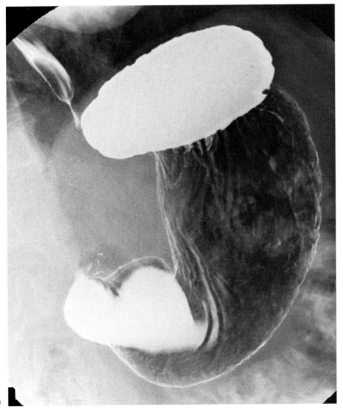

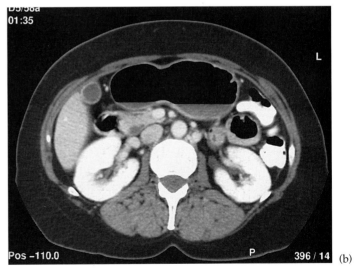

Fig. 3.2 Normal stomach. (a) Double-contrast barium meal (DCBM). The mucosa has been coated with barium, showing a normal rugal pattern, and the areae gastricae are visible. Normal gaseous distension of the lumen with CO_2 is apparent. (b) Spiral CT scan with IV contrast enhancement. The stomach has been distended with CO_2, using an oral gas-forming agent. The normal gastric wall is shown. This is usually about 3 mm in thickness and should not exceed 5 mm.

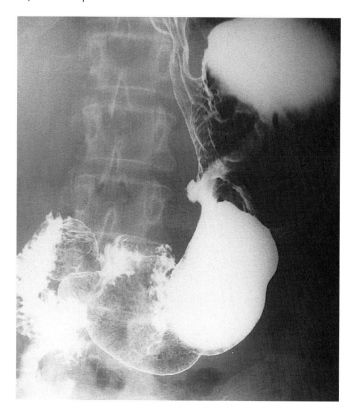

Fig. 3.3 Benign gastric ulcer. A 1.5 cm diameter, penetrating ulcer crater is seen to fill with barium on the lesser curve of the stomach. The adjacent greater curve of stomach is characteristically indrawn to form a transient incisura resulting from muscle spasm. The ulcer crater projects beyond the gastric wall and there is a well-defined ulcer collar.

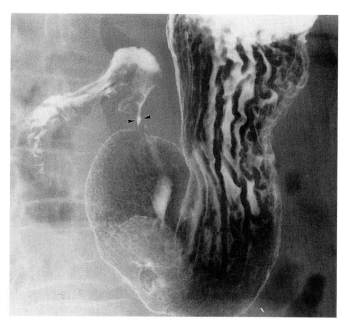

Fig. 3.5 Pyloric canal peptic ulcer, DCBM. There is a constant barium-filled crater within the pyloric canal (arrowheads) associated with considerable pyloroduodenal deformity, in keeping with long-standing peptic ulceration. The rugal mucosal pattern and the areae gastricae are well shown. The patient presented with recurrent abdominal pain, nausea and vomiting.

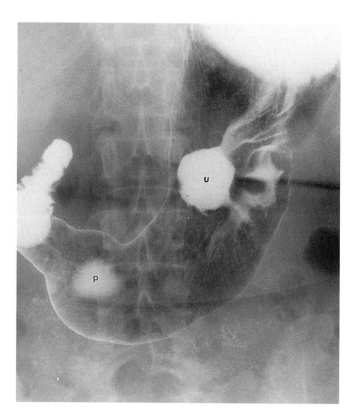

Fig. 3.4 Giant benign gastric ulcer. A very large ulcer crater, measuring almost 4 cm in diameter, is seen to fill with barium on the posterior wall of the body of the stomach. Thickened oedematous gastric folds are seen to radiate to the edge of the ulcer crater (u). A small pool of barium is visible in the antrum of the stomach (p). Fluoroscopy showed that this was inconstant and therefore of no pathological significance.

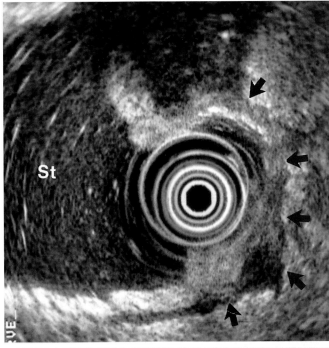

(a)

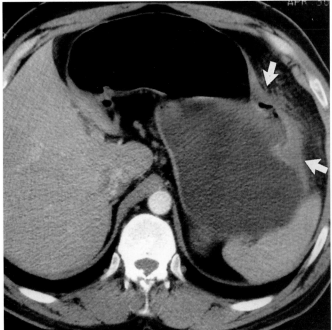

(b)

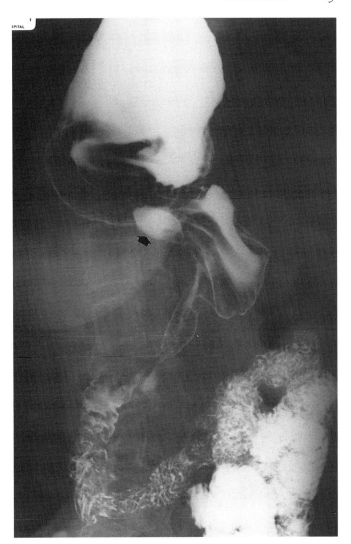

Fig. 3.7 Benign gastric ulcer associated with non-obstructive gastric volvulus. A 3.5 cm diameter ulcer crater is seen to fill with barium on the lesser-curve aspect of the stomach (arrowhead). Most of the stomach has undergone rotation and herniation into the mediastinum, but no obstruction was present.

Fig. 3.6 Benign gastric ulcer, endoscopic ultrasound. (a) The probe is lying within the ulcer crater. There is destruction of the layered structure (arrows), with irregularity of the serosal margin. No definite mass lesion has been identified. There are no reliable endoscopic US criteria to differentiate between a benign gastric ulcer and ulcerated malignancy. St, stomach. (b) A CT scan in the same patient shows the ulcer crater on the greater curve (between arrows). The stomach has been distended with water. (Courtesy of Dr Alison McLean.)

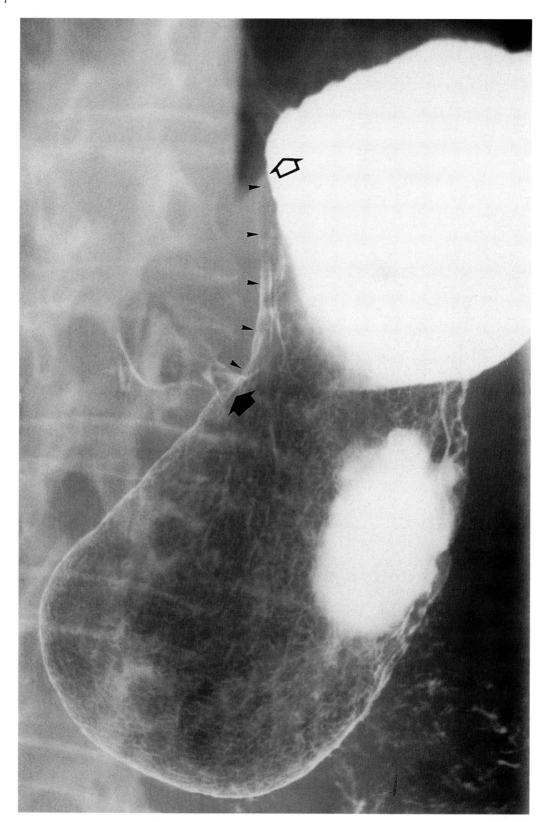

Fig. 3.8 Grossly contracted lesser curve of the stomach. This 62-year-old female patient had a long history of recurrent lesser-curve gastric ulcers, which has resulted in gross cicatrization and contraction of the lesser curve (small arrowheads), with resultant relative lengthening of the greater curve and apparent upward migration of the pylorus (large black arrowhead). There is no current gastric ulceration. The position of the oesophagogastric junction is indicated by the open arrowhead. There was no previous gastric surgery.

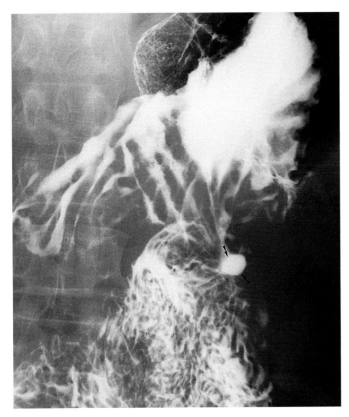

Fig. 3.9 Benign stomal ulceration. This middle-aged male patient had a previous vagotomy and gastrojejunostomy for duodenal ulceration. There was a recent history of recurrent abdominal pain and vomiting. The DCBM shows a constant, well-circumscribed, 1.5 cm ulcer crater (double arrowheads) straddling the gastrojejunostomy. The adjacent mucosal folds, particularly on the gastric side of the stoma, are markedly thickened, in keeping with oedema. The gastrojejunostomy was still patent.

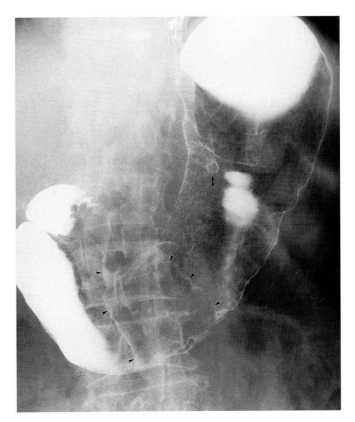

Fig. 3.10 Calcified coeliac artery. In this elderly patient, the abdominal aorta is displaced to the left and the calcified coeliac artery is projected end-on through the body of the stomach (double arrowhead). This should not be confused with a gastric ulcer. In addition, the DCBM shows a technical artefact in the antrum of the stomach, in which normal mucosal coating has been temporarily prevented by contact between the anterior and posterior walls of the stomach (arrowheads). This appearance should not be confused with a pathological filling defect.

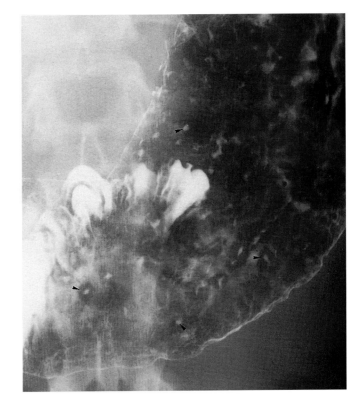

Fig. 3.11 Erosive gastritis. A DCBM showing multiple erosions affecting the gastric mucosa (arrowheads). These are depicted by very small collections of barium, surrounded by an oedematous halo. These non-specific lesions occurred in a 25-year-old female psychiatric patient with a 6-month history of epigastric pain, nausea and vomiting. She had made multiple attempts at self-poisoning. These lesions are indistinguishable from the aphthoid ulcers of Crohn's disease. However, endoscopic biopsy in this case revealed non-specific gastritis.

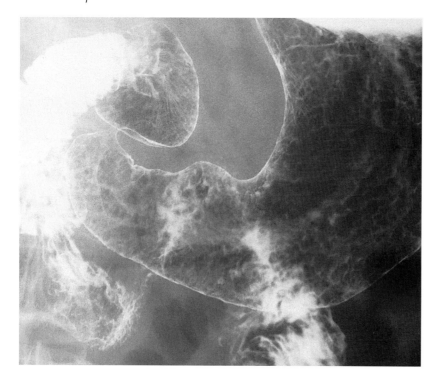

Fig. 3.12 Erosive gastritis. This 67-year-old female patient presented with non-specific dyspeptic symptoms. The DCBM shows normal gastric distensibility, but multiple gastric erosions are visible, particularly in the antrum.

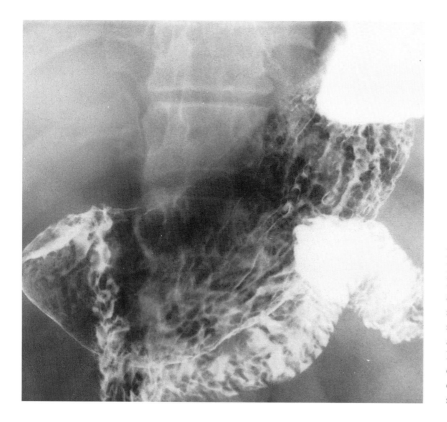

Fig. 3.13 Crohn's disease of the stomach. A DCBM in a 34-year-old male patient with histologically proved small-bowel Crohn's disease and non-specific dyspeptic symptoms. Numerous small rounded lesions are shown throughout the stomach, many with a central niche, typical, although not diagnostic, of aphthoid ulcers. Histology of the gastric mucosa confirmed non-caseating granulomata characteristic of Crohn's disease. The differential diagnosis includes non-specific erosive gastritis and multiple polyps.

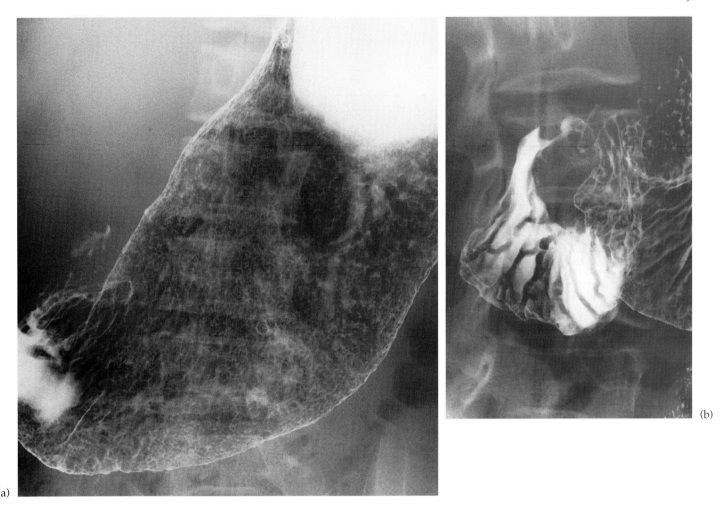

(a)

(b)

Fig. 3.14 Gastric sarcoidosis. (a) A DCBM in a 17-year-old male patient with several months' history of vomiting, 19 kg (3 stone) weight loss and diarrhoea. The distensibility of the stomach is normal, but there is a very widespread reticular pattern, which, together with an irregular stricture of the second part of the duodenum, was thought radiologically to represent Crohn's disease (b). The mucosal biopsies indicated epithelioid granulomata, suggestive of sarcoidosis.

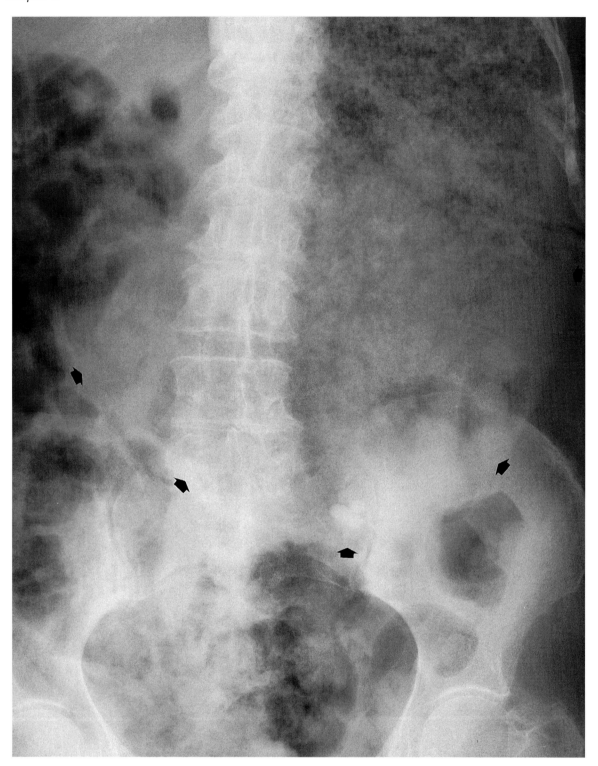

Fig. 3.15 Pyloric stenosis (postpeptic ulcer). This 62-year-old female patient has a long history of recurrent duodenal ulceration. For 3 months, vomiting was a prominent feature, and this included some items ingested several days previously. This plain abdominal X-ray shows a very extensive area of mottling, predominantly in the left upper quadrant, but extending to the right and into the left iliac fossa. This was due to a huge food residue in a markedly distended stomach, the greater curve being indicated by the arrowheads. The differential diagnosis includes gastric bezoar, pancreatic pseudocyst and splenomegaly.

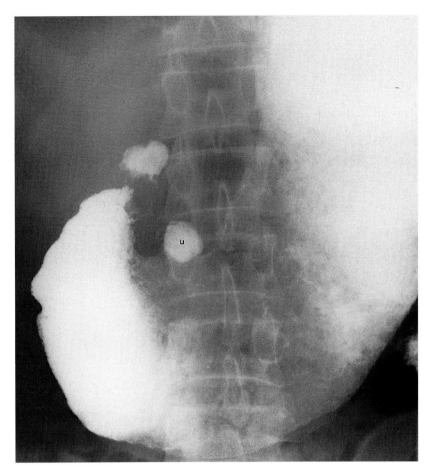

Fig. 3.16 Gastric-outlet obstruction (postpeptic ulceration) and gastric stasis ulcer. This elderly male patient had a very long history of periodic dyspepsia, epigastric pain and vomiting. The DCBM shows a hugely distended stomach, with a very large fasting residue. A large penetrating ulcer crater (u) is seen to arise from the lesser curve aspect of the gastric antrum. The pyloric canal is narrow, and gastric emptying was very slow.

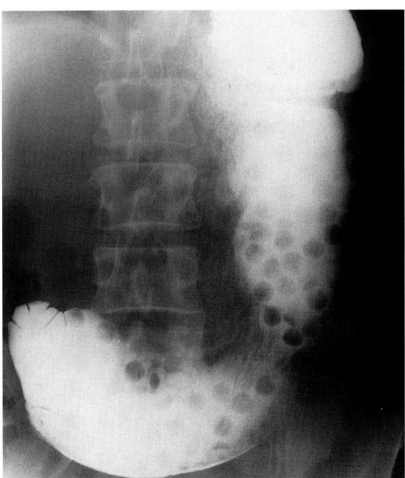

Fig. 3.17 Benign pyloric stenosis. This DCBM in a male patient with long-standing periodic dyspepsia shows numerous well-circumscribed filling defects throughout the stomach. These consisted of undigested codeine tablets, which the patient used for self-medication.

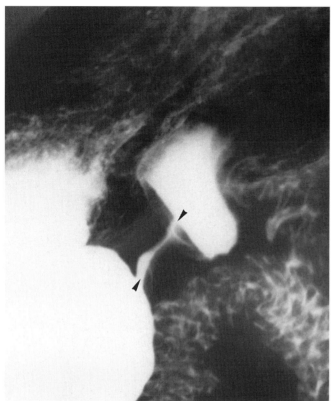

(a)

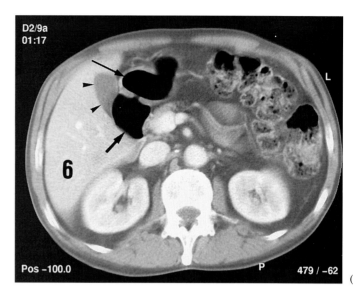

(b)

Fig. 3.18 (a) **Adult hypertrophic pyloric stenosis and pyloric carcinoma.** This 55-year-old male patient had a 12-year history of periodic dyspepsia and a recent history of vomiting. The DCBM shows a smooth stricture of the pyloric canal, which measures 20 mm in length and which fails to relax normally (normal pyloric canal length is 5–10 mm). The duodenum was normal. Histology of the resected specimen showed adult hypertrophic pyloric stenosis and also a small pyloric-canal carcinoma. **(b) Normal pyloric canal.** The CT scan shows a normal pyloric sphincter between the antrum of the stomach (long thin arrow) and duodenal bulb (short arrow). Both have been distended with CO_2. Arrowheads, gallbladder; 6, segment 6 of the liver.

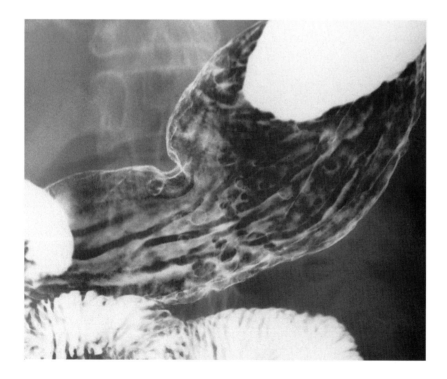

Fig. 3.19 **Hyperplastic gastric polyps.** This DCBM shows multiple, fixed filling defects on the gastric mucosa. There is normal gastric distensibility. The differential diagnosis includes food residue, hamartomatous polyps and multiple adenomata.

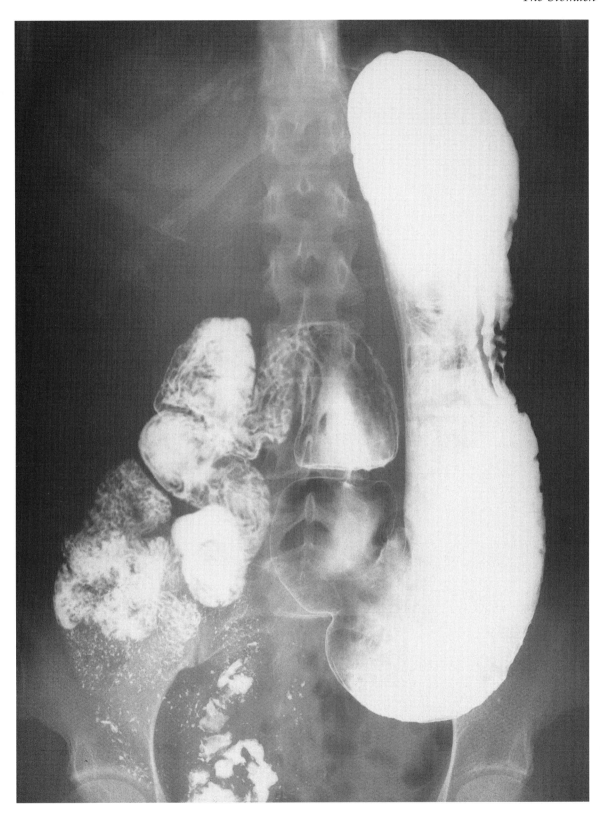

Fig. 3.20 Gastric pseudo-obstruction. A 21-year-old female patient with a long history of chronic constipation had been treated by colectomy and ileorectal anastomosis for slow transit. The DCBM shows marked gastric distension, which was slow to empty and which contained a substantial fasting residue. There was no evidence of any obstructing lesion in the stomach, duodenum or small bowel.

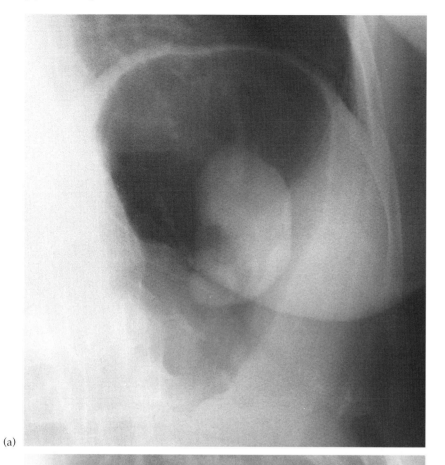

(a)

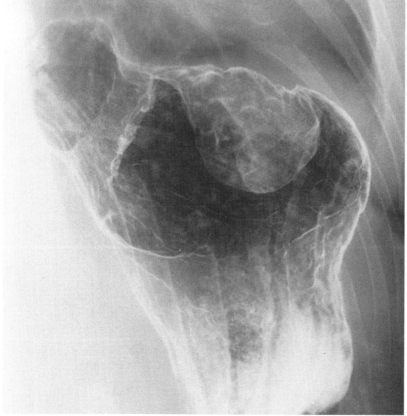

(b)

Fig. 3.21 Leiomyoma of the stomach. (a) A plain
film with the patient prone. A 7 cm smooth
opacity of soft-tissue density is outlined by gas in
the stomach. (b) An erect DCBM, which shows
the soft-tissue mass arising from the fundus of the
stomach. The endoscopic appearance was typical
of leiomyoma and mucosal biopsy was normal.

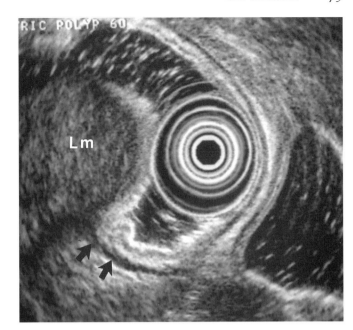

Fig. 3.22 Leiomyoma, endoscopic ultrasound. A large mass of intermediate reflectivity (Lm) arising from the muscularis propria (arrows) of the gastric wall. The layer of origin suggests that this is likely to be a leiomyoma. There are no reliable criteria on endoscopic US to distinguish between benign and malignant lesions. However, a size greater than 3 cm and a heterogeneous appearance are suspicious features of malignancy and warrant biopsy. (Courtesy of Dr Alison McLean.)

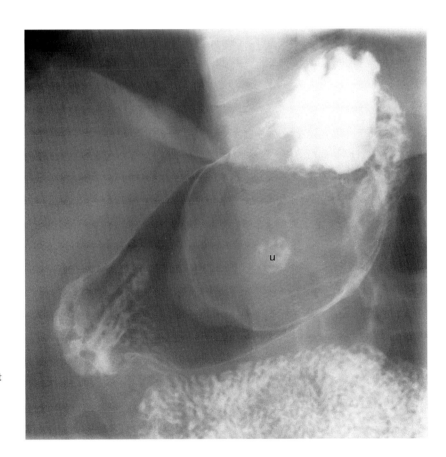

Fig. 3.23 Leiomyoma with ulceration. A middle-aged female patient presented with a recent haematemesis. The DCBM shows a very large, 12 cm, smooth filling defect occupying a large part of the body of the stomach. On the surface of the lesion there is a constant barium niche (u), consistent with ulceration. These findings were confirmed endoscopically.

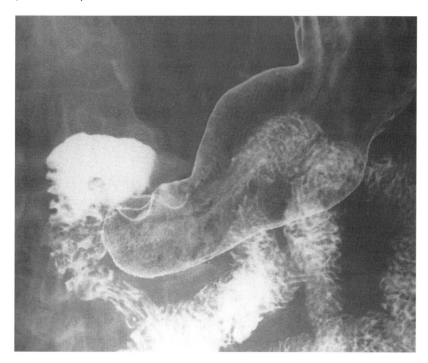

Fig. 3.24 Leiomyomata of gastric antrum. This 80-year-old female patient presented with non-specific dyspeptic symptoms. Two barium-meal examinations 12 months apart revealed identical findings. Two smooth filling defects are seen to arise from the lesser-curve aspect of the antrum. Endoscopic biopsy on two separate occasions revealed normal mucosa.

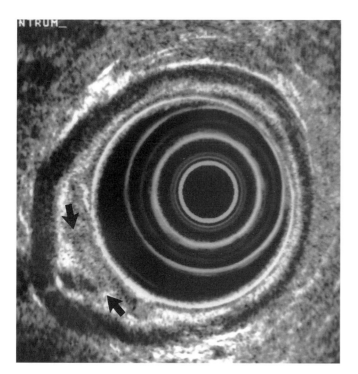

Fig. 3.25 Pancreatic rest in wall of stomach. Endoscopic ultrasound shows a slightly hypoechoic mass (arrows) deep to the mucosal layer, which contains a branching hypoechoic focus, suggesting a central primitive duct system, as seen on DCBM studies. (Courtesy of Dr Alison McLean.)

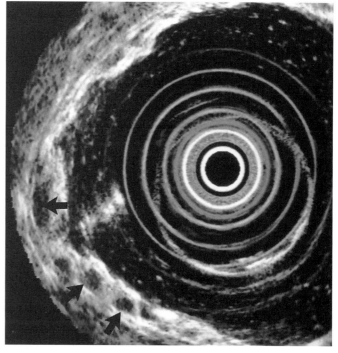

Fig. 3.26 Gastric varices. Endoscopic ultrasound shows multiple anechoic areas (arrows) within the submucosa (layer 3). The patient has a splenic vein thrombosis, with development of gastric varices. (Courtesy of Dr Alison McLean.)

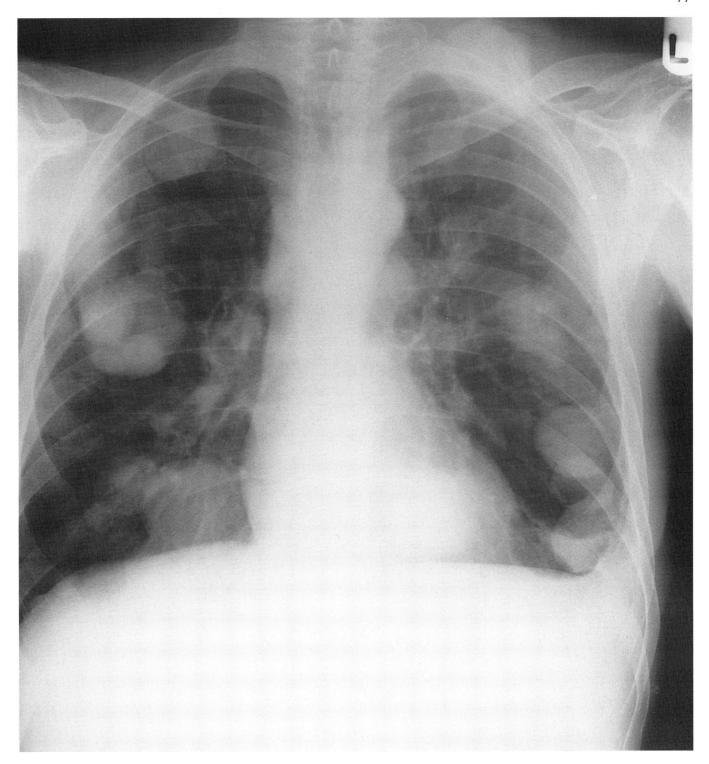

Fig. 3.27 Gastric carcinoma with metastatic spread. The chest X-ray shows numerous well-defined mass lesions within both lung fields, including one large lesion projected through the heart shadow at the left base, in keeping with pulmonary metastases. In addition, there is a well-defined supraclavicular mass lesion on the left side (Virchow's nodes) (Troisier's sign).

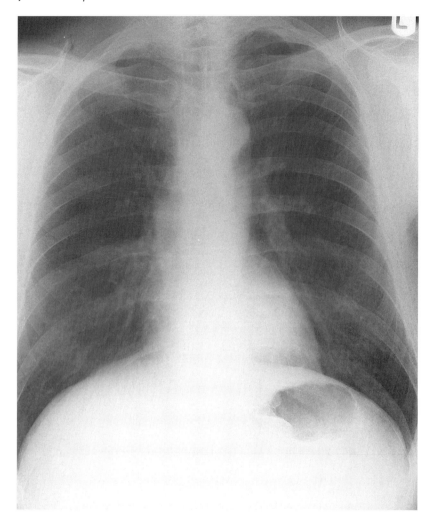

Fig. 3.28 Carcinoma of the cardia. This chest X-ray taken soon after a barium-meal examination shows an irregular filling defect in the gas bubble of the gastric fundus. A similar, but less obvious, abnormality may be apparent on a plain X-ray. Cancer of the stomach is the third most common alimentary tract malignancy.

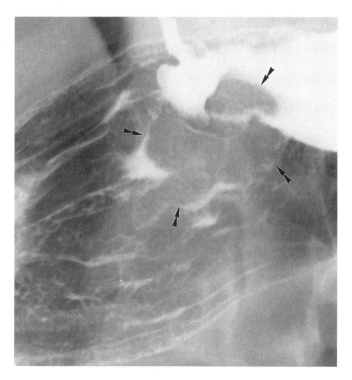

Fig. 3.29 Carcinoma of the cardia. A 67-year-old male patient experienced progressive dysphagia over a 4–6-week period. The DCBM shows a constant irregular filling defect involving the cardia and extending into the distal oesophagus. Minimal oesophageal dilatation was present. The margins of the lesion are indicated by double arrowheads. The detection of such lesions depends on adequate mucosal coating and careful fluoroscopy, utilizing the barium pool.

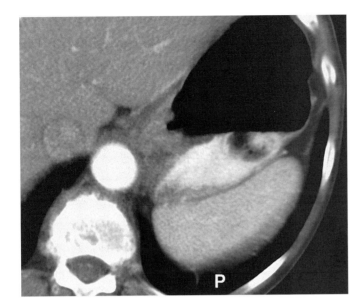

Fig. 3.30 Carcinoma of the cardia, spiral CT scan. The patient
has been given oral Gastrografin and a gas-forming agent to
distend the stomach. There is a constant, irregular filling defect
involving the cardia, in keeping with carcinoma. This was
confirmed by endoscopic biopsy. The mass encases the aorta for
about 180°.

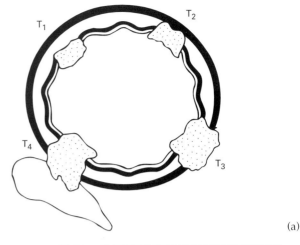

(a)

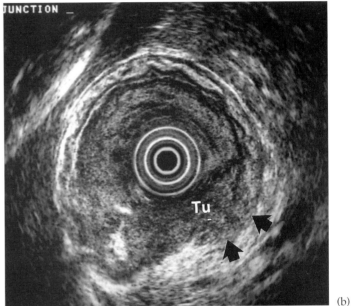

(b)

Fig. 3.31 Gastric carcinoma, endoscopic ultrasound. The ability
to resolve the layers of the bowel wall makes endoscopic US a
valuable tool for tumour staging. This is particularly valuable in
early disease, where the tumour may be limited to the submucosa
or muscularis propria. (a) Diagrammatic representation of T
staging of gastrointestinal cancer: T1 tumour limited to the
mucosa or submucosa; T2 tumour invading muscularis propria;
T3 tumour penetrates serosa (visceral peritoneum) without
invasion of the adjacent structures; T4 tumour invades adjacent
structures. (b) A polypoid tumour mass (Tu) at the gastric cardia
is projecting into the lumen of the stomach, with the normal wall
stretched around the tumour. At the point of origin, there is
destruction of the normal wall, with extension beyond the
muscularis (T3). (c) There is diffuse infiltration of the gastric
antrum with thickening and destruction of the layered pattern of
the wall. There is also a trace of ascites (straight arrow). The
tumour is seen to extend beyond the gastric wall into the
pancreas (P, curved arrows) (T4). An enlarged rounded
hypoechoic malignant node is identified, adjacent to the gastric
wall (N, thick arrow). L, liver. (Courtesy of Dr Alison McLean.)

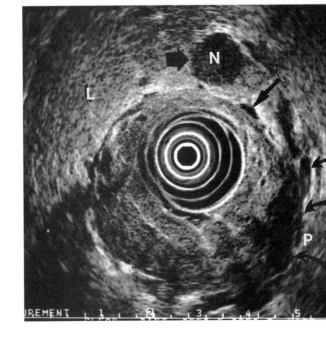

(c)

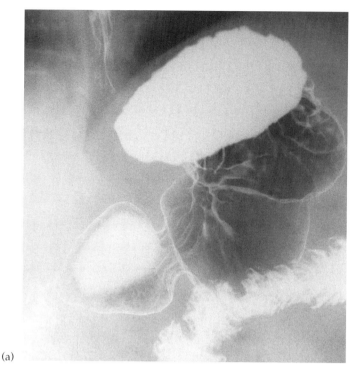

(a)

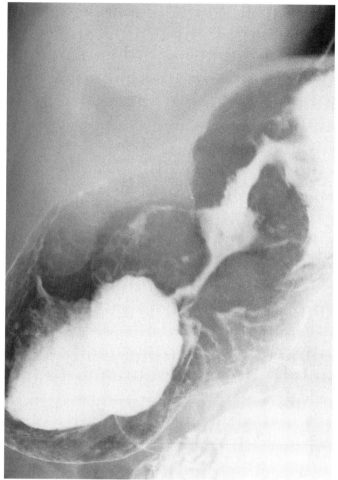

(b)

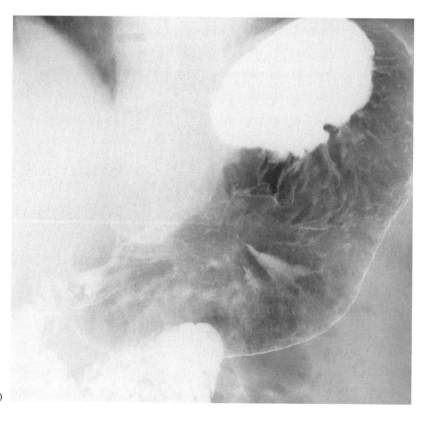

(c)

Fig. 3.32 Malignant gastric ulcer. (a) A 60-year-old male patient had a lesser-curve gastric ulcer diagnosed by DCBM. Multiple endoscopic biopsies at that time revealed no evidence of malignancy and the patient was treated for 2 years with an H_2-receptor antagonist. After an initial symptomatic improvement, the patient's symptoms recurred, he lost weight and the DCBM was repeated. (b and c) The second examination shows a very extensive ulcerated, lobulated tumour mass involving the lesser curve of the stomach and the anterior and posterior walls. Gastric carcinoma was confirmed endoscopically.

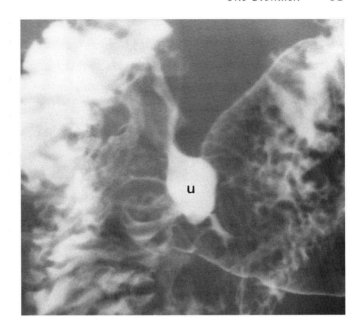

Fig. 3.33 Malignant gastric ulcer. A 64-year-old male patient presented with a short history of abdominal pain, nausea and vomiting. The DCBM shows a large, irregular ulcer crater (u) in the antrum of the stomach, with considerable mucosal irregularity adjacent to it. Endoscopic biopsy confirmed carcinoma. Predisposing factors to gastric cancer are chronic atrophic gastritis, pernicious anaemia, adenomatous polyps and previous gastric surgery, particularly gastrojejunostomy.

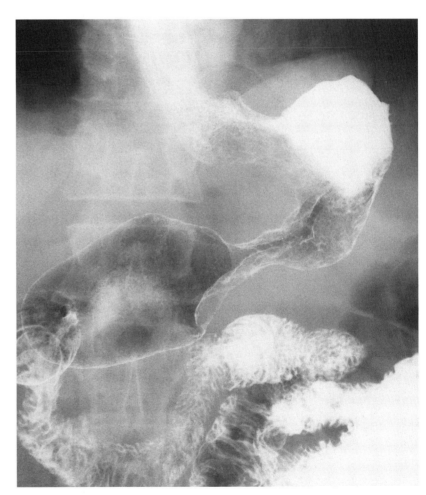

Fig. 3.34 Carcinoma of the fundus and the body of the stomach. The DCBM shows a marked loss of distensibility of the fundus and most of the body of the stomach, with marked irregularity of the mucosa in this region. The antrum of the stomach distends normally and the mucosa appears normal. Fluoroscopically, the affected stomach appears rigid. The differential diagnosis includes lymphoma and extension of malignancy from adjacent organs—in particular, the pancreas.

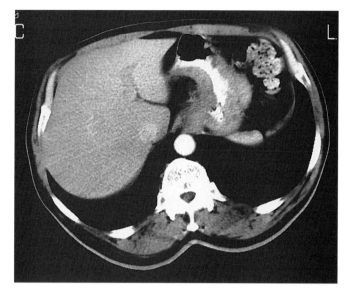

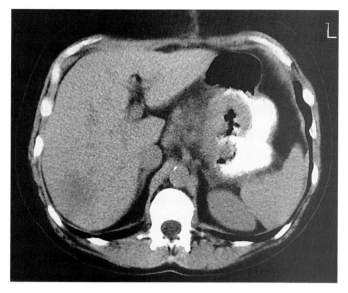

Fig. 3.35 Oesophagogastric carcinoma. A spiral CT scan in a 68-year-old male with 2 months' history of anorexia and 19 kg (3 stone) weight loss. There is evidence of massive tumour infiltration involving the distal oesophagus, the fundus and the body of the stomach. Enlarged retroperitoneal lymph nodes were apparent on the lower sections.

Fig. 3.37 Carcinoma of the stomach. A spiral CT scan in a 55-year-old male patient with anorexia, weight loss and anaemia. The examination was performed without IV contrast because of a prominent allergic history. A very large, irregular, ulcerated mass lesion is seen to affect much of the lesser curve of the stomach, with direct extension into coeliac lymph nodes. There is also evidence of metastatic liver disease on this unenhanced scan.

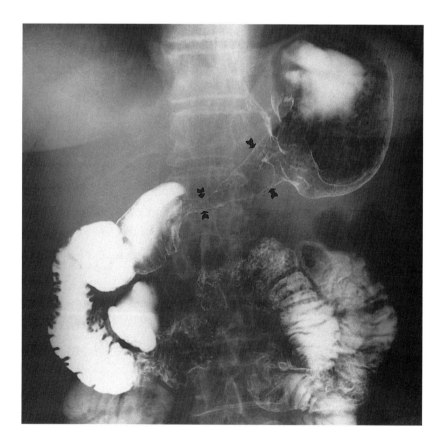

Fig. 3.36 Carcinoma of the body of the stomach. The DCBM shows marked loss of distensibility of the body and proximal antrum of the stomach (arrows). The fundus and proximal body and most of the antrum distend normally with gas. This 69-year-old female patient had a recent history of anorexia, weight loss and iron-deficiency anaemia.

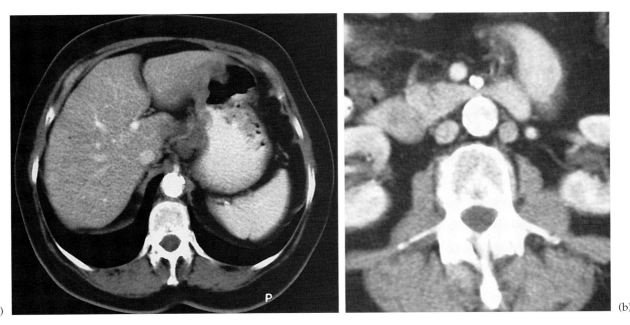

(a)   (b)

Fig. 3.38 Carcinoma of the stomach. (a) A spiral contrast-enhanced CT (CECT) scan in a 75-year-old female patient shows extensive tumour infiltration of the lesser-curve aspect of the stomach in continuity with lymphadenopathy affecting the left gastric nodes. (b) The patient is seen to have duplication of the inferior vena cava (IVC). The left IVC should not be confused with lymphadenopathy.

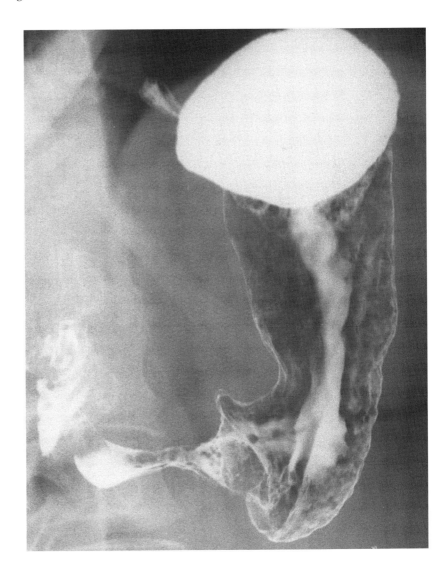

Fig. 3.39 Carcinoma of the stomach. A DCBM in a 73-year-old female patient with profound anorexia, weight loss, vomiting and anaemia. The antrum of the stomach shows marked loss of distensibility and mucosal irregularity, characteristic of carcinoma. The proximal edge of the lesion has a shouldered margin.

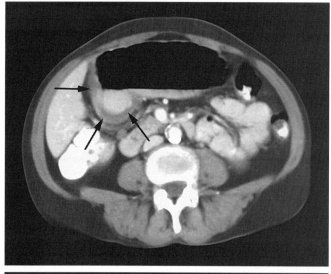

(a)

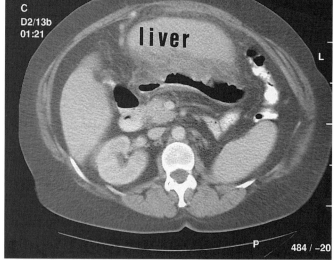

(c)

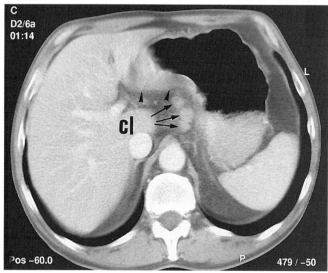

(b)

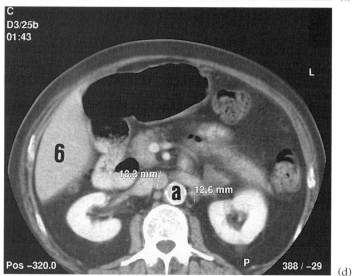

(d)

Fig. 3.40 Gastric carcinoma with spiral CECT. (a) There is diffuse thickening (>5 mm) of the antral wall and some loss of distensibility (arrows). The body of the stomach is of normal thickness and distends normally with CO_2. (b) The gastric antrum is thickened posteriorly (arrowheads). Enlarged left gastric lymph nodes are shown (>8 mm) (arrows). cl, caudate lobe of liver (segment 1). (c) There is diffuse infiltration characterized by irregular thickening of the stomach wall and marked loss of distensibility despite oral CO_2 and IV hyoscine. There is loss of definition of the anterior wall because of tumour infiltration of the gastrohepatic ligament (lesser omentum). (d) Retroperitoneal lymphadenopathy is apparent in this patient with proven gastric cancer. Nodes measuring 18 mm and 13 mm are shown. The primary lesion is not shown on this single section. a, aorta; 6, segment 6 of the liver.

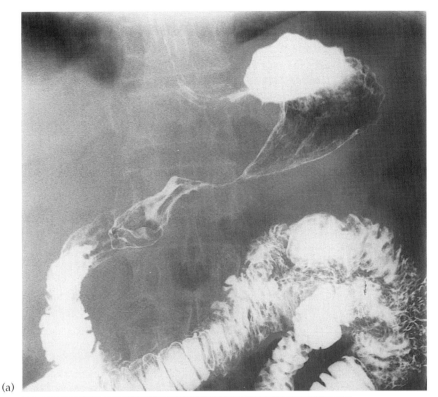

(a)

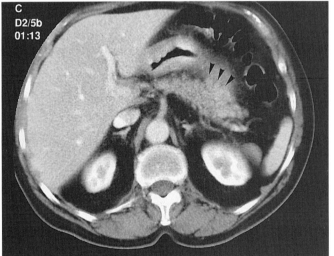

(b)

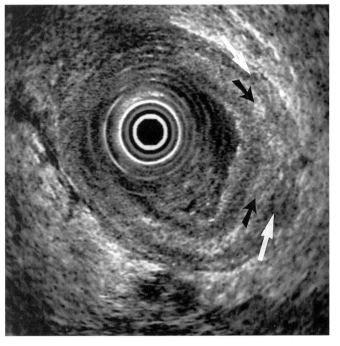

Fig. 3.41 Linitis plastica. (a) The DCBM shows a generalized loss of distensibility of the stomach, with a constant stricture involving the distal body. This was confirmed endoscopically, but endoscopic biopsies on two occasions revealed normal mucosa. (b) A CT of the upper abdomen with IV contrast enhancement confirms marked thickening of the body and antrum of the stomach, with evidence of direct extension of tumour across the lesser sac into the body of the pancreas (arrowheads). This feature was confirmed at operation and the tumour was unresectable.

Fig. 3.42 Linitis plastica, endoscopic ultrasound. Five to fifteen per cent of tumours are diffusely infiltrating, spreading predominantly in the submucosa and inciting a marked fibrotic response. Such tumours produce thickening of the gastric-wall layers, particularly layer 3 (submucosal; black arrows) and layer 4 (muscularis propria; white arrows), but preserving their layered appearance. As in the previous case, mucosal biopsy results were negative. On the basis of this ultrasound pattern, further deeper biopsies should be obtained. (Courtesy of Dr Alison McLean.)

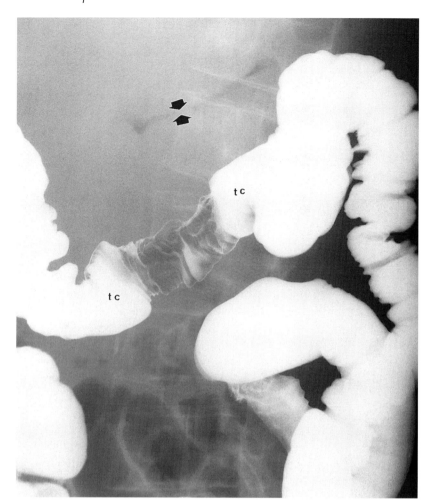

Fig. 3.43 Gastric cancer involving the transverse colon. The single-contrast barium enema in this patient with weight loss, anaemia and altered bowel habit demonstrates an unusual partial stricture of the transverse colon (tc), resulting from direct spread of gastric cancer via the greater omentum. The linear gas shadow (between arrowheads) indicates the contracted gastric lumen.

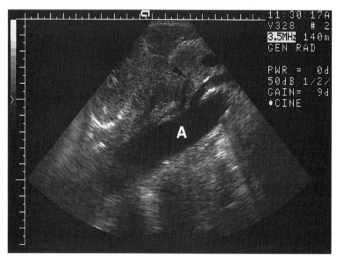

(a)

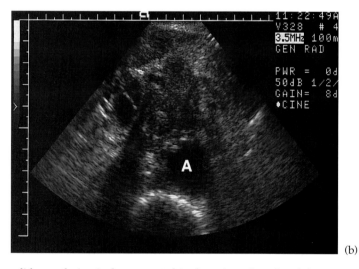

(b)

Fig. 3.44 Recurrent gastric carcinoma. (a) Sagittal and (b) transverse ultrasound scans (3.5 MHz) of the upper abdomen in a patient who, 12 months previously, had had a Polya gastrectomy for gastric carcinoma. There was recent profound weight loss. A solid mass lesion is demonstrated in the epigastrium, involving coeliac nodes and producing encasement of the coeliac artery (arrowhead) and its hepatic and splenic branches. The patient also had liver metastases. A, aorta.

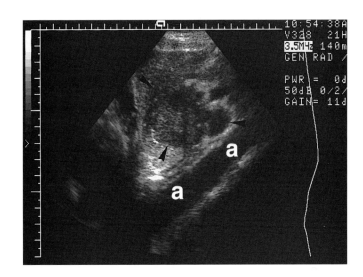

Fig. 3.45 Recurrent gastric carcinoma. Another example of local recurrence of gastric carcinoma (arrowheads) demonstrated by ultrasound postgastrectomy. a, aorta.

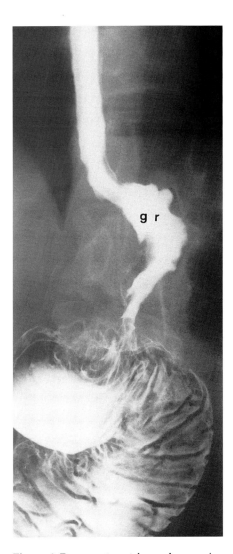

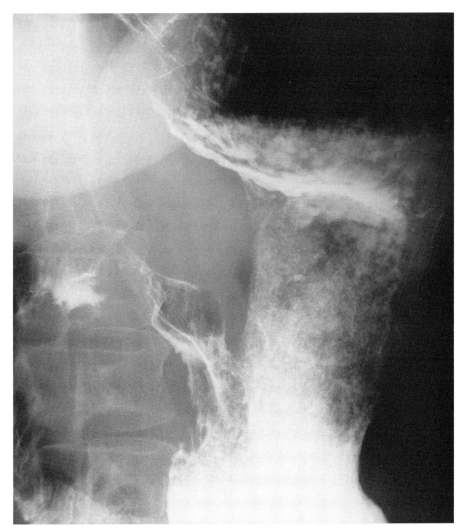

Fig. 3.46 Recurrent gastric carcinoma. A female patient who had had a previous subtotal gastrectomy with a Polya reconstruction had recent anorexia and weight loss. The DCBM shows a small grossly contracted and irregular gastric remnant (gr), with marked loss of distensibility. Tumour recurrence was confirmed endoscopically.

Fig. 3.47 Metastatic disease involving the stomach. This female patient had a previous history of mastectomy and recent vomiting. The DCBM shows a large fasting residue in the stomach, which is distended, and the antrum is irregularly contracted. Histology of the gastric lesion was identical to the patient's breast primary. The differential diagnosis includes primary gastric carcinoma and local spread of pancreatic carcinoma.

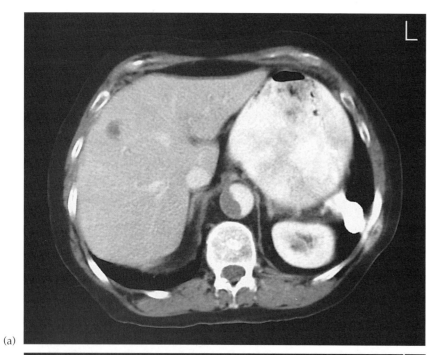

(a)

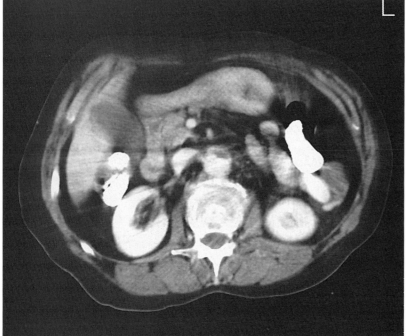

(b)

Fig. 3.48 Metastatic disease involving the stomach. A spiral CECT in a 71-year-old female patient with a previous mastectomy and recent vomiting and weight loss. (a) The fundus and proximal body of the stomach are obstructed, containing a large fasting food residue. (b) The distal body and antrum show diffuse thickening, consistent with tumour. This was found to be due to metastatic breast carcinoma. Metastatic liver disease was also present.

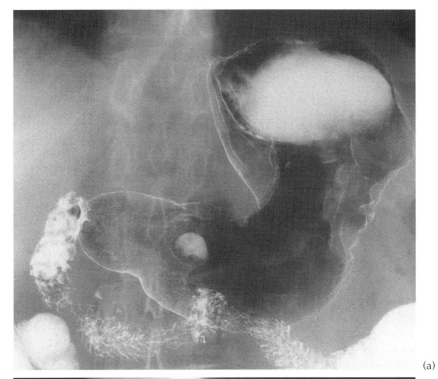

(a)

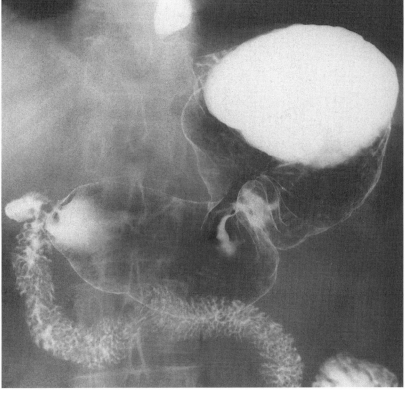

Fig. 3.49 Gastric lymphoma. A 69-year-old female patient with anorexia, weight loss and Hb 7.4 g. (a) Before treatment there was a very extensive filling defect involving the greater and lesser curves of the stomach, with a separate ulcerated lesion in the antrum. Histology indicated lymphoma. (b) A very substantial improvement is seen after 4 months of chemotherapy, with some residual deformity and partial loss of distensibility of the mid-portion of the body. The ulcerated antral lesion has disappeared.

(b)

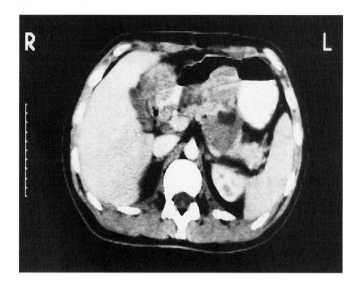

Fig. 3.50 Leiomyosarcoma. Incremental CT scan in a young adult male with recurrent haematemesis and melaena. A very extensive, lobulated, solid mass lesion is seen to affect a large part of the stomach, with backward extension into the pancreas and lateral extension into the porta hepatis. Histology indicated leiomyosarcoma. The differential diagnosis includes primary gastric cancer, lymphoma and extension of pancreatic carcinoma [5, 12].

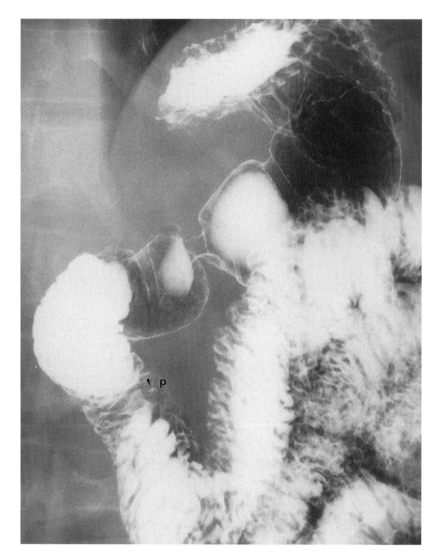

Fig. 3.51 Pyloroplasty. The DCBM shows widening of the pyloric canal following previous surgery. The duodenal papilla is indicated (p, arrowhead).

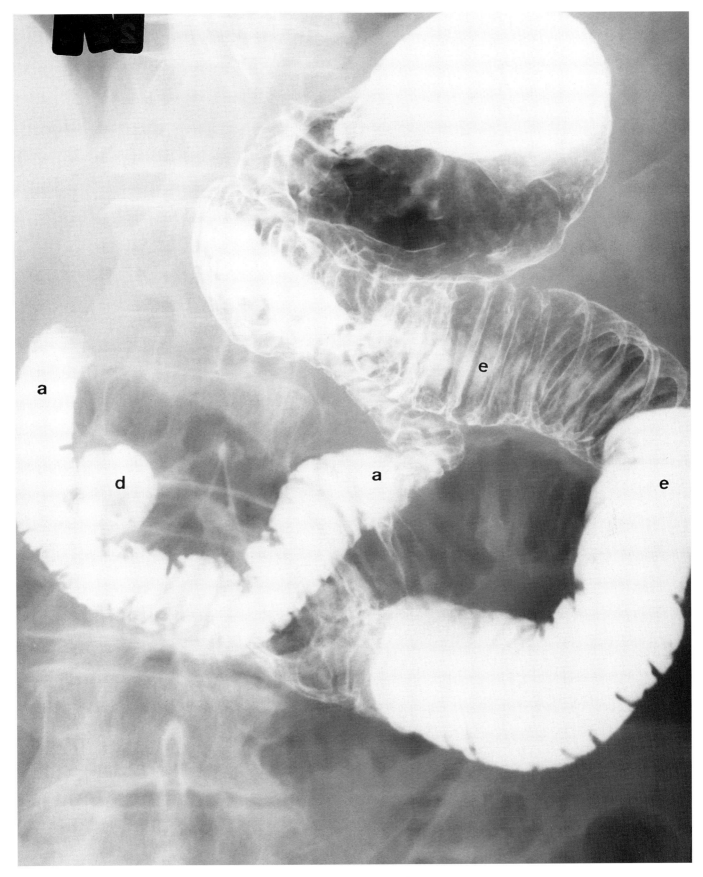

Fig. 3.52 Partial gastrectomy (Polya reconstruction). The end-to-side anastomosis is seen to be widely patent and both afferent (a) and efferent (e) loops are seen to fill with contrast. A duodenal diverticulum is shown (d).

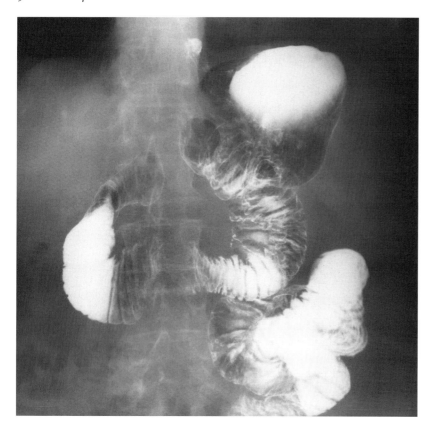

Fig. 3.53 Partial gastrectomy (Polya reconstruction). The DCBM shows normal filling of the afferent and efferent loops. There is normal extrinsic compression of the third part of the duodenum, where it crosses the abdominal aorta. The closed end of the duodenal loop is shown. Multiple calcified gallbladder calculi are visible.

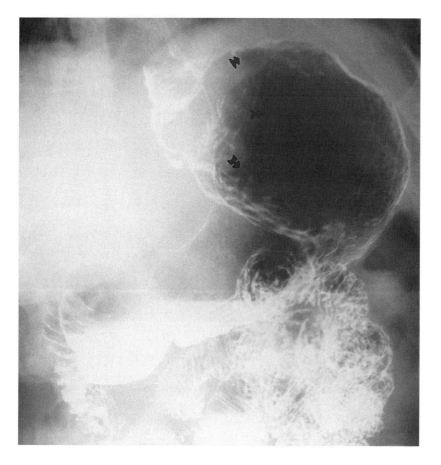

Fig. 3.54 Nissen fundoplication, antireflux surgery. The DCBM shows a constant filling defect (arrows) involving the cardia. This should not be confused with pathology in the proximal stomach, e.g. carcinoma [13, 14].

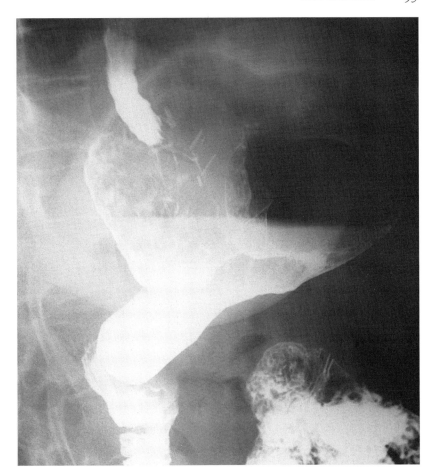

Fig. 3.55 Nissen fundoplication, antireflux surgery. The DCBM lateral view of the stomach shows a large soft-tissue filling defect involving the cardia and fundus posteriorly. Numerous surgical clips are apparent, which, together with eliciting a relevant history, should indicate the diagnosis.

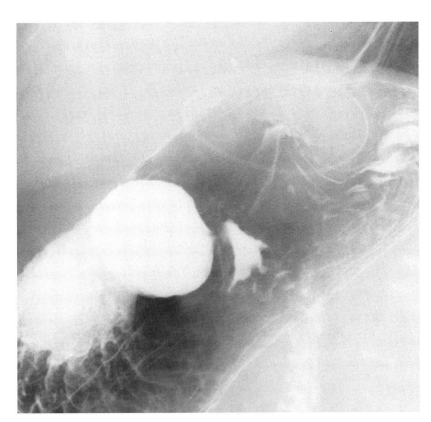

Fig. 3.56 Angelchik prosthesis, antireflux surgery. The prosthesis is seen as an opaque collar surrounding the cardia. The stomach is otherwise normal.

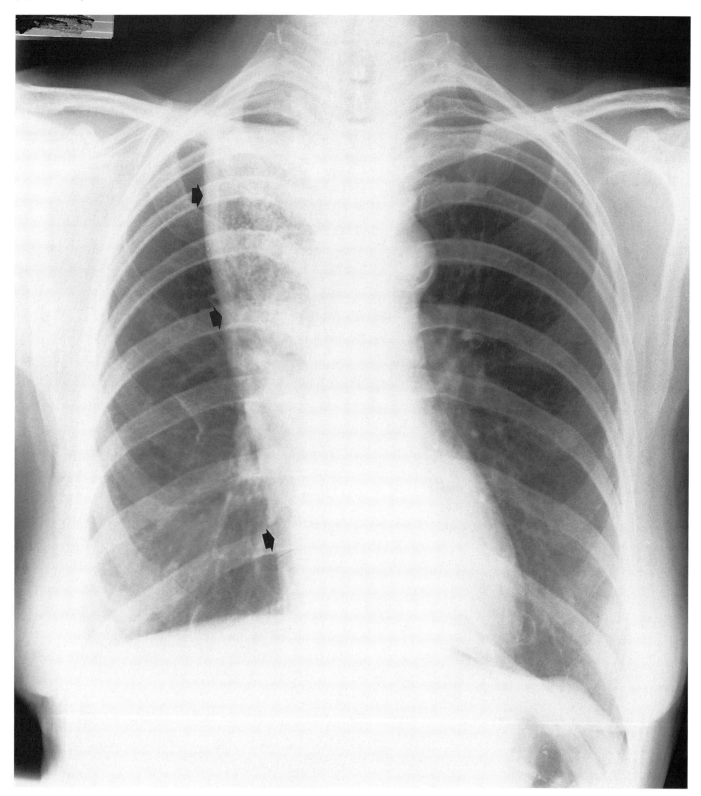

Fig. 3.57 Oesophagectomy and gastric pull-through. This PA chest X-ray shows marked widening of the mediastinal contour on the right side, the well-defined margin (arrows) being formed by the wall of the stomach. A fluid level is just visible at the level of the thoracic inlet.

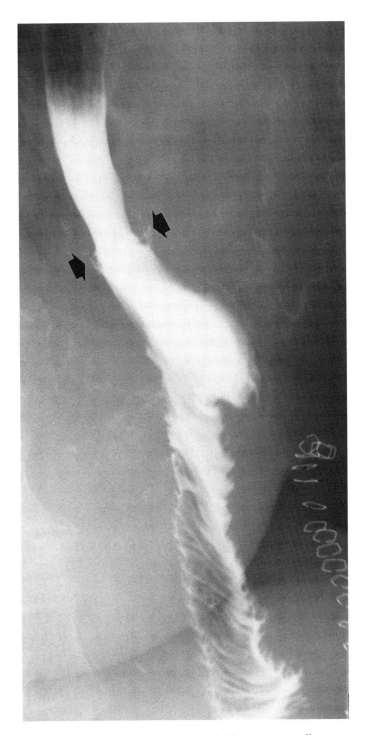

Fig. 3.58 Total gastrectomy. A water-soluble contrast swallow demonstrates patency of the oesophagojejunal anastomosis (marked by surgical clips and arrowheads), 72 h after operation. There is no leakage of contrast from the anastomosis.

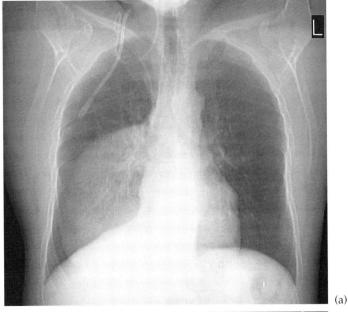

(a)

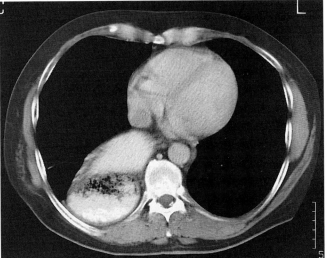

(b)

Fig. 3.59 Oesophagogastrectomy for carcinoma with gastric pull-through. (a) An unusual, well-circumscribed, homogeneous shadow can be seen in the right mid and lower zones, the silhouette of the right heart border and right hemidiaphragm being preserved. This indicates that the opacity lies posteriorly in the chest. (b) A spiral CECT with oral contrast shows the mobilized stomach in the right hemithorax. Enlarged lymph nodes were demonstrated below the diaphragm on lower sections.

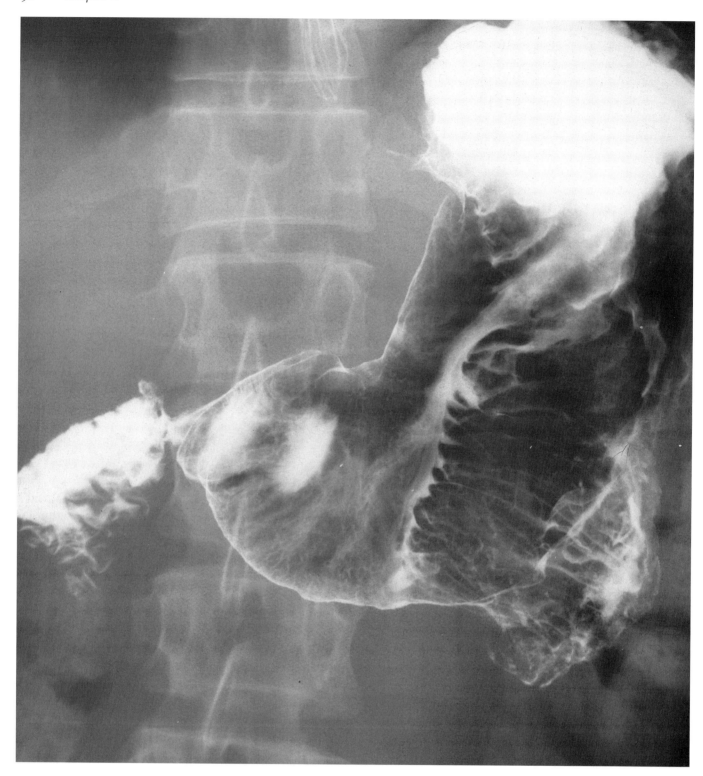

Fig. 3.60 Gastrojejunostomy with intussusception of the efferent loop [13, 15, 16]. This middle-aged male patient had had a previous vagotomy and gastrojejunostomy for chronic duodenal ulceration, with recent recurrent vomiting. The DCBM shows a large, fixed filling defect in the body of the stomach, the surface of which has a transverse linear pattern, characteristic of the mucosa of jejunum. This was confirmed endoscopically. The differential diagnosis includes leiomyoma, carcinoma, lymphoma, bezoar and blood clot.

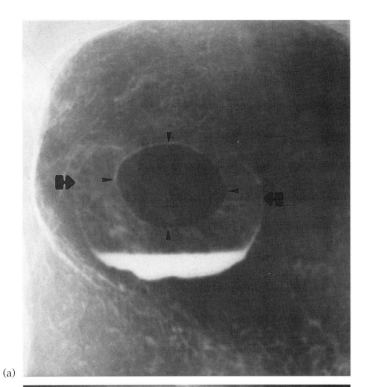

(a)

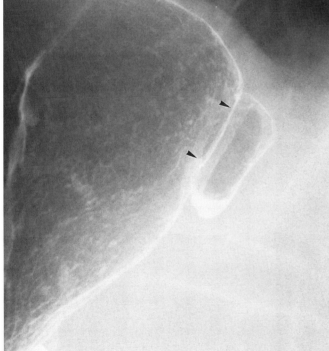

(b)

Fig. 3.61 Congenital gastric diverticulum. The DCBM, (a) AP and (b) lateral views, shows a well-defined wide-mouthed diverticulum arising from the posterior aspect of the fundus of the stomach. The body of the diverticulum is indicated by arrows and the neck by arrowheads. Three-quarters of such lesions occur in the vicinity of the cardia, 15–20% in the prepyloric region and less than 5% on the greater curve. Diverticula need to be distinguished from large, penetrating ulcer craters. In the former, the mucosa is intact with very clearly defined margins and there is no suggestion of oedema or radiating folds [17, 18].

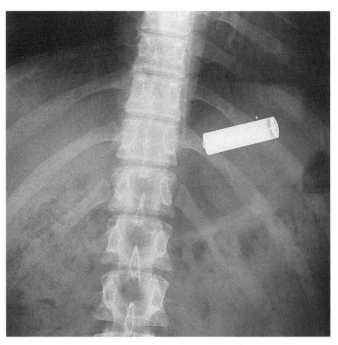

Fig. 3.62 Ingested foreign body. A densely opaque battery is projected within the stomach in a mentally disturbed psychiatric patient.

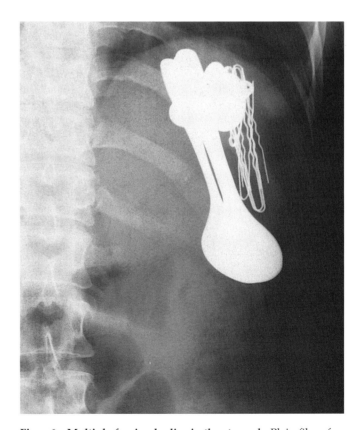

Fig. 3.63 Multiple foreign bodies in the stomach. Plain film of upper abdomen shows numerous metallic foreign bodies, apparently within the stomach, of a psychiatric patient.

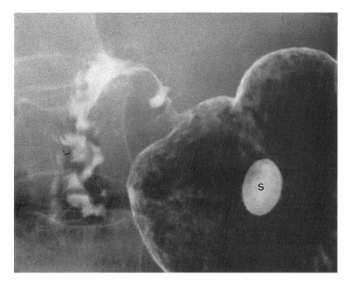

Fig. 3.64 Foreign body in the stomach. The DCBM shows a radio-opaque coin (sixpence, s), which had been ingested 43 years previously. There is marked pyloroduodenal deformity, in keeping with long-standing peptic ulceration.

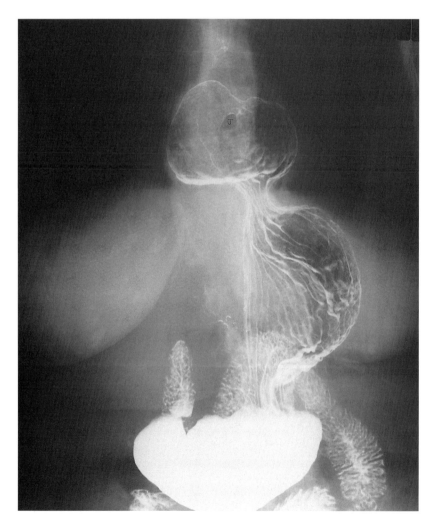

Fig. 3.65 Fixed sliding hiatus hernia. This erect view of a DCBM shows a relatively large sliding hiatus hernia, which is fixed in the erect position. The oesophagogastric junction is indicated (J). The stomach is otherwise normal.

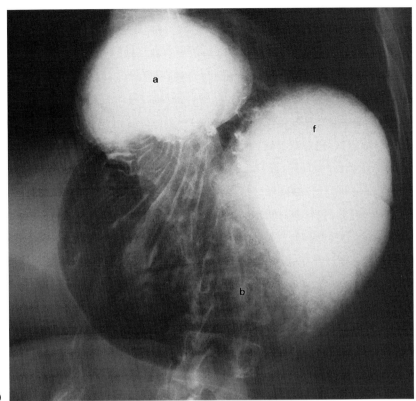

(a)

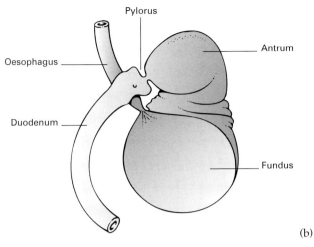

(b)

Fig. 3.66 Gastric volvulus. (a) Female patient with sudden onset of severe epigastric pain and vomiting. In this mesenteroaxial volvulus, the stomach is seen to have rotated around an axis extending from the lesser to the greater curvature. a, antrum; b, body; f, fundus. (Courtesy of Dr R.D. Edwards.) (b) A diagram depicting a mesenteroaxial volvulus.

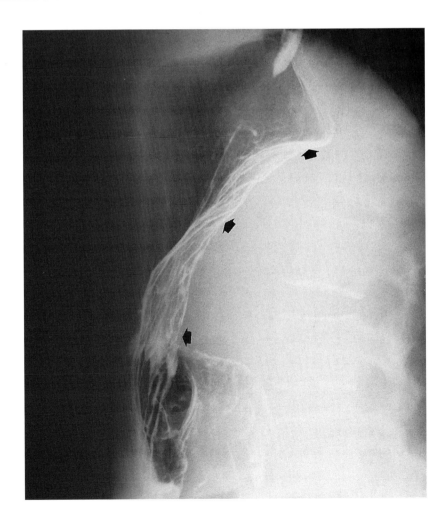

Fig. 3.67 Extrinsic compression and displacement of the stomach by adrenal metastases. A lateral DCBM shows marked compression and forward displacement of the posterior wall of the stomach (arrowheads) by a large retroperitoneal mass lesion. This was subsequently shown to be due to adrenal metastases from a bronchial carcinoma.

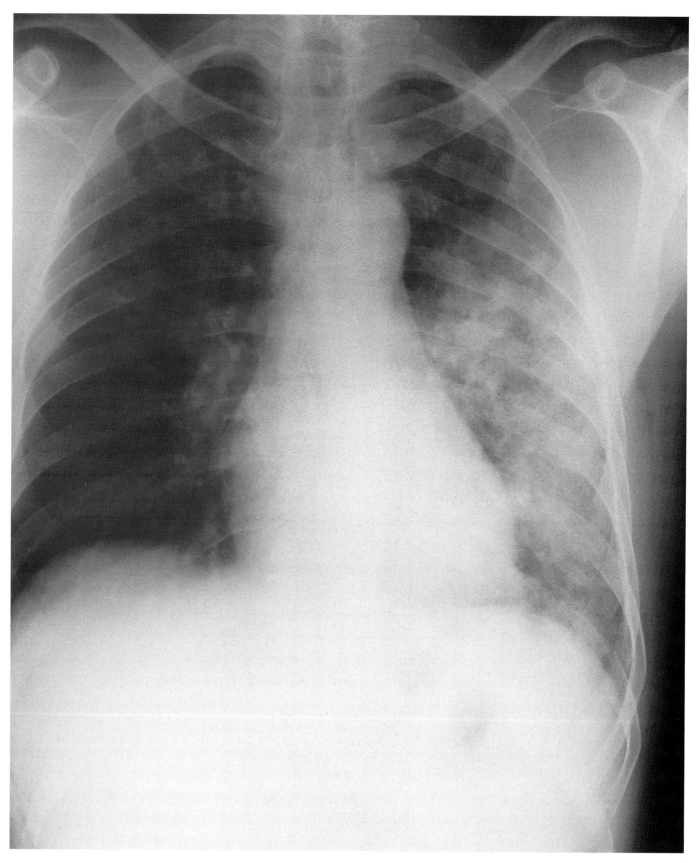

Fig. 3.68 Severe aspiration pneumonia. A PA chest X-ray in a young male patient 1 h following a diagnostic endoscopy. Extensive consolidation is shown in the left lung field, consistent with aspiration pneumonia.

4: The Duodenum

Anatomy

The Romans observed that the duodenum is 12 inches long and hence evolved the term duodenum from duodecim (personal communication). Anatomically the shortest portion of the small bowel, the duodenum in practice is considered part of the upper alimentary tract. It occupies a strategic position on the abdomen, with close relationships with the stomach, pancreas, lesser sac, right kidney, gallbladder, common bile duct, portal vein, superior mesenteric artery and vein and transverse colon. Because it is mostly extraperitoneal, its position is relatively fixed and, together with the commencement of the jejunum, the duodenum is more susceptible to trauma than other parts of the small bowel [1].

The duodenum is arbitrarily divided into four parts. The first part passes upwards, to the right and posteriorly from the pylorus and largely consists of the duodenal bulb or cap, because of its shape on barium studies. The descending or second part passes downwards intimately related to the head of the pancreas medially, the right kidney laterally and the transverse colon anteriorly. The third (horizontal) part straddles the inferior vena cava and aorta, passing posterior to the superior mesenteric vein and artery and the root of the small-bowel mesentery. The fourth part is directed upwards and is covered anteriorly and on its left side by an extension of the left leaf of the mesentery, the right aspect of the fourth part being attached to the upper limit of the root of the mesentery. The junction of the duodenum and jejunum, the duodenojejunal flexure, is fixed and marked by a band of thick fibrous tissue, called the ligament of Treitz. The hepatoduodenal ligament is the lower part of the lesser omentum, connects the porta hepatis with the proximal duodenum and forms the anterior margin of the foramen of Winslow. This ligament contains the portal vein, the hepatic artery and the common hepatic and common bile duct and it is a common site for the spread of biliary tract and gallbladder malignancy.

The mucosal pattern in the duodenal cap is variable. Spiral, longitudinal or transverse folds may be seen and they can normally be effaced by gaseous distension of the duo-denum. Valvulae conniventes, or transverse folds, are visible in the second and third parts, which are not effaceable by gaseous distension. The second part also includes the ampulla of Vater [2], which can be seen in about two-thirds of routine double-contrast barium meals [3]. A hooded fold and a distal longitudinal fold typically mark the position of the ampulla, which is normally not more than 1.5 cm in diameter. In one-quarter of examinations, the accessory pancreatic duct of Santorini (the primitive dorsal duct) may be seen [3]. The duodenum has a rich blood supply, derived from both the coeliac and the superior mesenteric arteries. The gastroduodenal artery is formed by the bifurcation of the common hepatic artery and it supplies the duodenum via the anterior and posterior superior pancreaticoduodenal branches, which anastomose with corresponding anterior and posterior inferior pancreaticoduodenal branches of the superior mesenteric artery. The right gastric artery makes a small contribution to the duodenum.

Plain film radiography

As a rule, plain abdominal X-rays are of very little value in duodenal disease. In specific situations, however, useful information may be obtained—for example, in duodenal ulcer perforation, obstruction and cholecystoduodenal fistula resulting in gallstone ileus.

Barium studies

The double-contrast barium-meal study of the upper gastrointestinal tract, unlike endoscopy, normally includes a thorough examination of the whole of the duodenum. This is particularly useful if disease is suspected beyond the first part. Satisfactory relaxation of the duodenal loop normally requires intravenous hyoscine (Buscopan) or glucagon, and multiple projections are obtained under fluoroscopic control once the duodenum has been coated with high-density, low-viscosity barium and distended with an oral gas-forming agent. Barium is contraindicated in the presence of upper gastrointestinal haemorrhage, in which endoscopy is the investigation of choice, so that, if arteriography is required, the field will not be obscured by a persistent residue of barium. Similarly, barium should be avoided if there is likely to be an urgent need for CT scanning. With the widespread use of H_2-receptor antagonists and proton-pump inhibitors, the need for barium studies in patients with non-specific dyspeptic symptoms has sharply diminished, particularly in young patients.

Water-soluble contrast studies

If duodenal ulcer perforation is suspected or in the post-operative period following gastroduodenal surgery, water-soluble contrast, e.g. meglumine diatrizoate (Gastrografin), should be used in preference to barium.

Computerized tomography scanning

In detecting free intraperitoneal air, CT is superior to plain films. The air is seen to collect beneath the anterior abdominal wall in the mid-abdomen [4]. The wall of the duodenum is normally about 1 mm thick, and thickening can result from duodenitis or pancreatitis. Duodenal tumours are uncommon and CT is useful in defining and staging these lesions [5]. False-positive results may be produced by incomplete distension of the duodenum [6]. Because of its situation and relatively fixed normal position, the duodenum, distended with positive contrast, or even with water or gas, may be a useful marker of disease in adjacent organs—for example, the pancreas, retroperitoneal lymph nodes and even the abdominal aorta [7]. Computerized tomography is useful in defining duodenal rupture resulting from trauma [8–10].

Angiography

This technique is not routinely used in investigation of duodenal disease, but selective catheterization of the coeliac and superior mesenteric arteries and their branches may be invaluable in the diagnosis and management of severe duodenal haemorrhage.

References

1 Dahnert W. (1996) *Radiology Review Manual*, 3rd edn. Baltimore: Williams & Wilkins, 574.

2 Ferrucci J.T., Benedict K.T., Page D.L., Fleischli D.J. & Eaton S.B. (1970) Radiographic features of the normal hypotonic duodenogram. *Radiology* 96, 401–408.

3 Stevenson G.W., Somers S. & Virjee J. (1980) Routine double contrast barium meal: appearance of the normal duodenal papillae. *Diagnostic Imaging* 49, 6–14.

4 Burgener F.A. & Kormano M. (1996) *Differential Diagnosis in Computed Tomography*. Stuttgart: Thieme Medical Publishers, 311.

5 Cwikiel W. & Andre-Sanberg A. (1991) Diagnostic difficulties with duodenal malignancies: a new strategy. *Gastro-intestinal Radiology* 16, 301–304.

6 Scatarige J. & di Santis D.J. (1989) CT of the stomach and duodenum. *Radiological Clinics of North America* 27, 687–706.

7 Megibow A.J. (1986) Duodenum. In: Megibow A.J. & Balthazar E.J. (eds) *Computed Tomography of the Gastro-intestinal Tract*. St Louis: Mosby, 175–216.

8 Gore R.M. (1994) Cross-sectional imaging. In: Gore R.M., Levine M.S. & Laufer I. (eds) *A Textbook of Gastro-intestinal Radiology*. Philadelphia: W.B. Saunders, 310.

9 Megibow A.J. (1994) The gastro-intestinal tract. In: Haaga J.R., Lanzieri C.E., Sartoris D.J. *et al.* (eds) *Computed Tomography and Magnetic Resonance Imaging of the Whole Body*, 3rd edn. St Louis: Mosby, 866–867.

10 Carnaze J.C., Sheedey P.F., Stephens D.H. *et al.* (1981) Computed tomography in duodenal rupture due to blunt abdominal trauma. *Journal of Computer Assisted Tomography* 5, 267–269.

11 Nolan D.J. (1997) The duodenum. In: Grainger R.G. & Allison D.J. (eds) *Grainger and Allison's Diagnostic Radiology*, 3rd edn. New York: Churchill Livingstone, 973–983.

12 Levine M.S. (1994) Peptic ulcers. In: Gore R.M., Levine M.S. & Laufer I. (eds) *A Textbook of Gastro-intestinal Radiology*. Philadelphia: W.B. Saunders, 562–597.

13 Ball R.P., Segal A.L. & Golden R. (1948) Post-bulbar ulcers of the duodenum. *American Journal of Roentgenology* 59, 90–99.

14 Edwards R.H. & Foster J.H. (1962) Pneumoperitoneum in perforated duodenal ulcer. *American Journal of Surgery* 104, 551–554.

15 Reeders J.W.A.J. & Rosenbusch G. (1994) Radiology of benign and malignant diseases of the duodenum. In: Freeny P.C. & Stevenson G.W. (eds) *Margulis and Burhenne's Alimentary Tract Radiology*, 5th edn. St Louis: Mosby, 467–511.

16 Pugash R.A., O'Brien S.C. & Stevenson G.W. (1990) Perforating duodenal diverticulitis. *Gastro-intestinal Radiology* 15, 156.

17 Murfitt J. (1993) The pancreas. In: Sutton D. (ed.) *A Textbook of Radiology and Imaging* 5th edn. Edinburgh: Churchill Livingstone, 991–1022.

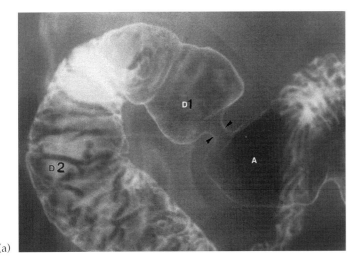

(a)

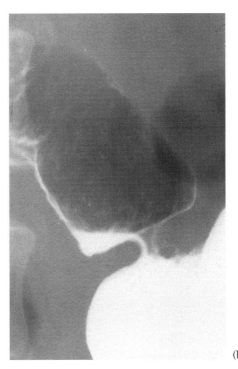

(b)

Fig. 4.1 Normal duodenum. (a) A double-contrast barium meal (DCBM) shows a normally distended antrum (A), duodenal cap (D1) and second part of the duodenum (D2). The pyloric canal, surrounded by the pyloric sphincter, normally measures no more than 10 mm in length (arrowheads). RAO position. (b) Normal duodenal cap. The DCBM in erect oblique position shows normal mucosal coating and normal gaseous distension of the first part.

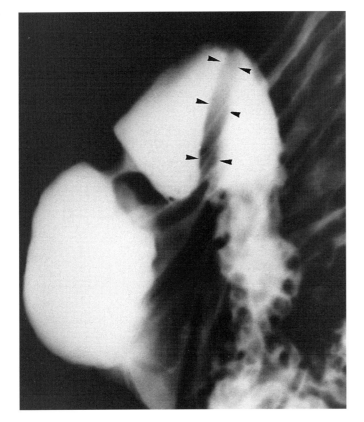

Fig. 4.2 Normal duodenum. The DCBM shows supine oblique projection of the barium-filled duodenum. An oblique extrinsic compression of the first part of the duodenum (arrowheads) is caused by the common bile duct.

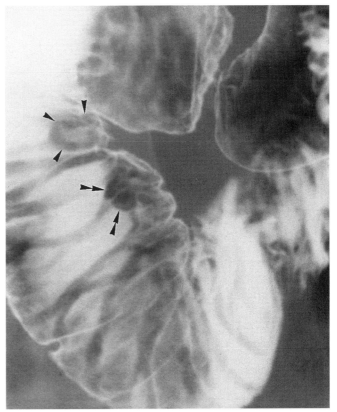

Fig. 4.3 Normal duodenum (second part). The normal circular fold pattern is apparent and the major papilla is indicated by the double arrowheads. This is normally not more than 1.5 cm in diameter. An accessory papilla (single arrowheads), which is present in approximately 60% of cases, is indicated 2 cm more proximally, also on the concave aspect.

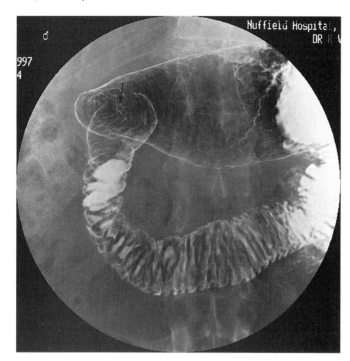

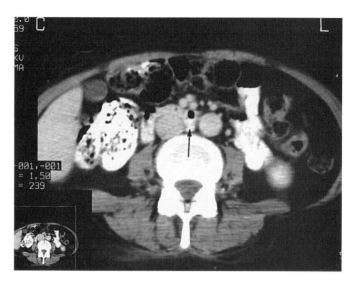

Fig. 4.4 Normal duodenal loop. A DCBM in a subject with a horizontal stomach and posteriorly placed duodenal cap (bulb). The pyloric canal, seen end-on (arrow), should not be confused with an ulcer crater. The normal circular fold pattern of the second, third and fourth parts is shown. This is not effaced by normal gaseous distension.

Fig. 4.5 Normal duodenum (third part). This normal spiral CT scan with IV contrast enhancement and with oral contrast (Gastrografin) shows part of the third part of the duodenum (arrow) interposed between the inferior vena cava (IVC) and the aorta as it passes behind the mesenteric vessels. Had this segment not been opacified with contrast, it could have been mistaken for lymphadenopathy. This phenomenon may be seen in patients following retroperitoneal lymph-node dissection, but this patient had had no previous abdominal surgery.

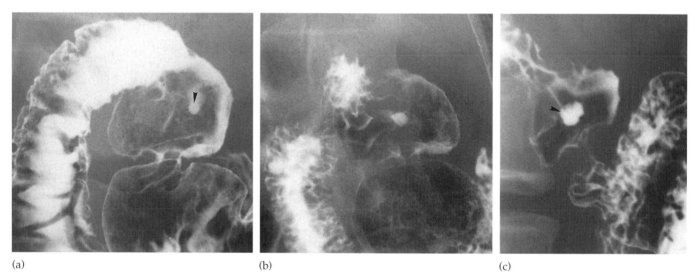

(a)   (b)   (c)

Fig. 4.6 Duodenal peptic ulcer (first part posterior). (a) In this patient, the duodenal bulb distends normally and the mucosa is essentially normal, apart from a 5 mm niche of barium (arrowhead) indicating an ulcer crater. This appearance needs to be constant and reproducible. (b) In a second patient, there is a 7 mm posterior central ulcer crater, with normal distension of the cap, but with evidence of thickening of the mucosa, in keeping with duodenitis. (c) In a third patient, there is a 10 mm posterior ulcer crater close to the base of the duodenal cap, and mucosal folds are seen radiating from it. The contour of the cap is also moderately deformed, in keeping with some cicatrization. Approximately one-quarter of duodenal ulcers are posteriorly located.

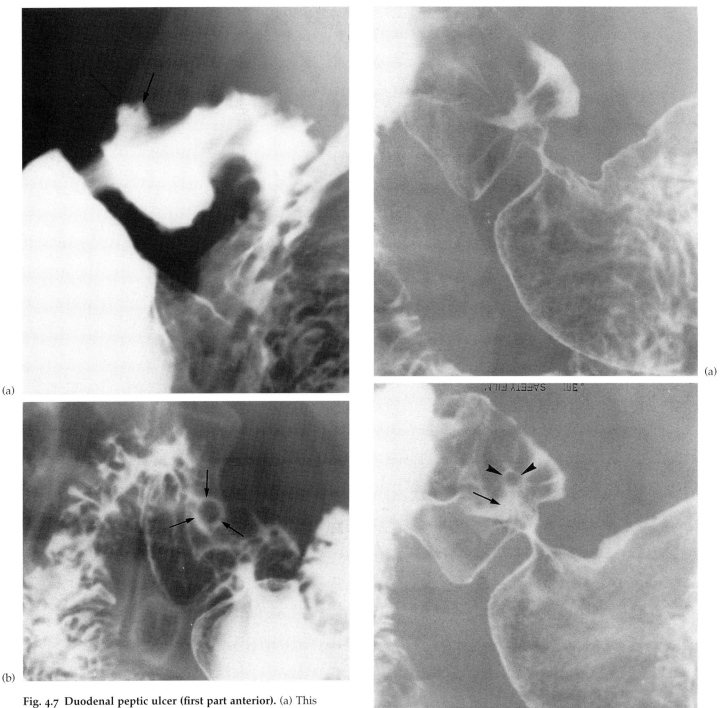

(a)

(b)

(a)

(b)

Fig. 4.7 Duodenal peptic ulcer (first part anterior). (a) This profile view of the barium-filled duodenum shows a persistent irregular niche (arrow), indicating an 8 mm ulcer crater on the anterior wall of the duodenum. (b) A supine, oblique compression view in another patient shows a ring shadow (arrows), which was readily reproducible, indicating the margin of an ulcer crater on the anterior wall of the duodenum. Approximately half of duodenal ulcers are on the anterior wall, almost one-quarter are inferior and one in 20 are on the superior aspect.

Fig. 4.8 Multiple duodenal peptic ulcers. (a) In this patient, initially a stellate posterior ulcer was apparent. (b) When compression was also applied, a reproducible ring shadow also became apparent, indicating an anterior ulcer crater (arrowheads). Arrow, posterior ulcer.

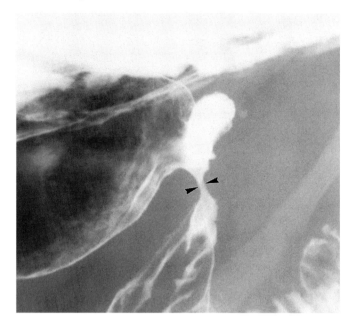

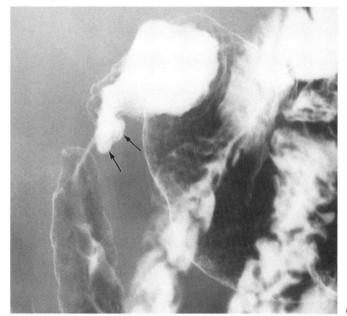

(a)

Fig. 4.9 Duodenal scarring secondary to peptic ulceration. In this patient, with a long history of periodic dyspepsia, the normal anatomy of the pyloroduodenal region is no longer recognizable because of gross deformity resulting from scar tissue, and there is a persistent stenosis (arrowheads) unrelieved by Buscopan.

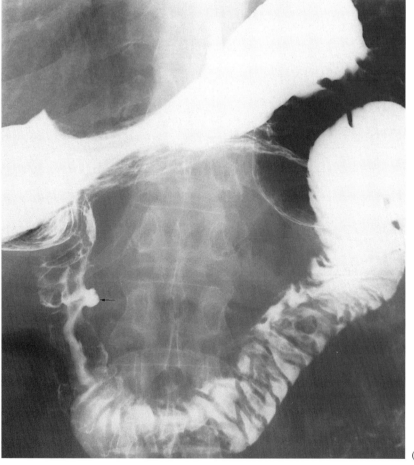

(b)

Fig. 4.10 Duodenal peptic ulcer (postbulbar).
(a) The DCBM shows marked duodenal deformity (arrows), with a large persistent niche of barium almost 15 mm in diameter in the proximal second part. The patient had a history of relapsing dyspepsia and recent back pain [11]. In these patients, haemorrhage is a significant feature and may occur in 40–80% of patients. (b) Another patient, in whom the DCBM shows a 10 mm penetrating ulcer crater more distally in the second part (arrow) and with an incisura on the opposite wall of the duodenum [12, 13]. A further tiny ulcer crater is shown more proximally in the second part.

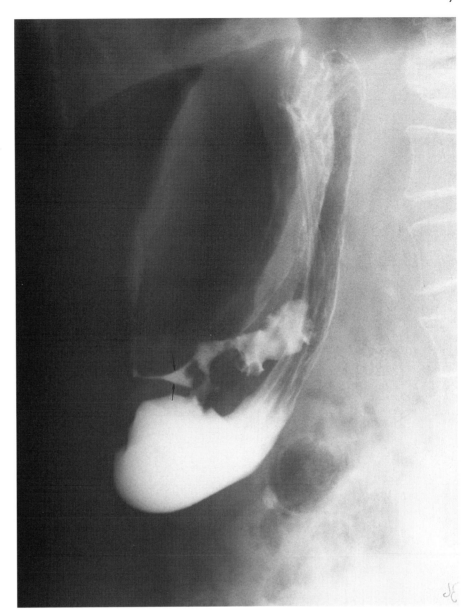

Fig. 4.11 Anterior duodenal ulcer perforation. A lateral view of the stomach and duodenum after oral Gastrografin shows marked duodenal deformity, with free spillage of contrast (arrows) into the peritoneal cavity. A large volume of air is also shown in the subphrenic space anteriorly. Pneumoperitoneum is not a constant feature of perforated duodenal ulcers, in one study only two-thirds of patients exhibiting this sign [14].

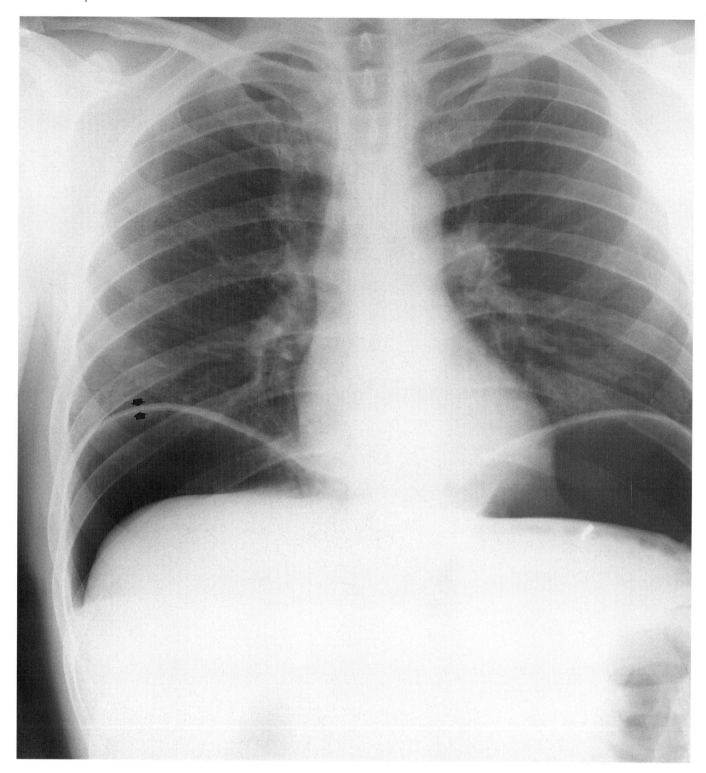

Fig. 4.12 Duodenal ulcer perforation, pneumoperitoneum.
This erect chest X-ray shows a large volume of free air in the peritoneal cavity in a patient with a duodenal ulcer perforation. The presence of a pneumoperitoneum and the volume of air that accumulates depend on how quickly the ulcer seals off spontaneously [12]. The line depicted by the arrowheads consists of visceral pleura, parietal pleura, diaphragm and parietal peritoneum.

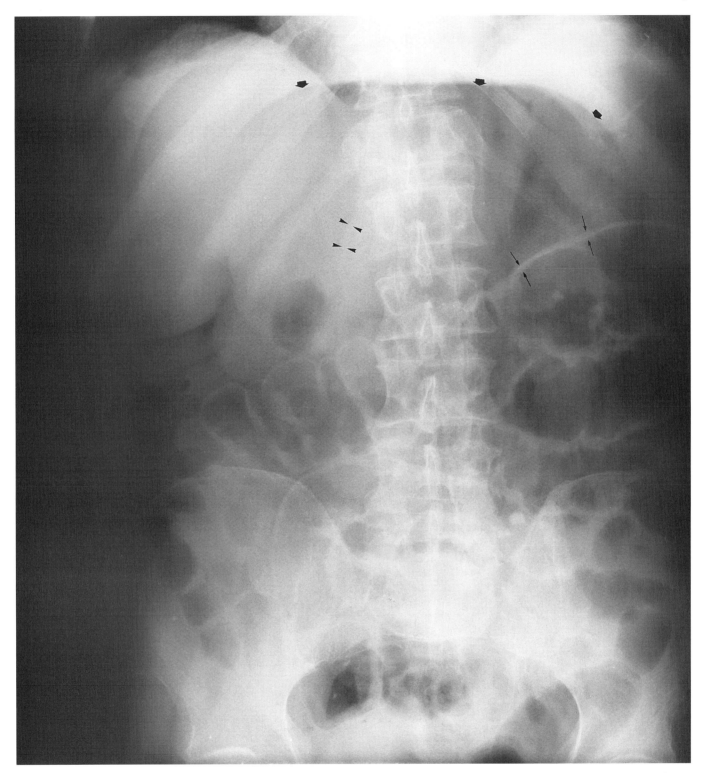

Fig. 4.13 Duodenal ulcer perforation, pneumoperitoneum. This supine abdominal film shows a large volume of free air within the peritoneal cavity (large arrowheads). In addition, both the mucosal and the serosal surfaces of the transverse colon are outlined by gas—Rigler's sign (arrows). Part of the falciform ligament, which is normally invisible on a plain film, is outlined by air in the right and left subphrenic spaces (small arrowheads). Air is also visible in Morrison's pouch.

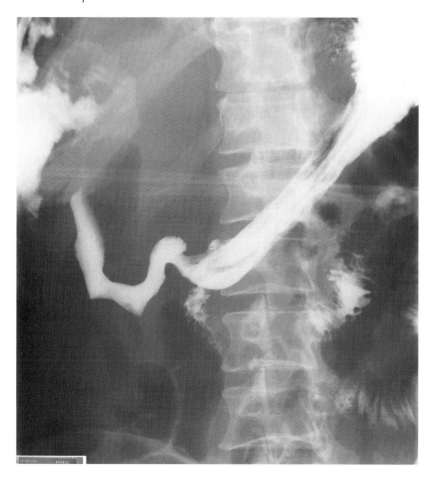

Fig. 4.14 Duodenal ulcer perforation, contrast study. A large volume of Gastrografin is seen escaping from a perforation more than 1 cm in diameter in the first part of the duodenum. The contrast is seen tracking into the right subphrenic space of the peritoneal cavity.

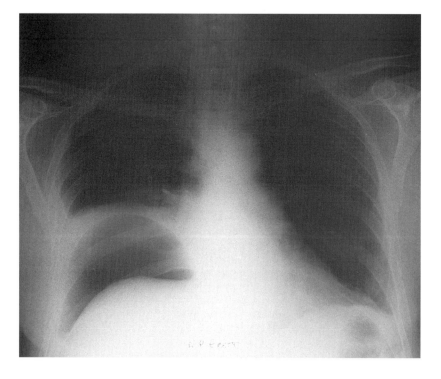

Fig. 4.15 Subphrenic abscess complicating duodenal ulcer perforation. In this patient, duodenal ulcer perforation was not initially suspected. The patient became pyrexial and an erect chest X-ray shows a large volume of gas under the markedly elevated right hemidiaphragm. There is a reactive small pleural effusion and right basal atelectasis. The volume of pus in the abscess was relatively small compared with the volume of gas.

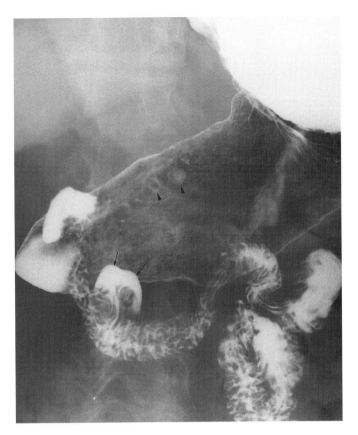

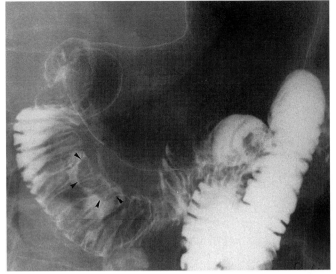

(a)

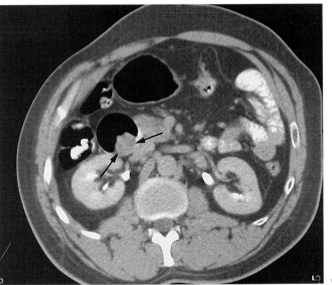

(b)

Fig. 4.16 Duodenal diverticulum. This DCBM shows a moderate-sized diverticulum (arrows) arising from the concave aspect of the second part of the duodenum, in which the muscosa had a normal appearance. These are found in 1–6% of all upper gastrointestinal barium studies [15]. However, post-mortem studies indicate a much higher incidence [16]. This patient also has signs of erosive gastritis (arrowheads) and there is a small hiatus hernia.

Fig. 4.18 (a) Carcinoma of the ampulla of Vater. This 70-year-old female patient presented with a 4-week history of increasing jaundice, pale stools and pruritis. The DCBM shows a constant, lobulated filling defect on the concave aspect of the duodenum (arrowheads) measuring 3 cm in length. Endoscopic confirmation [17]. **(b) Non-ampullary primary duodenal carcinoma.** A spiral CECT with oral CO_2 and IV Buscopan 20 mg of a 49-year-old male patient with iron-deficiency anaemia. It shows a constant solid filling defect in the posteromedial aspect of the second part of the duodenum (arrows). Histological confirmation. Treatment by Whipple's pancreatico-duodenectomy.

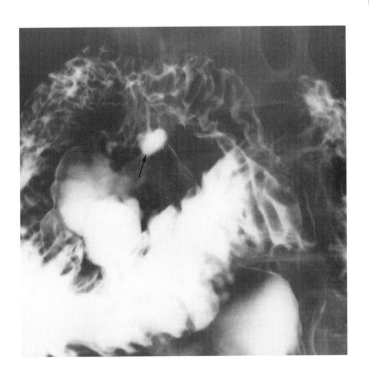

Fig. 4.17 Duodenal diverticulum complicated by peptic ulcer. There is a large diverticulum arising from the postbulbar part of the first part of the duodenum and filling a large part of the concavity of the duodenal sweep. A constant ulcer crater, measuring almost 10 mm, is seen in the neck of the diverticulum (arrow) [15]. Other complications of duodenal diverticula include abscesses or fistulae, haemorrhage and perforation.

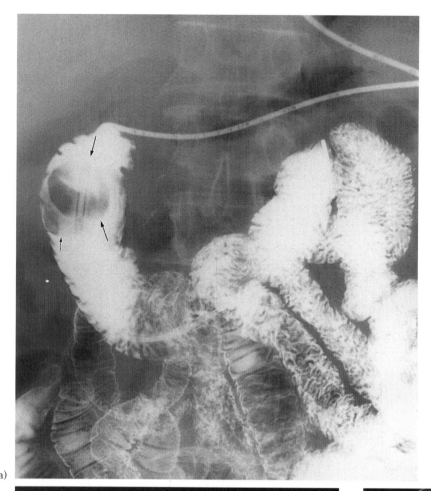

(a)

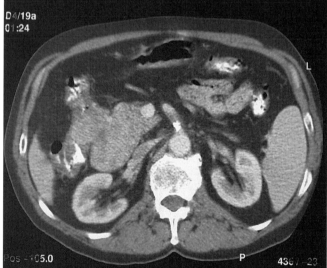

(b)

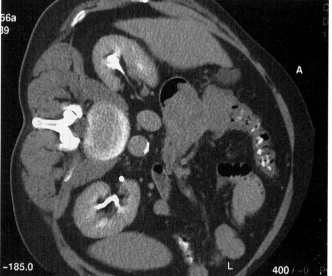

(c)

Fig. 4.19 Stromal tumour of the hepatic flexure invading the duodenum. A 65-year-old male patient presented with a haematemesis. Endoscopy at that time failed to demonstrate a bleeding source in the upper gastrointestinal tract. The patient responded to conservative management, and an out-patient small-bowel enema (a) revealed no abnormality in the jejunum or ileum, but there was a constant, lobulated filling defect in the second part of the duodenum, measuring 4.5 cm in diameter (arrows). (b) In the same patient, a spiral CT scan with contrast enhancement demonstrates a mass lesion in the hepatic flexure of the colon, extending into the second part of the duodenum. (c) The examination was repeated with the patient right side raised with further Carbex. This confirms a large duodenal filling defect contiguous with the mass in the hepatic flexure, with no fat plane between the two.

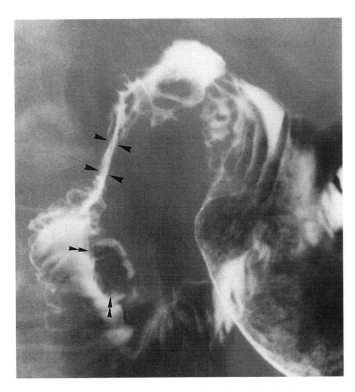

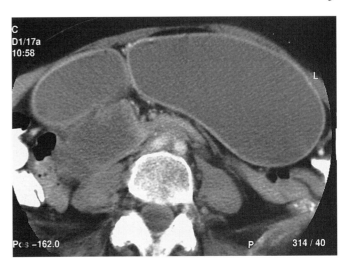

Fig. 4.21 Duodenal obstruction secondary to pancreatic cancer. A spiral CT scan with contrast enhancement in a 77-year-old female patient with copious vomiting and abdominal distension shows massive dilatation of the fluid-filled stomach and first and second parts of the duodenum. The third part of the duodenum is grossly constricted and infiltrated by a carcinoma of the uncinate process of the pancreas. The fat between the aorta and the IVC is also seen to be involved.

Fig. 4.20 Carcinoma of the pancreas invading the duodenum. There is gross deformity of the first and second parts of the duodenum, despite a muscle relaxant. A persistent duodenal stricture (arrowheads) is caused by duodenal encasement. The ampulla of Vater (double arrowheads) is apparently not involved in the infiltrative process.

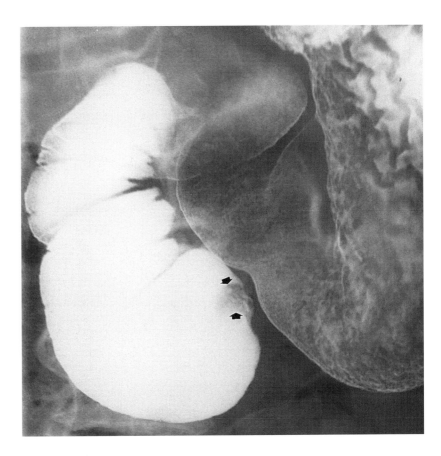

Fig. 4.22 Pancreatic carcinoma obstructing the third part of the duodenum. A second patient with gross duodenal obstruction, caused by a pancreatic cancer (arrowheads) encasing the third part of the duodenum. The diagnosis was confirmed surgically. (Courtesy of Dr Laura M. Wilkinson.)

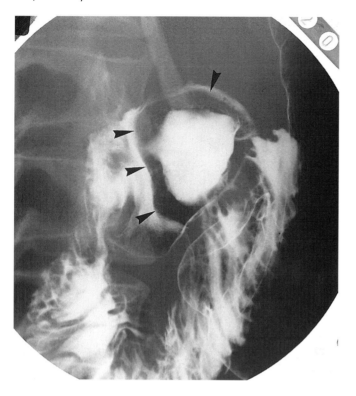

Fig. 4.23 Duodenal metastatic disease. A 30-year-old female patient had a malignant melanoma excised from her face. A local recurrence of the tumour was treated surgically 5 years later. She subsequently developed profound iron-deficiency anaemia. This DCBM shows a constant, relatively smooth filling defect in the first part of the duodenum (arrowheads), on the surface of which a large ulcer crater was detected. Metastatic melanoma was confirmed endoscopically.

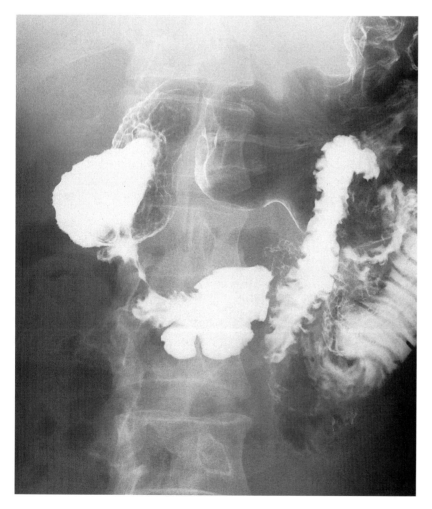

Fig. 4.24 Crohn's disease of the duodenum. A 33-year-old male patient presented with several months' history of upper abdominal pain and vomiting. The DCBM shows a constant, fairly tight, irregular stricture of the second part of the duodenum, with mucosal oedema and ulceration. A trace of the barium is seen to reflux into the ampulla of Vater.

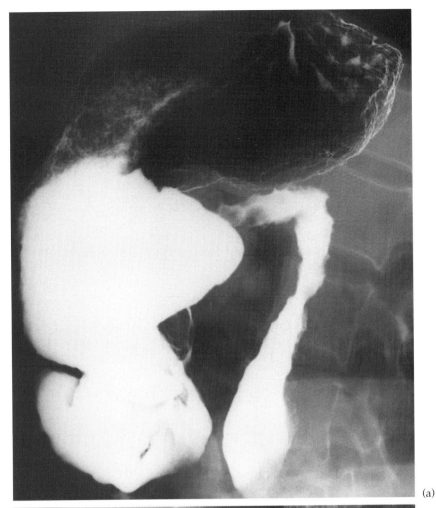

(a)

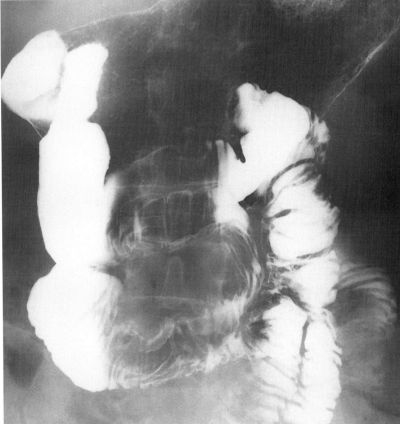

(b)

Fig. 4.25 Crohn's disease of the stomach and duodenum. This 60-year-old female patient had increasing upper abdominal pain for several weeks. The DCBM shows diffuse ulceration of the stomach and duodenum, which also shows reduced distensibility. In addition, there is a marked degree of extrinsic compression of the third part of the duodenum and sections of the proximal jejunum, in keeping with lymphadenopathy. The diagnosis was confirmed histologically.

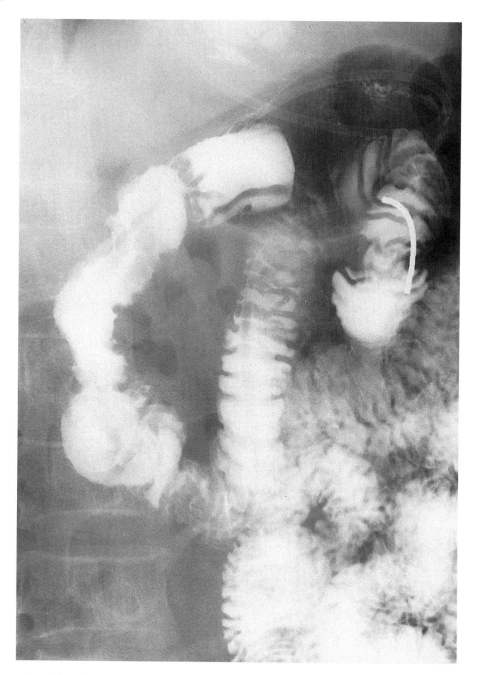

Fig. 4.26 Coeliac disease involving the duodenum. A male patient had a previous history of ileal stricture, which was thought to be due to Crohn's disease, without histological confirmation. A recent small-bowel enema failed to confirm jejunal or ileal strictures or ulceration, but the circular fold pattern in the second part of the duodenum was abolished and the mucosa is seen to be distinctly irregular, suggestive of mucosal swelling, without definite ulceration. Microscopy of the duodenal biopsies showed subtotal villous atrophy and increased intraepithelial lymphocytes. The changes were consistent with coeliac disease.

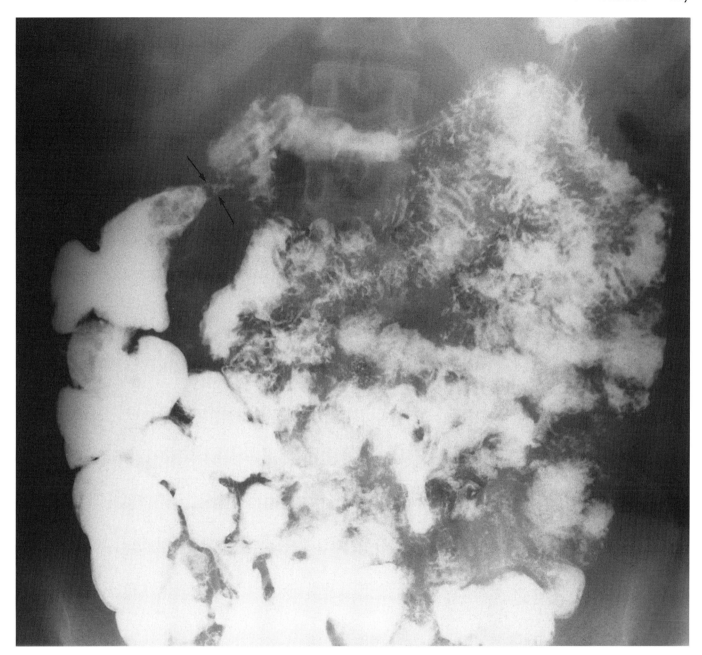

Fig. 4.27 Tuberculosis of the duodenum. A 29-year-old patient from Africa presented with several weeks' history of nausea, non-specific abdominal pain and weight loss. The barium-meal follow-through shows an obvious fistula (arrows) between the anterolateral border of the second part of the duodenum and the hepatic flexure of the colon. The fistula was confirmed endoscopically and tuberculosis was confirmed bacteriologically. The patient also had a colonic stricture at her splenic flexure (not shown).

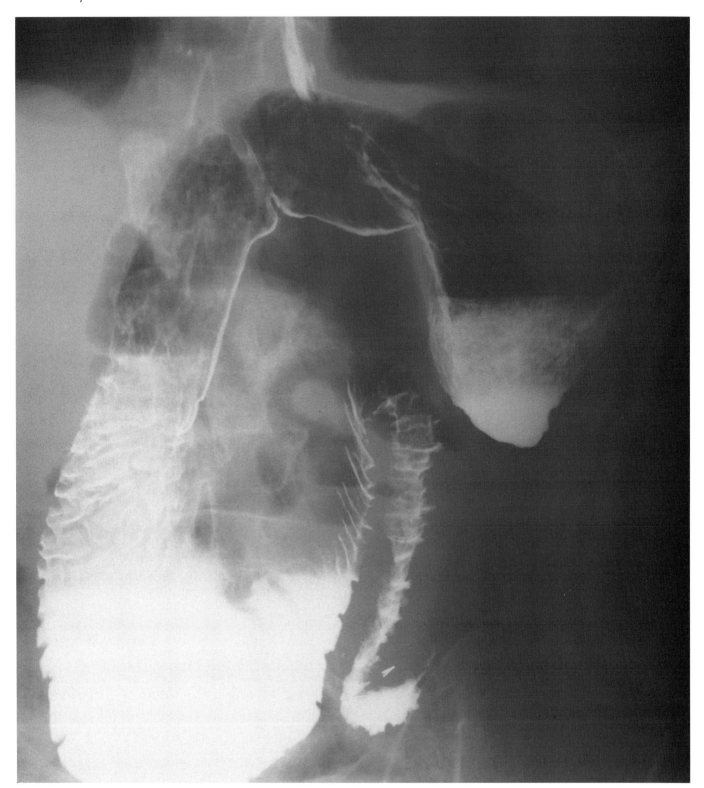

Fig. 4.28 Radiation damage to the duodenum and jejunum.
A middle-aged male patient had had previous radiotherapy to the left renal area for what was originally thought to be a renal carcinoma. He subsequently developed severe diarrhoea and malabsorption. He later developed a palpable testicular swelling, the histology of which was seminoma. Review of the original histology was compatible with seminoma. The stomach and duodenum are seen to be distended on this erect view and there is marked fold thickening in the fourth part of the duodenum and the jejunum, which also show a loss of distensibility. The differential diagnosis includes intramural haemorrhage, lymphoma, serosal metastases and Crohn's disease.

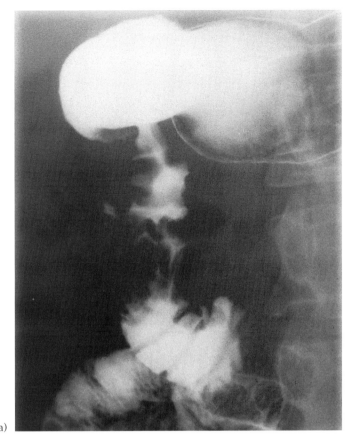

(a)

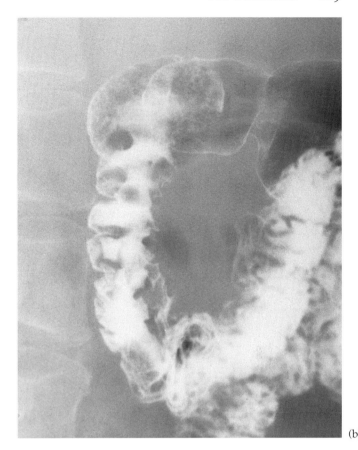

(b)

Fig. 4.29 Duodenal ischaemia. A 44-year-old male patient with a history of upper abdominal pain who had had three major cerebrovascular accidents as well as peripheral vascular disease. Duodenal endoscopy, multiple biopsies and laparotomy revealed no evidence of Crohn's disease or neoplasm. Angiography demonstrated occlusion of the coeliac artery and superior mesenteric artery. Only tiny collateral vessels were demonstrated in this area. (a) The DCBM shows marked persistent deformity and reduced distensibility of the duodenal loop, in keeping with ischaemia. (b) Similar changes were still present on a repeat examination 1 year later. (Reproduced from *British Journal of Radiology* **56**, 136–138, with permission.)

Fig. 4.30 Duodenal obstruction caused by congenital peritoneal band (Ladd's band). A middle-aged male patient gave a history of intermittent vomiting. The barium meal shows marked dilatation and obstruction of the duodenal loop, with a very abrupt change in calibre in the distal end of part three, beyond which the bowel is collapsed. However, the mucosa shows no evidence of intrinsic pathology. The congenital peritoneal band was confirmed surgically and the patient was cured by surgical division of it.

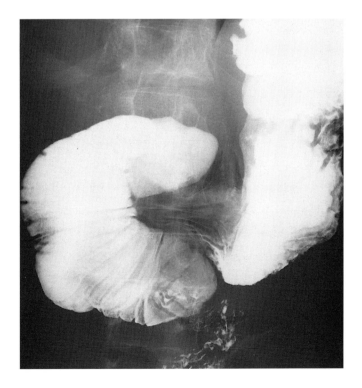

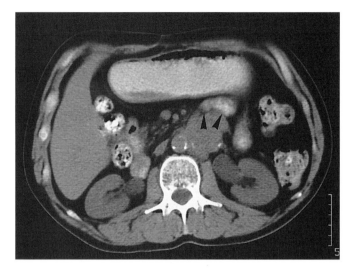

Fig. 4.31 Duodenal displacement and compression by phaeochromocytoma. This spiral CT scan shows a slightly calcified para-aortic mass lesion, which is seen to displace the fourth part of the duodenum anteriorly (arrowheads). This was caused by an extra-adrenal phaeochromocytoma in a 47-year-old male.

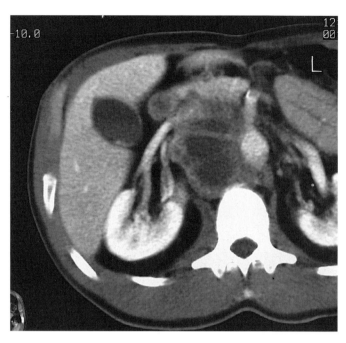

Fig. 4.33 Duodenal displacement and compression by metastatic teratoma. A spiral CT scan in a 39-year-old male patient with a germ-cell testicular tumour shows marked anterior displacement by a large, partly cystic, retroperitoneal mass lesion, which is seen to extend behind the abdominal aorta. The renal artery and vein are seen to be elevated and attenuated.

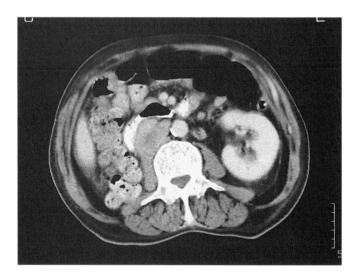

Fig. 4.32 Duodenal compression and displacement by recurrent renal carcinoma. A contrast-enhanced CT scan in a patient with a previous nephrectomy for carcinoma and known pulmonary, liver and bone metastases. The second part and proximal third part of the duodenum were seen to be displaced laterally and forwards by a paracaval mass lesion. The right kidney is absent.

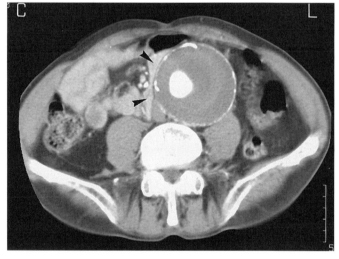

Fig. 4.34 Duodenal compression and attenuation by abdominal aortic aneurysm. An enhanced spiral CT scan demonstrates a large (7.2 cm diameter) abdominal aortic aneurysm. The second part of the duodenum is seen to be stretched and compressed (arrowheads) between the wall of the aneurysm medially and the gallbladder containing gallstones laterally.

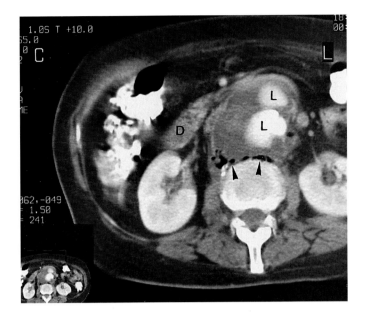

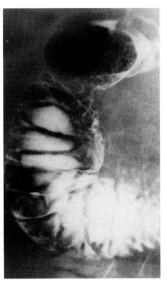

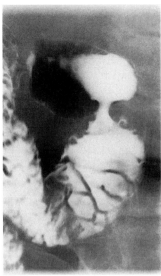

Fig. 4.35 Duodenal compression and displacement by a mycotic abdominal aortic aneurysm. A 62-year-old female patient had *Salmonella* septicaemia and a mycotic aneurysm of the abdominal aorta. The spiral CT scan shows gas bubbles in the wall of the aneurysm (arrowheads) and the second and third parts of the duodenum (D) were seen to be displaced upwards and laterally. Contrast in the false lumen of the aneurysm is shown (L). (Courtesy of Dr Alasdair Taylor.)

Fig. 4.36 Duodenal compression caused by an annular pancreas. A 63-year-old female patient had no symptoms or signs of duodenal obstruction. The DCBM shows supine and prone views of the duodenal loop, in which there is a constant smooth constriction of the second part of the duodenum, characteristic of an annular pancreas.

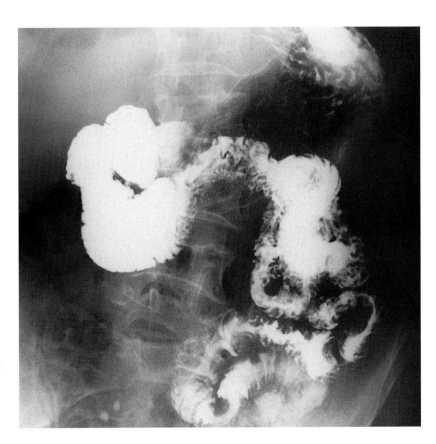

Fig. 4.37 Duodenal compression and displacement by haematoma. A 64-year-old male patient complained of vomiting 4 weeks after an aortic bifurcation graft. The DCBM shows constant extrinsic compression and displacement of the fourth part of the duodenum and the duodenojejunal flexure. This was due to a retroperitoneal haematoma related to the proximal graft anastomosis, which was resolved by conservative measures.

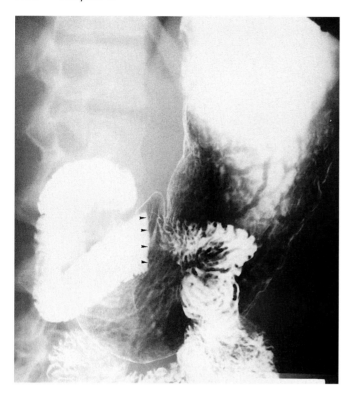

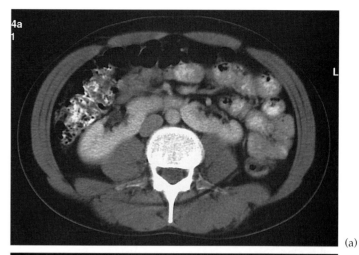

(a)

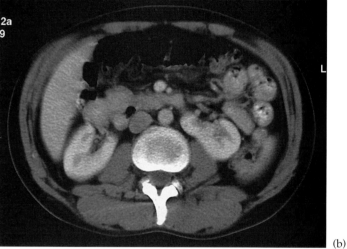

(b)

Fig. 4.38 Duodenal ileus. A steep RAO projection of this DCBM shows a sharp cut-off in the third part of the duodenum (arrowheads) at the level of the superior mesenteric artery, associated with partial duodenal obstruction. The mucosa is seen to be normal.

Fig. 4.40 Horseshoe kidney (bipolar fusion). A normal spiral CT study is shown in a patient with a horseshoe kidney. The contrast-enhanced nephrogram of the isthmus (a) should not be confused with the contrast-enhanced third part of duodenum (b).

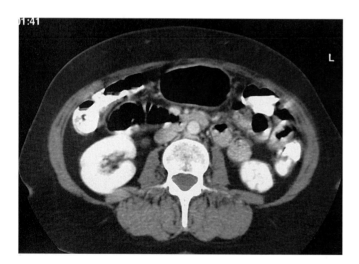

Fig. 4.39 Duodenal ileus. A spiral CT scan with contrast enhancement in a female patient aged 52, who had a similar appearance on DCBM to the patient in Fig. 4.38. The spiral CT scan shows proximal duodenal dilatation, with gaseous distension as far as the point at which the duodenum passes between the superior mesenteric artery and the aorta.

5: The Small Bowel

Anatomy

Anatomically, the ligament of Treitz marks the beginning of the small intestine at the duodenojejunal flexure and it ends at the ileocaecal valve, measuring approximately 5 m in length. The attachment of the small bowel to the posterior abdominal wall by a long wide mesentery means that it is remarkably mobile and entirely intraperitoneal. The proximal two-fifths of the small bowel is referred to as the jejunum and the distal three-fifths constitute the ileum, but there is no abrupt morphological transition between the two. The blood supply is delivered by many branches of the superior mesenteric artery. Circular folds, plicae circulares or valvulae conniventes are numerous in the jejunum, four to seven per 2.5 cm, and these gradually become more widely separated in the ileum, two to four per 2.5 cm, based on measurements using the small-bowel infusion technique (*vide infra*) [1]. The folds are also deeper and thicker, 1.9–2.0 mm, in the jejunum and shallower and thinner in the ileum, approximately 1.0 mm. However, the accuracy of the measurements depends on adequate distension of the lumen. The wall thickness is normally 1–2 mm and the diameter decreases from a maximum of 4.5 cm in the proximal jejunum to a maximum of 3.5 cm in the ileum, again based on measurements using the barium infusion technique. There is no exact consensus for a maximum diameter in the small bowel under physiological conditions, but figures of 3.0 cm [2] and 2.5 cm [3] have been cited.

Plain film radiography

Only a small volume of gas is normally present in the small bowel. Short fluid levels are not abnormal, three fluid levels not exceeding 2.5 cm in length being acceptable. More than two fluid levels in dilated small bowel (greater than 2.5 cm) are abnormal and usually indicate a mechanical obstruction or paralytic ileus [3, 4]. Fluid levels will be visible only if a horizontal beam technique is used. Meteorism refers to the accumulation of gas in slightly distended small-bowel loops with relatively little fluid content, resulting from an increased ingestion of swallowed air. This is associated with severe pain or respiratory embarrassment. Plain X-rays of the abdomen may be of value in detecting free air in the peritoneal cavity, opaque foreign bodies or intestinal obstruction—for example, resulting from an incarcerated hernia or impaction of a gallstone (gallstone ileus)

Barium follow-through

The barium-meal follow-through (BMFT) is the most widely used method for imaging the small bowel. Most commonly, it is performed as an adjunct to an upper gastrointestinal barium-meal series, but it may also be carried out as a dedicated small-bowel meal study [5]. Sequential films are taken at approximately 15–30 min, depending on the progress of the ingested barium. Spot films of the terminal ileum and of any suspicious areas are taken. Depending on the transit time, the procedure may vary in length—for example, 2–4 h—but this process may be accelerated by a variety of methods, including oral or IV metoclopramide (Maxolon). The BMFT or dedicated small-bowel meal technique may be modified to produce a double-contrast study by giving a gas-forming agent to generate up to 1 l carbon dioxide [6].

Small-bowel enema (enteroclysis)

The small-bowel enema (SBE) infusion method is a highly accurate technique in expert hands, with a sensitivity of 93% and specificity of 97%, based on a series of almost 1500 cases [7]. The method involves the rapid infusion of a barium sulphate suspension, either as a relatively dilute single-contrast study (using, for example, 1000 ml of 20% w/v barium) or alternatively a biphasic study, using a combination of a smaller volume (for example, 150–200 ml of higher-density barium 100% w/v) followed by a much larger volume (for example, 1–2 l of 0.5% aqueous solution of methylcellulose or magnesium sulphate) to produce a double-contrast effect. In this way, the whole length of the small bowel may be visualized fluoroscopically and representative films taken. Testing the distensibility of the lumen is the most important aspect of enteroclysis [1]. A further modification of this method uses air as well as 350–500 ml of barium sulphate 50–70% w/v in order to produce the double-contrast effect [8]. The main disadvantage of these infusion methods is the need for duodenal intubation, but the recent introduction of smaller-calibre catheters—12 F and, more recently, 10 F—has reduced patient discomfort [9]. In expert hands, the radiation dose to the patient compares well with other barium techniques. In Nolan's series [10], the mean effective patient dose was 1.0 mSv and this was markedly less than the average patient dose received during abdominal CT studies (7.0–8.0 mSv) [11]. The choice between the infusion methods and follow-through studies varies markedly from one centre to another, depending not least on the personal preference of the radiologist. Ideally, the accuracy of the two methods should be established by a prospective comparison, but in the literature there is a conspicuous lack of direct comparison, on account of the unjustifiable radiation dose incurred if both methods were to be used in the same patient [1]. In one series of 88 patients examined by enteroclysis, of whom 52 also had a BMFT, Gurian *et al.* [12] reported an overall accuracy of 96% for the infusion technique, compared with 65% for the follow-through method. However, a final diagnosis was established by endoscopy or surgery in only 27 of the 88 cases. In a study by Ott *et al.* [13], no difference was detected in overall accuracy between the two techniques, although adhesions were more easily detected using SBE. In another study of 370 SBEs, Diner *et al.* [14] found no significant difference in accuracy between the two methods. Maglinte *et al.* [15] reviewed 42 cases in which small-bowel pathology had been demonstrated by enteroclysis and confirmed surgically in each case, but which were not detected by the follow-through method. Technical factors appeared to be responsible for most of the missed diagnoses.

Oral pneumocolon

Whenever demonstration of the terminal ileum is impaired using BMFT or SBE methods, a much clearer view can be obtained by introducing air via a rectal catheter. This distends the caecum and terminal ileum, thus producing a double-contrast effect [16]. Success of this modification depends on the patient having a relatively clean colon.

Ileostomy enema

The distal small bowel may be examined satisfactorily in patients with an ileostomy by retrograde infusion of barium, with or without air, introduced via a Foley catheter [17].

Computerized tomography scanning

A new generation of much faster CT scanners, employing volume data acquisition, using the spiral (helical) method [18, 19] rather than incremental slices, has resulted in a more detailed display of the anatomy and pathology of the small bowel. The whole of the abdomen may be examined during a single breath-hold. Consequently, very useful information about the extraluminal component of intestinal disease and the effects of pathology on adjacent tissues and organs, including lymph nodes, can be obtained very rapidly and with virtually no discomfort to the patient. This is particularly important in seriously ill or injured patients. Particular applications include small-bowel infarction [20, 21], the complications of inflammatory bowel disease [22], the detection and analysis of intestinal obstruction [23–25] and the staging of neoplasms. In many centres, where small-bowel ischaemia, abscesses, Crohn's disease or obstruction are clinically suspected, CT is the first-choice imaging modality [26]. In the evaluation of intestinal obstruction, CT has the advantage over conventional infusion methods in avoiding the need for oral contrast medium. The bowel wall may be enhanced by giving IV contrast—for example, 100 ml at a rate of 3 ml/s, commencing 50–70 s before the start of the scan. In this context, CT also provides extraluminal information, on, for example, lymphadenopathy and metastatic liver disease, ascites or hydronephrosis. According to Gleeson, this information has made the greatest clinical impact in small-bowel CT scanning, together with its ability to indicate the most suitable biopsy site [16]. In the absence of overt clinical obstruction, oral contrast is normally given—200–1000 ml in different centres—some departments preferring a dilute barium suspension to Gastrografin. The luminal diameter is normally 2–3 cm and the most significant disease indicators are thickening of the wall, increased attenuation of the mesenteric fat ('dirty fat') and an increased number of mesenteric vessels [17]. The bowel wall is normally less than 3 mm thick when distended with contrast, and the fold thickness is not more than 3 mm [27]. The analysis of small-bowel disease demands careful opacification of the lumen, so that misinterpretation of undistended loops can be avoided [28]. In the jejunum, valvulae conniventes are commonly seen, but these are usually not visible in the ileum [29]. The surrounding mesentery should have a fat density of less than -75 Hounsfield units.

Ultrasound

The clinical value of ultrasound in the small bowel has generally been underestimated, very useful information being available using modern, high-resolution, real-time equipment. Obstructed small bowel may be readily recognized by this method [30] and, in the 6% of patients with small-bowel obstruction who have a 'gasless' abdomen on plain films, ultrasound may establish the diagnosis [26]. Real-time scanning is a rapid, non-invasive, radiation-free, inexpensive means of demonstrating thickening of the bowel wall in inflammatory bowel disease [31, 32] and malignancy [33]. This is particularly obvious in the presence of ascites, which affords a natural acoustic window. The role of ultrasound, however, is limited by bowel gas and obesity.

Angiography

The blood supply to the small bowel can be readily demonstrated by selective injection of contrast medium into the superior mesenteric artery; the technique is enhanced by using the digital-subtraction technique and in expert hands is a very safe procedure. If acute or chronic ischaemia is suspected, it is important to obtain a lateral view of the abdominal aorta, so that the origins of the coeliac, superior mesenteric and inferior mesenteric arteries may be profiled. Despite rapid improvements in CT scanning, angiography remains the method of choice in the evaluation of acute [34] and chronic [35] ischaemia, as well as in the diagnosis and management of lesions responsible for haemorrhage into the small bowel [36]. There is likely to be a major role in the future for MR angiography enhanced with IV gadolinium.

References

1 Herlinger H. (1994) Barium examinations. In: Gore R.M., Levine M.S. & Laufer I. (eds) *A Textbook of Gastro-intestinal Radiology*. Philadelphia: W.B. Saunders, 766–788.

2 Dahnert W. (1996) *Radiology Review Manual*, 3rd edn. Baltimore: Williams & Wilkins, 573.

3 Field S. (1997) The plain abdominal radiograph. In: Grainger R.D. & Allison D.J. (eds) *Diagnostic Radiology*, 3rd edn. New York: Churchill Livingstone, 885–907.

4 Gammill S.L. & Nice C.M. (1972) Air fluid levels: the occurrence in normal patients and their role in the analysis of ileus. *Surgery* **71**, 771–780.

5 Nolan D.J. (1997) The small intestine. In: Grainger R.G. & Allison D.J. (eds) *Diagnostic Radiology*, 3rd edn. New York: Churchill Livingstone, 985–1008.

6 Fraser G.M. & Preston P.G. (1983) The small bowel barium follow through enhanced with oral effervescent agent. *Clinical Radiology* **34**, 673–679.

7 Dixon P.M., Roulston M.E. & Nolan D.J. (1993) The small bowel enema: a ten year review. *Clinical Radiology* **47**, 46–48.

8 Yao T. (1994) Double contrast enteroclysis with air. In: Freeny P.C. & Stevenson G.W. (eds) *Margulis and Burhenne's Alimentary Tract Radiology*, 5th edn. St Louis: Mosby, 548–551.

9 Traill Z.C. & Nolan D.J. (1995) Technical note: intubation fluoroscopy times using a new enteroclysis tube. *Clinical Radiology* **50**, 339–340.

10 Hart D., Haggett P.J., Boardman P., Nolan D.J. & Wall B.F. (1994) Patient radiation doses from enteroclysis examinations. *British Journal of Radiology* **67**, 997–1000.

11 Shrimpton P.C., Jones D.G., Hillier M.C. *et al.* (1991) *Survey of CT Practice in the UK, Part II: Dosimetric Aspects*, NRPB—R249. London: HMSO.

12 Gurian L., Gentdrzejewski J., Katon R. *et al.* (1982) Small bowel enema: an under utilised method of small bowel examination. *Digestive Diseases and Sciences* **27**, 1101–1108.

13 Ott D.J., Chen Y.M., Gelfand D.W. *et al.* (1985) Detailed per-oral small bowel examination v. enteroclysis. *Radiology* **155**, 29–34.

14 Diner W.C., Hoskins E.O.L. & Navab F. (1984) Radiological examination of the small intestine: review of four hundred and two cases and discussion of indications and methods. *Southern Medical Journal* **77**, 68–74.

15 Maglinte D.D.T., Burney B.T. & Miller R.E. (1982) Lesions missed on small bowel follow through: analysis and recommendations. *Radiology* **144**, 737–739.

16 Gleeson J.A. (1993) The small intestine. In: Sutton D. (ed.) *A Textbook of Radiology and Imaging*, 5th edn. Edinburgh: Churchill Livingstone, 829–856.

17 Somers S. & Stevenson G. W. (1994) The small bowel. In: Freeny P.C. & Stevenson G.W. (eds) *Margulis and Burhenne's Alimentary Tract Radiology*, 5th edn. St Louis: Mosby, 512–532.

18 Brink J.A. (1995) Technical aspects of helical (spiral) CT. *Radiologic Clinics of North America* **33** (5), 825–841.

19 Brink J.A. (1997) Spiral CT. *Clinical Radiology* **52**, 489–503.

20 Federle M.P., Chun G., Jeffery R.B. & Rayor R. (1984) Computed tomographic findings in bowel infarction. *American Journal of Roentgenology* **142**, 91–95.

21 Smerud M.J., Johnson C.D. & Stevens D.H. (1990) Diagnosis of bowel infarction: a comparison of plain films and CT scan in twenty-three cases. *American Journal of Roentgenology* **154**, 99–103.

22 Goldberg H.I., Gore R.M., Margulis A.R. *et al.* (1983) Computed tomography in the evaluation of Crohn's disease. *American Journal of Roentgenology* **140**, 277–282.

23 Frager D., Medwid S.W., Baer J.W. *et al.* (1994) CT of small bowel obstruction: value in establishing the diagnosis and determining the degree and cause. *American Journal of Roentgenology* **162**, 37–41.

24 Balthazar E.J. (1994) CT of small bowel obstruction. *American Journal of Roentgenology* **162**, 255–261.

25 Gazelle G.S., Goldberg M.A., Whittenberg J. *et al.* (1994) Efficacy of CT in distinguishing small bowel obstruction from other causes of small bowel dilatation. *American Journal of Roentgenology* **162**, 43–47.

26 Vecchioli A., Franco A., Maresca G. *et al.* (1994) Cross-sectional imaging of the small bowel. In: Gore R.M., Levine M.S. & Laufer I. (eds) *A Textbook of Gastro-intestinal Radiology*. Philadelphia: W.B. Saunders, 789–801.

27 Burgener F.A. & Kormano M. (1996) *Differential Diagnosis in Computed Tomography*. Stuttgart: Thieme Medical Publishers, 293.

28 Megibow A.J. (1994) The gastro-intestinal tract. In: Haaga J.R., Lanzieri C.E., Sartoris D.J. *et al.* (eds) *Computed Tomography and Magnetic Resonance Imaging of the Whole Body*, 3rd edn. St Louis: Mosby, 855–895.

29 Desai R.K., Tagliabue J.R., Wegryn S.A. *et al.* (1991) CT evaluation of wall thickening in the alimentary tract. *Radiographics* **11**, 771–783.

30 Scheible W. & Goldberger L.E. (1979) Diagnosis of small bowel obstruction: the contribution of diagnostic ultrasound. *American Journal of Roentgenology* **133**, 685–688.

31 Dubbins P.A. (1984) Ultrasound demonstration of bowel wall thickness in inflammatory bowel disease. *Clinical Radiology* **35**, 227–231.

32 Dubbins P.A. (1993) The small bowel and colon. In: Cosgrove D.O., Meire H. & Dewbury K. (eds) *Abdominal and General Ultrasound*. Edinburgh: Churchill Livingstone, 765–776.

33 Bin W., Jianguo L. & Baowei D. (1992) The sonographical appearances of small bowel tumours. *Clinical Radiology* **46**, 30–33.

34 Clark R.A. & Gallant T.E. (1984) Acute mesenteric ischaemia: angiographic spectrum. *American Journal of Roentgenology* **142**, 555–562.

35 Stanton P.E., Jr, Hollier P.A., Seidel T.W. *et al.* (1986) Chronic intestinal ischaemia: diagnosis and therapy. *Journal of Vascular Surgery* **4**, 338–344.

36 Allison D.J. (1997) Gastro-intestinal angiography. In: Grainger R.G. & Allison D.J. (eds) *Diagnostic Radiology*, 3rd edn. New York: Churchill Livingstone, 1091–1108.

37 Adam A., Roddie M.E. & Bowley N.B. (1997) The biliary tract. In: Grainger R.G. & Allison D.G. (eds) *Grainger and Allison's Diagnostic Radiology*, 3rd edn. New York: Churchill Livingstone, 1201–1234.

38 Swift S.E. & Spencer J.A. (1998) Gallstone ileus CT findings. *Clinical Radiology* **53**(6), 451–454.

39 Aleman S. (1948) Jejuno-gastric intussusception: a rare complication of the operated stomach. *Acta Radiologica* **29**, 383–395.

Suggested further reading

Buckley J.A., Jones B. & Fishman E.K. (1997) Small bowel cancer, imaging features and staging. In: Gore R.M. (ed.) *Staging Gastrointestinal Malignancy*. Radiologic Clinics of North America, Vol. 35(2). Philadelphia: W.B. Saunders, 381–402.

Maglinte D.D.T. & Reyes B.L. (1997) Small bowel cancer radiologic diagnosis. In: Gore R.M. (ed.) *Staging Gastrointestinal Malignancy*. Radiologic Clinics of North America, Vol. 35(2). Philadelphia: W.B. Saunders, 361–380.

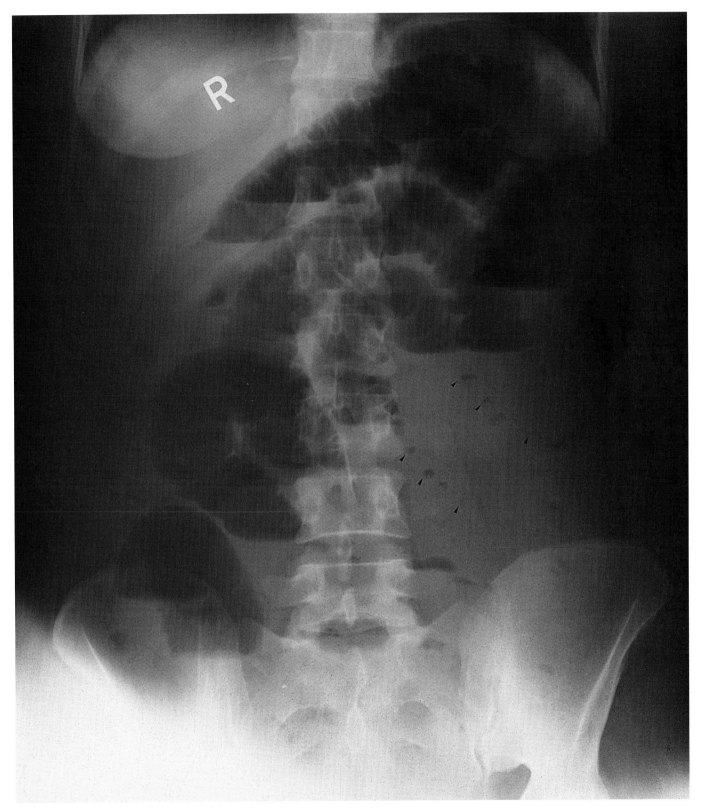

Fig. 5.1 Mechanical small-bowel obstruction due to adhesions.
An erect abdominal plain X-ray shows gaseous and fluid distension of multiple small-bowel loops, with multiple fluid levels, which may be demonstrated only by a horizontal X-ray beam. The circular-fold pattern is shown, clearly identifying the small-bowel loops. In addition, the 'string-of-beads' sign is evident. This is caused by small pockets of gas being trapped between circular folds in fluid-distended small bowel (arrowheads) [3]. Postoperative adhesions are the commonest cause of mechanical small-bowel obstruction in the Western world. Virtually no gas is present in the large bowel.

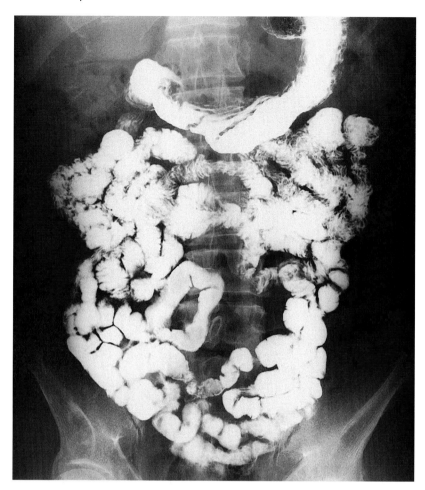

Fig. 5.2 Normal barium follow-through study of the small bowel. The normal filling pattern at 45 min shows normal segmentation in the jejunum and ileum, due to peristalsis.

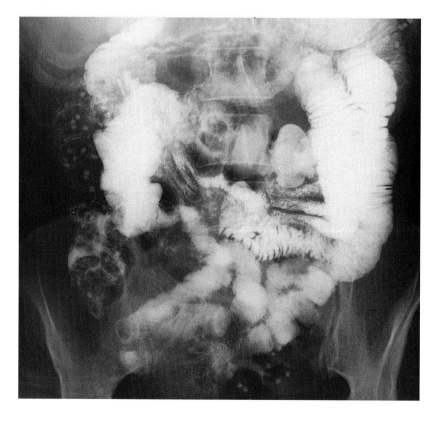

Fig. 5.3 Postoperative fibrous adhesions. A delayed film in a barium follow-through study shows considerable deformity, with abrupt changes in calibre of the small bowel and angulation, due to multiple adhesions. On fluoroscopy, the small-bowel loops had a relatively fixed appearance, but the mucosa appeared normal. There is relatively mild proximal dilatation of the small bowel, and the head of the barium column has reached the colon. Multiple opaque markers are shown in the large bowel as a result of a previous transit study.

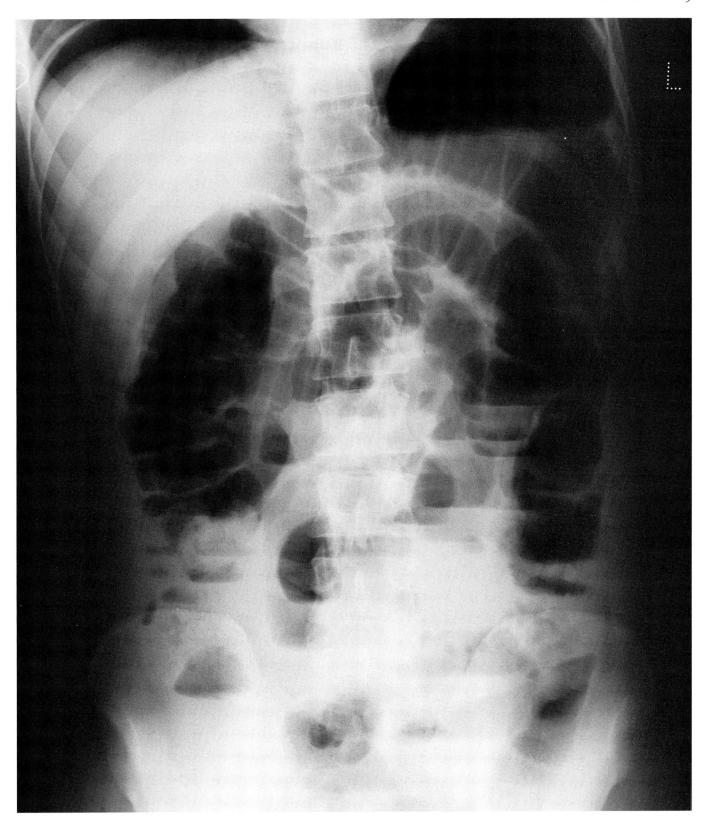

Fig. 5.4 Postoperative paralytic ileus and pneumoperitoneum. A 25-year-old male patient had generalized abdominal distension 4 days following a right hemicolectomy and ileal resection for Crohn's disease. This erect abdominal film shows a moderate amount of free air under the right hemidiaphragm and there is generalized gaseous distension of the stomach, the small bowel and, to a lesser extent, the large bowel, with numerous fluid levels. More than half of all patients within a few days of laparotomy will have evidence of a pneumoperitoneum [3].

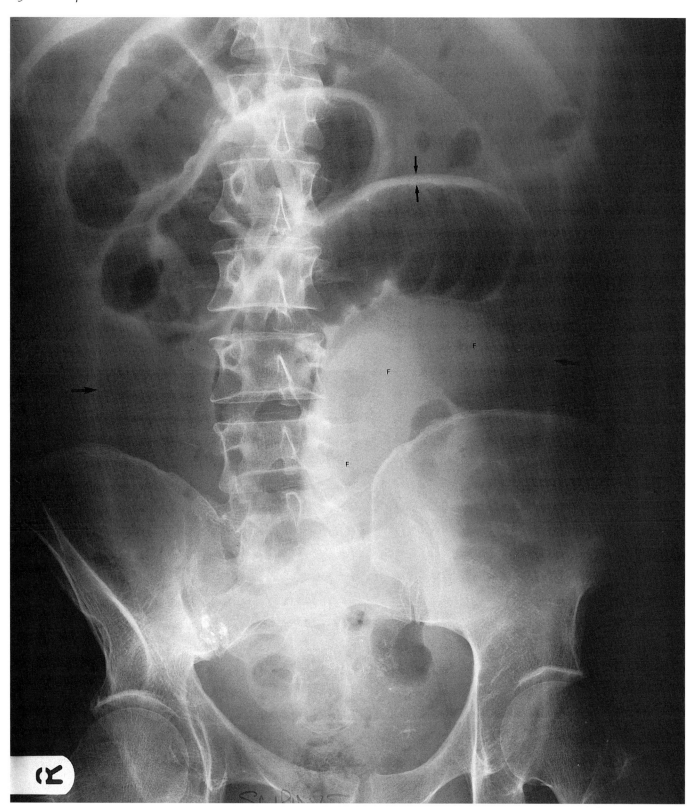

Fig. 5.5 Small-bowel obstruction and perforation leading to peritonitis. Supine abdominal X-ray shows a large volume of free air in the peritoneal cavity, together with a large volume of fluid, the fluid margin being indicated in both flanks by the larger arrows. There is considerable gaseous distension of the small-bowel loops and one loop is distended entirely by fluid (F). Gas is seen on both sides of the bowel wall (between small arrows), which is a sign of pneumoperitoneum. There is also evidence of slight thickening of the small-bowel wall. At laparotomy, pneumoperitoneum and peritonitis were confirmed, resulting from a small-bowel perforation. The patient had had previous radiotherapy for a colonic carcinoma and had extensive small-bowel radiation damage and adhesion formation, leading to partial obstruction.

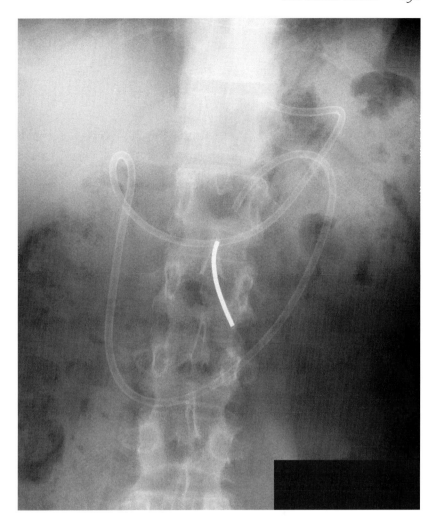

Fig. 5.6 Small-bowel enema. This control film (not routine) shows the starting position, with the leading end of the infusion catheter (10 F Merck) advanced well round the duodenum into the proximal jejunum.

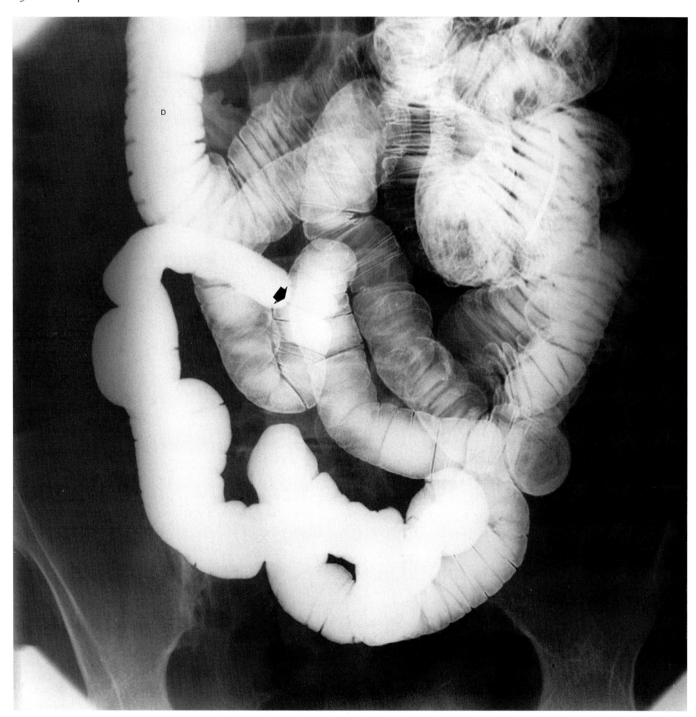

Fig. 5.7 Normal small-bowel enema. The barium column has advanced well into the ileum, having been propelled by a large volume of water containing magnesium sulphate. Numerous circular folds are visible in the jejunum and are much less numerous in the ileum, which is also of smaller calibre. D, duodenum; arrowhead, head of barium column.

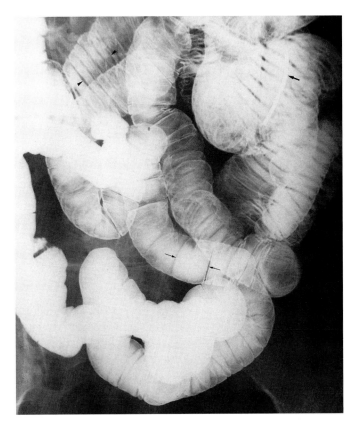

Fig. 5.8 Normal small-bowel enema. In the jejunum, five folds per 2.5 cm are present (between arrowheads), the normal range being four to seven. In the ileum, three folds per 2.5 cm are apparent (between arrows), the normal range being two to four [1]. Single arrow, tip of infusion catheter.

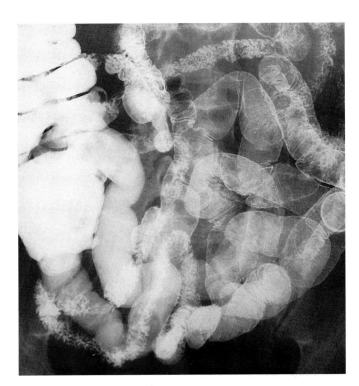

Fig. 5.9 Normal small-bowel enema. In some normal subjects, the ileum may be almost completely devoid of circular folds.

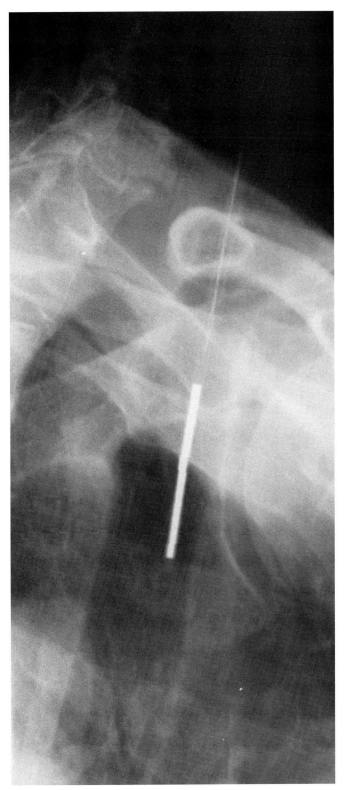

Fig. 5.10 Misplaced small-bowel enema tube. In this older patient, with prominent cervical osteophytes, the SBE tube is seen to have entered the trachea on this lateral projection of the thoracic inlet.

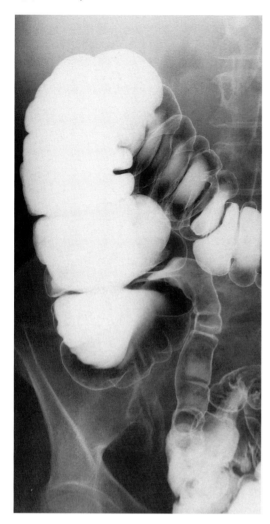

Fig. 5.11 Normal distal small bowel. In the majority of patients, the terminal ileum may be demonstrated during a double-contrast colonic enema, particularly if the patient is given a muscle relaxant, e.g. hyoscine or glucagon.

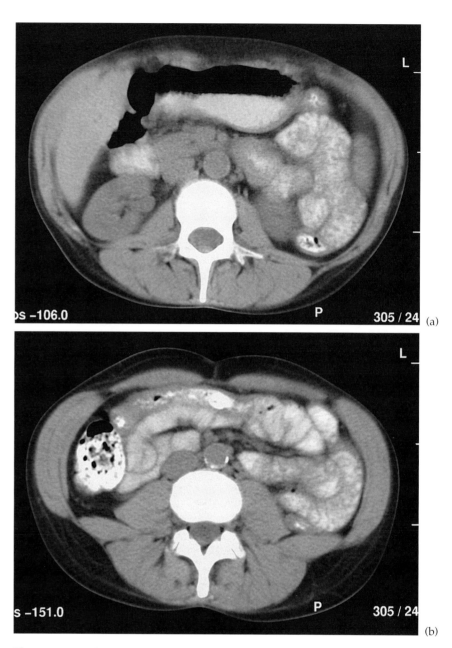

(a)

(b)

Fig. 5.12 Normal small-bowel CT study. (a) The feathery pattern of the normal jejunal mucosa is visible. (b) A more distal section shows contrast filling of the jejunum, ileum, caecum and transverse colon.

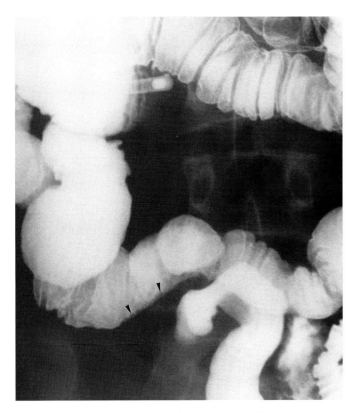

Fig. 5.13 Crohn's disease of the jejunum. An SBE in a 20-year-old female patient with several weeks' history of diarrhoea with non-caseating granulomata in the rectal biopsy. Part of the jejunum shows disruption of the circular fold pattern, moderate loss of distensibility and a very fine eccentric cobblestone pattern (arrowheads), in keeping with Crohn's disease.

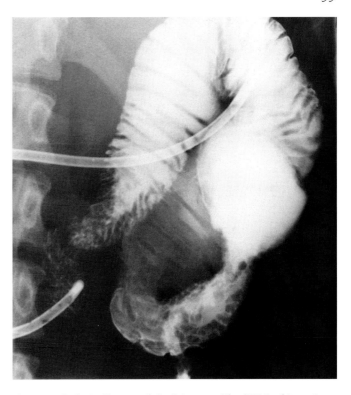

Fig. 5.15 Crohn's disease of the jejunum. The SBE in this patient shows a more extensive involvement of the jejunum, with a more marked cobblestone pattern, which is the result of focal mucosal oedema interspersed by longitudinal and transverse ulceration. There is also segmental loss of distensibility and proximal dilatation.

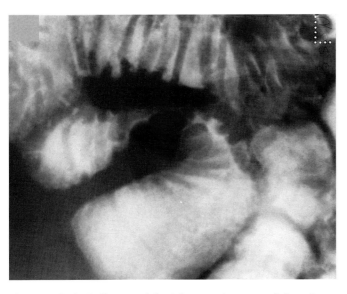

Fig. 5.14 Crohn's disease of the jejunum. A young adult male patient with diarrhoea and colicky abdominal pain. The SBE revealed thickening and nodularity of the circular fold pattern, together with a loss of distensibility of a 3 cm segment.

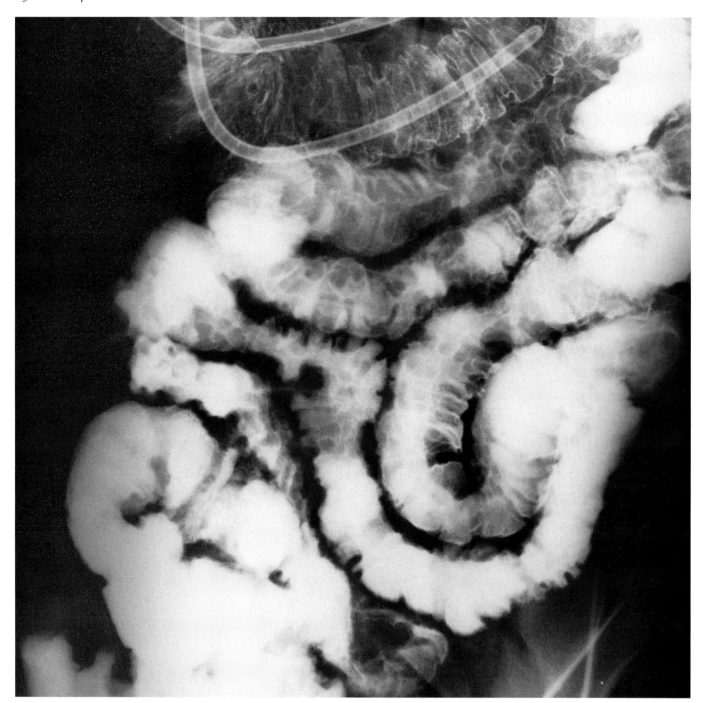

Fig. 5.16 Crohn's disease of the jejunum. An SBE in a 15-year-old male with severe diarrhoea and weight loss. There is very extensive jejunal disease, characterized by varying degrees of loss of distensibility, thickening of the small-bowel wall and gross disruption of the circular fold pattern, which is largely replaced by a marked cobblestone pattern. Histological confirmation.

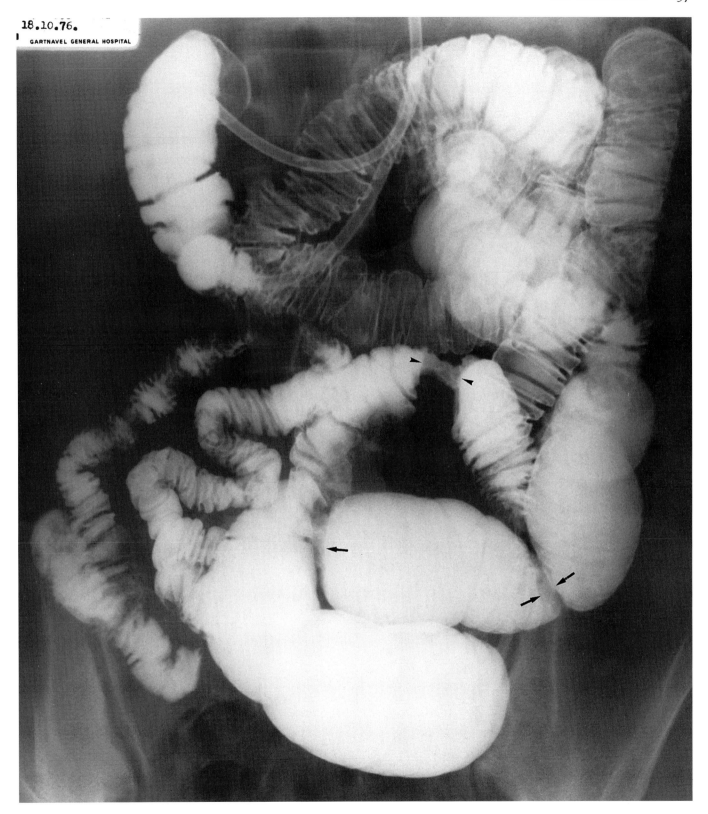

Fig. 5.17 Crohn's disease of the jejunum. The SBE shows a normal proximal jejunum, but there is a well-defined, irregular, constant stricture 1.5 cm in length (between arrowheads) and further shorter strictures between dilated segments more distally in the jejunum (arrows).

(a)

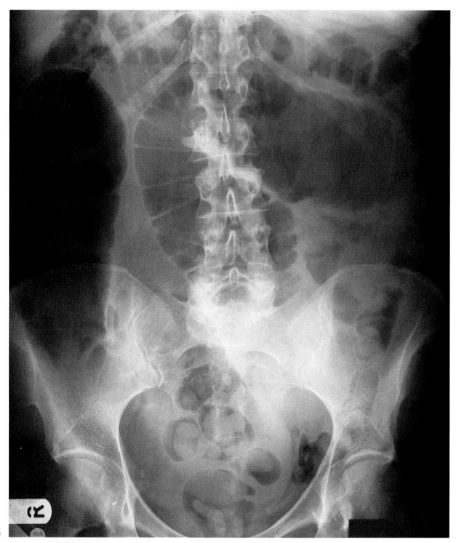

(b)

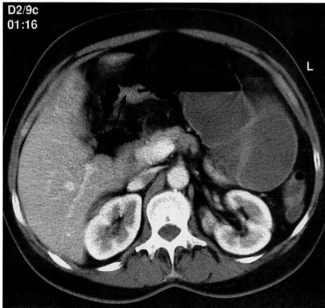

Fig. 5.18 Crohn's disease of the jejunum causing small-bowel obstruction. A 51-year-old female patient with a 4-month history of diarrhoea and borborygmi and profound weight loss (19 kg). (a) A supine abdominal X-ray shows gross distension of the small bowel, one segment measuring 9 cm in diameter. This has valvulae conniventes rather than a haustral pattern, indicating that it is small bowel and not a distended sigmoid loop. (b) A spiral contrast-enhanced CT (CECT) of the same patient confirms a gross degree of small-bowel obstruction, proximal to a 2 cm long stenotic lesion (arrow). This has a non-specific appearance, but histology of the surgically resected specimen indicated Crohn's disease.

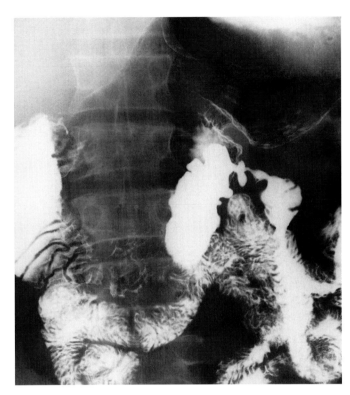

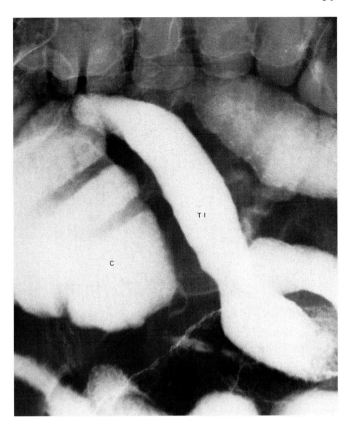

Fig. 5.19 Crohn's disease of the jejunum. A BMFT in a 60-year-old male patient with a 6-month history of nausea, weight loss and more recent vomiting. A succussion splash was clinically present. The duodenum was found to be partly obstructed by a tight irregular stricture at the duodenojejunal flexure. Pathology of the resected specimen indicated postinflammatory fibrosis, in keeping with Crohn's disease. The differential diagnosis includes direct spread of pancreatic carcinoma into small bowel and primary small-bowel malignancy, e.g. lymphoma.

Fig. 5.21 Crohn's disease of the ileum. The SBE in this patient with marked diarrhoea, weight loss and iron-deficiency anaemia shows very extensive but relatively superficial ulceration and fine nodularity, in keeping with mucosal oedema. There is no evidence of stricture. C, caecum; TI, terminal ileum.

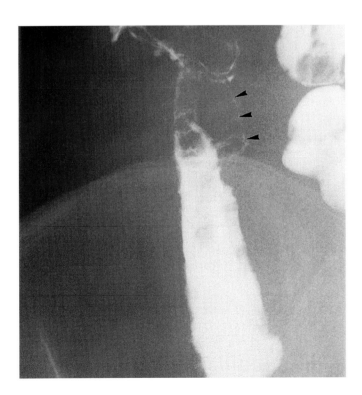

Fig. 5.20 Crohn's disease of the ileum. The last part of the BMFT in this 35-year-old female patient with right iliac fossa pain and diarrhoea shows fine marginal irregularity of the terminal ileum, in keeping with ulceration, together with much more penetrating interconnected fissure ulceration (arrowheads) extending for 1 cm from the mucosal surface. There is also considerable loss of distensibility and caecal deformity.

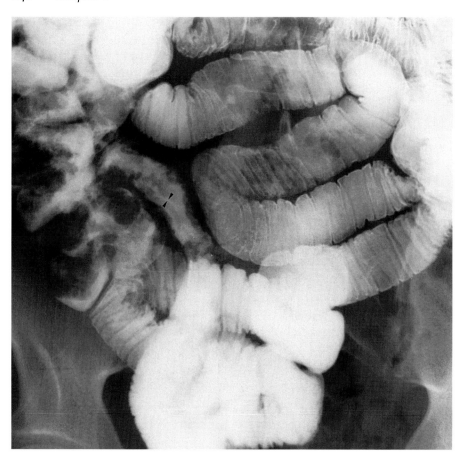

Fig. 5.22 Crohn's disease of the ileum.
An SBE in a 42-year-old female patient
with right iliac fossa pain without colonic
preparation. The distal 7 cm of the ileum
shows slight loss of distensibility, a
widespread cobblestone pattern and
linear ulceration (arrowheads), in keeping
with Crohn's disease.

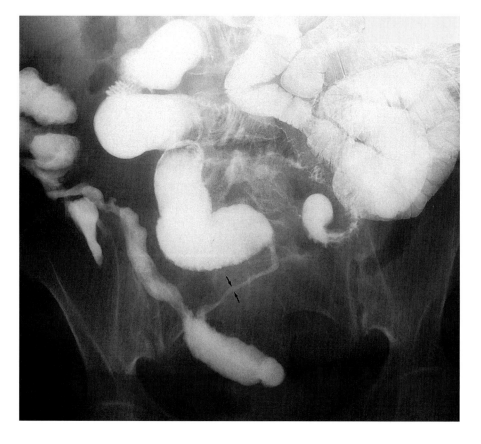

**Fig. 5.23 Crohn's disease of the ileum
with stricture formation.** The SBE of
this 63-year-old female patient with
intermittent colicky abdominal pain and
diarrhoea shows a 25 cm segment of distal
ileum, which is irregular in outline with
segmental loss of distensibility. Proximal
to this section, there is an 8 cm long
stricture (arrows) representing the string
sign of Kantor, proximal to which the
small bowel is partly obstructed. The mid
small bowel shows fold thickening,
nodularity and partial loss of
distensibility, also in keeping with
Crohn's disease.

(a)

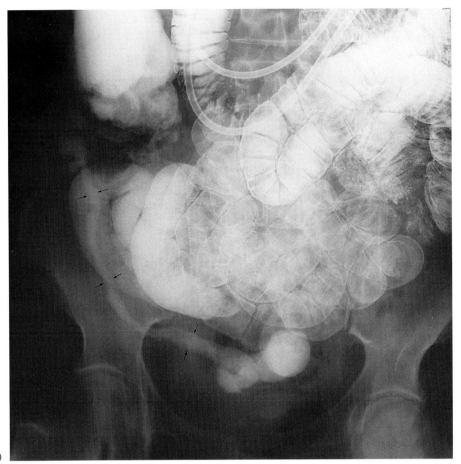

(b)

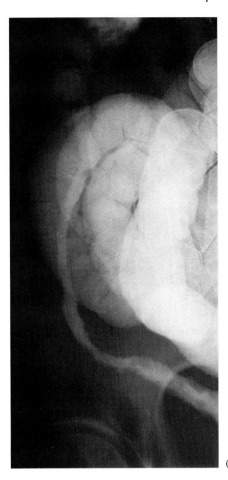

Fig. 5.24 Crohn's disease of the ileum. (a) An overview of the SBE shows that most of the small bowel distends normally and shows no mural thickening or ulceration, but the last 20 cm segment is grossly contracted and irregular in outline (arrows).

(b) A spot view of the right iliac fossa shows this segment in more detail. There is very widespread ulceration as well as loss of distensibility.

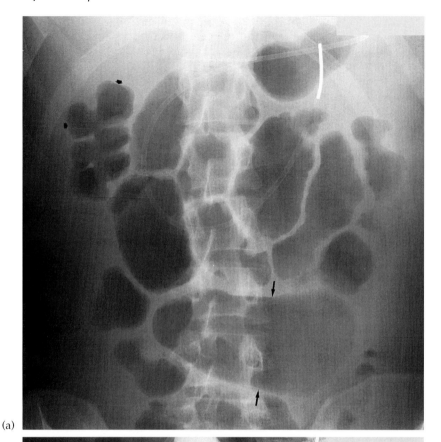

(a)

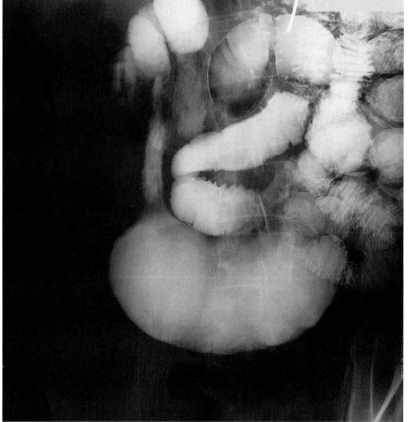

(b)

Fig. 5.25 Diffuse Crohn's disease of the small bowel. A 25-year-old male patient had severe weight loss over several months, iron-deficiency anaemia and marked hypoalbuminaemia. (a) A plain film (not routine) at the start of the SBE shows a grossly abnormal small-bowel pattern, consisting of multiple markedly dilated segments (one of which is marked by long arrows), a virtually complete loss of the circular fold pattern and some marginal irregularity. The normal gas-filled hepatic flexure is shown (arrowheads). (b) The SBE confirms the widespread changes of Crohn's disease, characterized by cobblestone ulceration and markedly dilated featureless loops. Histological confirmation of Crohn's disease.

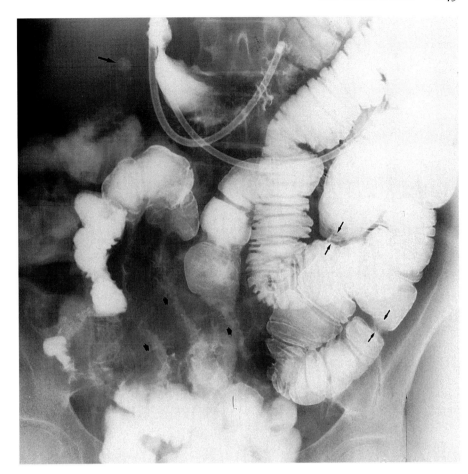

Fig. 5.26 Crohn's disease of the small bowel with multiple strictures. The proximal small bowel in this patient revealed two short jejunal strictures (small arrows). Much more extensive Crohn's disease was apparent in the ileum, where multiple loops revealed gross ulceration, mural thickening and stricture formation (arrowheads). The most important single function of enteroclysis is to test the distensibility of the small bowel. Multiple calcified gallstones are also shown (large arrow).

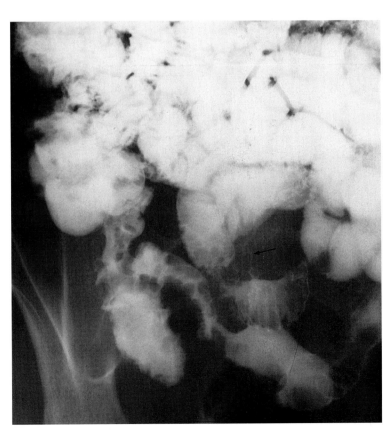

Fig. 5.27 Crohn's disease of the ileum with internal fistula. An SBE in a 17-year-old female patient with a 2-year history of colicky abdominal pain and diarrhoea. The SBE shows gross changes of Crohn's disease in the distal small bowel, characterized by marked deformity and gross cobblestone ulceration, and a fistulous track between adjacent segments of the small bowel is shown (arrow). The caecum is also seen to be grossly contracted and ulcerated. The patient died of anaphylactic shock shortly after an IV contrast-medium injection to assess the status of her urinary tract prior to bowel surgery.

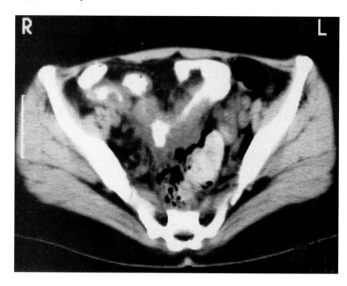

Fig. 5.28 Crohn's disease of the ileum. An incremental CT scan shows a constricted segment of small bowel in the pelvis, with a marked degree of mural thickening. The patient was known to have Crohn's disease.

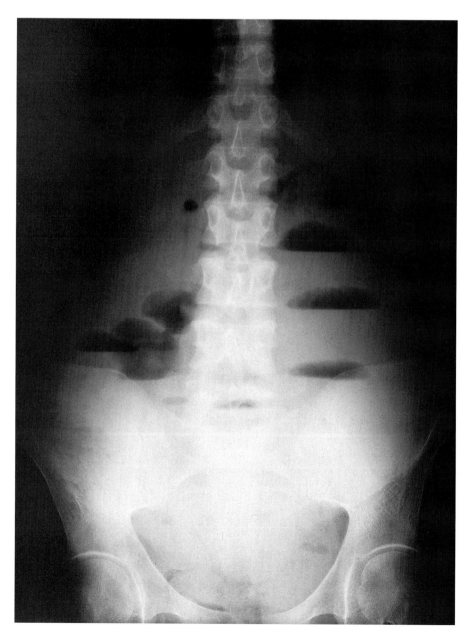

Fig. 5.29 Crohn's disease with small-bowel obstruction. A 23-year-old female patient had a 4-year history of periodic diarrhoea and abdominal pain, and proved Crohn's disease; there was also recent exacerbation of colicky pain and abdominal distension. This erect plain abdominal film shows multiple loops of small bowel distended with gas and fluid levels. There is virtually complete loss of colorectal gas. On plain films, the cause of mechanical small-bowel obstruction is not usually apparent.

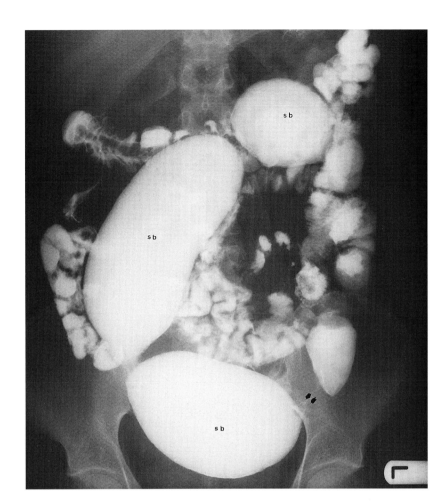

Fig. 5.30 Chronic small-bowel obstruction due to Crohn's disease. A BMFT in a female patient with a history of previous resection of right hemicolon and distal small bowel for Crohn's disease. Three markedly distended segments of small bowel (sb) are shown between strictures, one of which is marked by arrowheads. The dilated segments are completely lacking in a circular fold pattern and some marginal ulceration is visible. The potential for bacterial colonization of these segments is obvious.

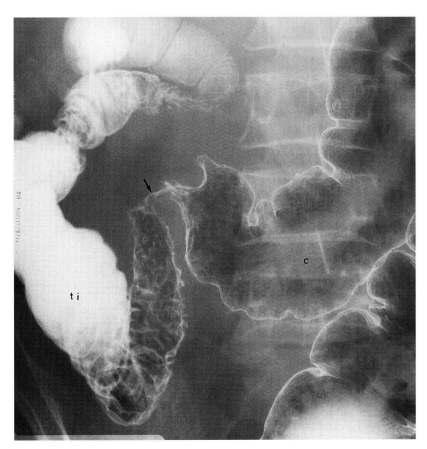

Fig. 5.31 Recurrent Crohn's disease at ileocolic anastomosis. Aphthoid ulcers are seen to affect the 'neoterminal ileum' and the colonic mucosa adjacent to the ileocolic anastomosis in a patient who had had a previous extensive colonic resection for Crohn's disease. A tight stricture is also apparent at the site of anastomosis (arrow), in keeping with recurrent disease. The patient also has sacroiliitis. ti, terminal ileum; c, colon.

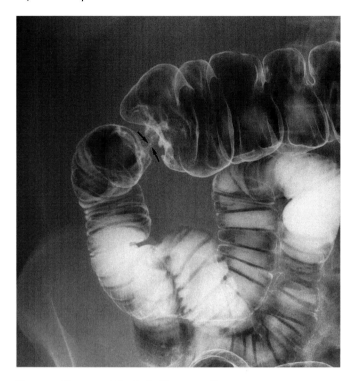

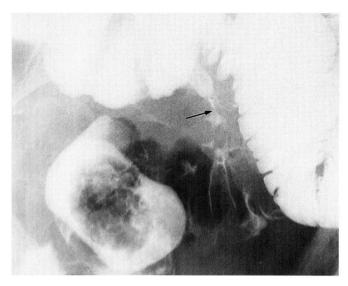

Fig. 5.33 Crohn's disease with ileosigmoid fistula. An SBE in a patient known to have small-bowel Crohn's disease with worsening diarrhoea. An irregular fistula 3 cm in length is shown between the ileum and sigmoid colon (arrow).

Fig. 5.32 Recurrent Crohn's disease at ileotransverse anastomosis. A very short, very tight stricture is demonstrated at the ileotransverse anastomosis (arrows) in a female patient having had a previous right hemicolectomy for Crohn's disease. The stricture has a rather shouldered margin and, on purely radiological grounds, it is not possible to exclude malignancy. Histology confirmed that this was a postinflammatory stricture.

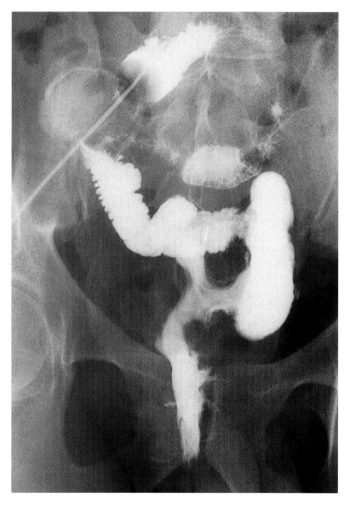

Fig. 5.34 Recurrent Crohn's disease in an ileal pouch. A water-soluble contrast study following sphincter-saving proctocolectomy and ileal pouch shows loss of distensibility of the distal portion of the pouch, with deep, penetrating, fissure ulceration.

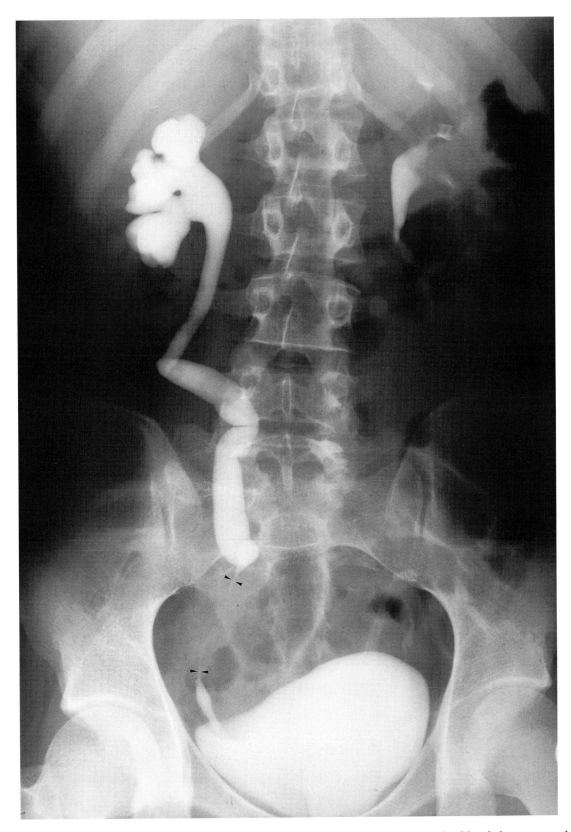

Fig. 5.35 Crohn's disease of the ileum causing ureteric obstruction. An IV urogram in a 14-year-old male patient known to have Crohn's disease, who developed a pelvic inflammatory mass, associated with right ureteric obstruction. The right renal pelvis and ureter are seen to be dilated above a smooth stricture 6 cm in length (arrowheads) in the right side of the pelvis, beyond which it is of normal calibre.

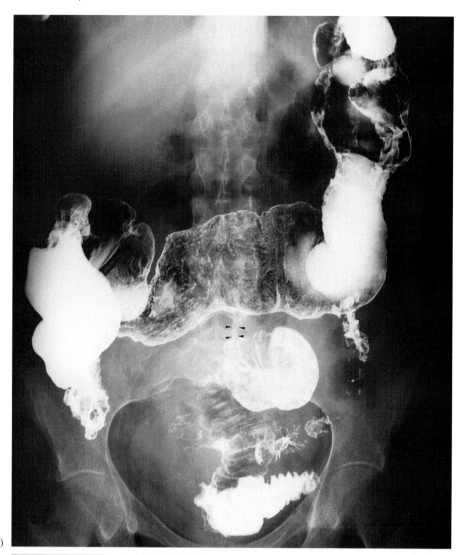

(a)

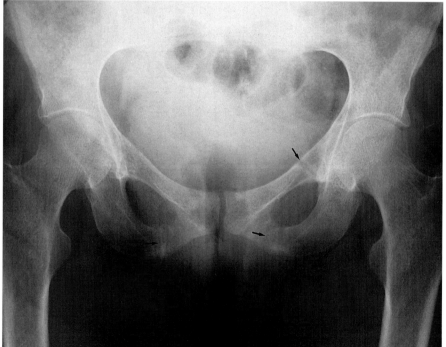

(b)

Fig. 5.36 Osteomalacia complicating enterocolic fistula in Crohn's disease.
(a) This postevacuation double-contrast barium enema shows a fistula between the transverse colon and the small bowel (arrowheads). Faintly calcified gallstones are also visible in the gallbladder.
(b) Anteroposterior view of the pelvis shows multiple Looser's zones (arrows) affecting the pubic bones. These are characteristic of osteomalacia.

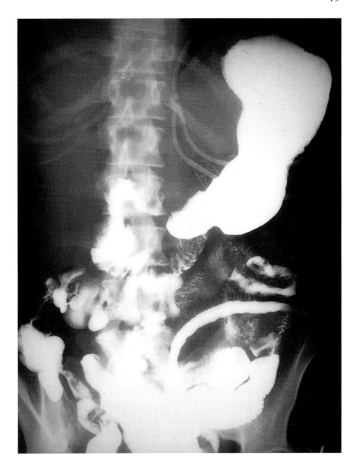

Fig. 5.37 Graft-versus-host disease. A barium follow-through examination shows segmental areas of ribbon-like luminal narrowing of the small bowel, with evidence of wall thickening. This appearance is seen in the subacute phase of graft-versus-host disease. This condition may develop after allogenic bone-marrow transplantation. It is due to the immunological response which is mounted by the foreign-donor lymphoid graft. (Courtesy of Dr Richard D. Edwards.)

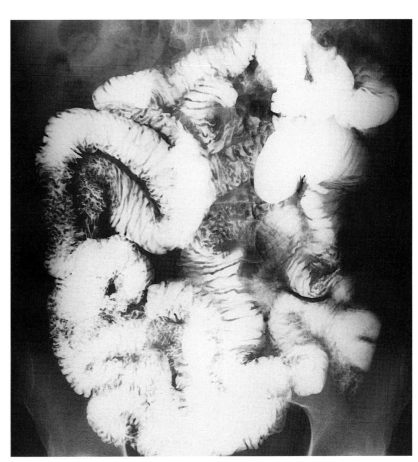

Fig. 5.38 Coeliac disease. A BMFT in a male patient with malabsorption shows dilatation of the small bowel loops, up to 4 cm. The upper normal limit is not more than 3 cm. In addition, the circular fold pattern in the ileum is similar to the jejunum (so-called jejunization of ileum). This condition is due to wheat-gluten sensitivity. This results in villous atrophy and a reduction in the absorptive surface of the small-bowel mucosa.

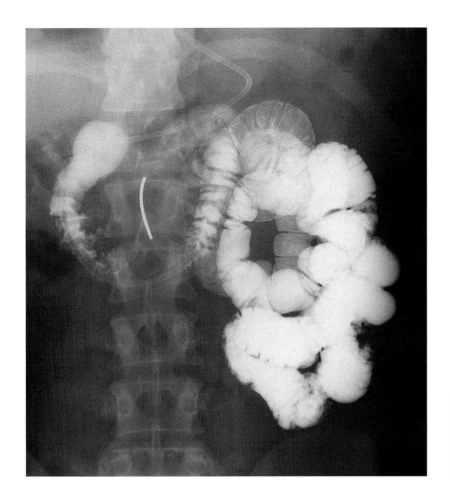

Fig. 5.39 Coeliac disease. The SBE in this patient with malabsorption shows a reduced number of jejunal folds, resembling a haustral pattern. In this condition, there is an increased risk of lymphoma in 8% and of small-bowel adenocarcinoma in 6% [2].

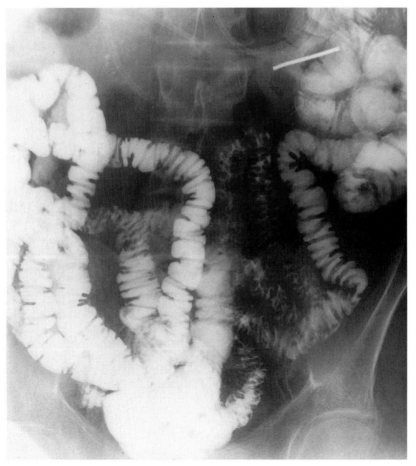

Fig. 5.40 Coeliac disease. An SBE was done to confirm or exclude malignancy in a 66-year-old male patient with proved coeliac disease, with a good initial response to gluten-free diet, but recent relapse. No neoplasm was found. However, there is a reduced number of proximal jejunal folds, the jejunal fold thickness is increased in keeping with oedema, there is an increased number of ileal folds (more than four per 2.5 cm) and there is an increased thickness of ileal folds (greater than 1 mm).

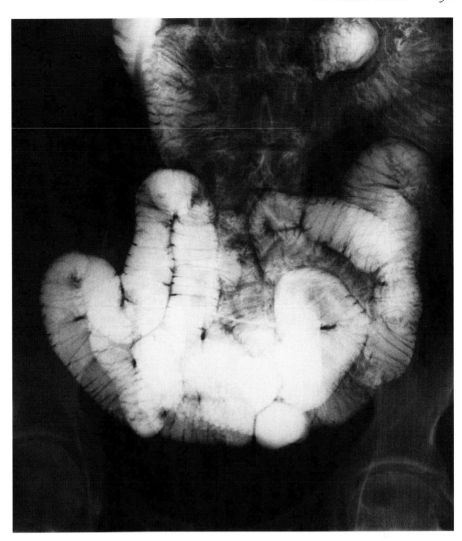

Fig. 5.41 Coeliac disease. The definitive
diagnosis in this condition depends on
jejunal biopsy. However, the 'jejunization
pattern' seen in this SBE is typical of
coeliac disease.

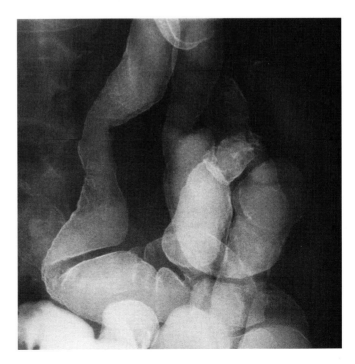

Fig. 5.42 Coeliac disease with total villous atrophy. The SBE in
this 64-year-old female patient with malabsorption shows a total
loss of the circular fold pattern in the jejunum. There is a fine
1–2 mm mesh of grooves in the mucosa outlining a mosaic of
islands in the mucosa.

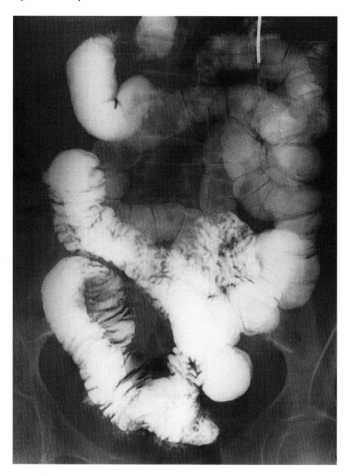

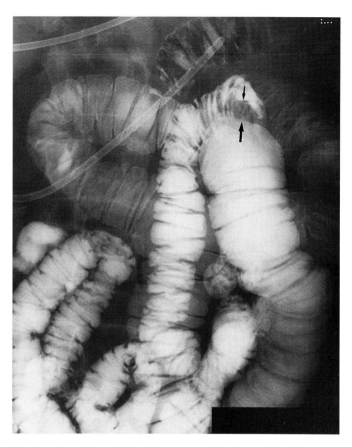

Fig. 5.43 Coeliac disease. A 64-year-old female patient known to have coeliac disease for 26 years, who had adhered to her gluten-free diet, has recently become jaundiced. The SBE shows changes typical of coeliac disease, a marked reduction in jejunal folds and a typical jejunal pattern in the ileum. No small-bowel tumour pathology was demonstrated. A CT scan demonstrated lymphadenopathy in the porta hepatis, which was shown to be non-Hodgkin's lymphoma.

Fig. 5.44 Lymphocytic lymphoma complicating coeliac disease. A 72-year-old male patient had a long history of coeliac disease. A previous jejunal perforation had been repaired, but there was no evidence of tumour at that time. Four years later, he developed colicky abdominal pain and the SBE shows an irregular filling defect in the jejunum; the large arrow is at the proximal end of the lesion and the small arrow at the distal end, where there is an abrupt change in calibre of the small bowel. Histology of the resected specimen indicated histiocytic lymphoma. This tumour accounts for 40% of all primary malignant neoplasms of the small bowel [5].

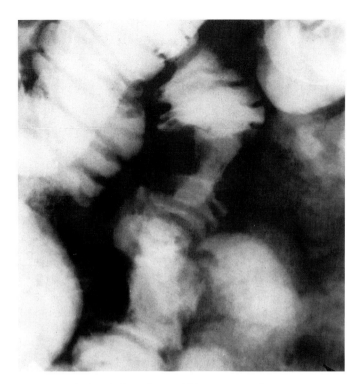

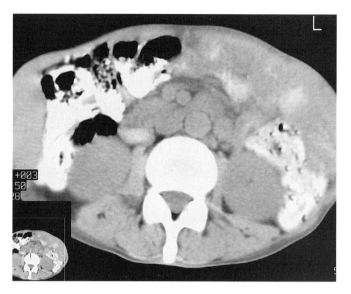

Fig. 5.46 Non-Hodgkin's lymphoma in a patient with coeliac disease. A 58-year-old male patient with known coeliac disease complained of recent abdominal pain and weight loss and clinically had hepatomegaly and splenomegaly. This spiral CT scan without contrast enhancement shows extensive para-aortic lymphadenopathy, and the liver and spleen are diffusely enlarged. Non-Hodgkin's lymphoma was confirmed histologically.

Fig. 5.45 Histiocytic lymphoma. This patient with no previous history of small-bowel pathology presented with colicky abdominal pain. The SBE shows one of several annular strictures, with evidence of mucosal destruction. Histology indicated hystiocytic lymphoma.

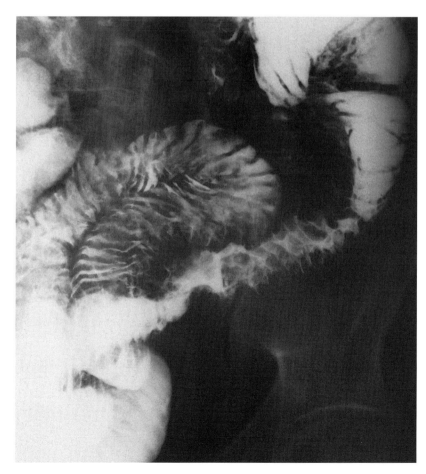

Fig. 5.47 Lymphoma of the ileum. The patient presented with a left inguinal hernia. At surgery, the hernial sac was found to contain ascitic fluid. A subsequent SBE shows a 16 cm stricture of ileum, with fissure ulceration remarkably similar to Crohn's disease. There is also marked deformity of an adjacent loop of small bowel. Laparotomy confirmed an extensive small-bowel tumour and histology confirmed lymphoma.

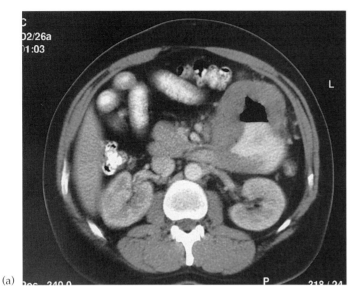

(a)

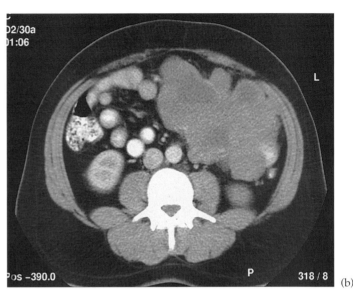

(b)

Fig. 5.48 Leiomyosarcoma of the small bowel. A 41-year-old male patient presented with vague left upper-quadrant pain and clinical examination revealed a palpable swelling in the left side of the abdomen. Ultrasound demonstrated a large solid mass of indeterminate origin. This spiral CECT shows a 16 cm lobulated solid mass lesion, with a central cavity containing gas and contrast medium. At operation, the tumour was found to arise from the fourth part of the duodenum and the proximal jejunum and histology of the resected specimen indicated leiomyosarcoma. (b) is 5 cm distal to (a).

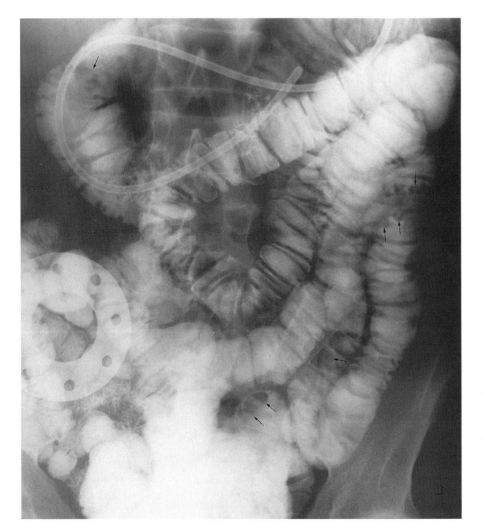

Fig. 5.49 Polyposis of the duodenum and small bowel. A 65-year-old male patient with iron-deficiency anaemia had a total proctocolectomy at age 36 for polyposis coli. The SBE shows multiple filling defects in the duodenum (confirmed endoscopically) and the small bowel, consistent with adenomatous polyps (arrows).

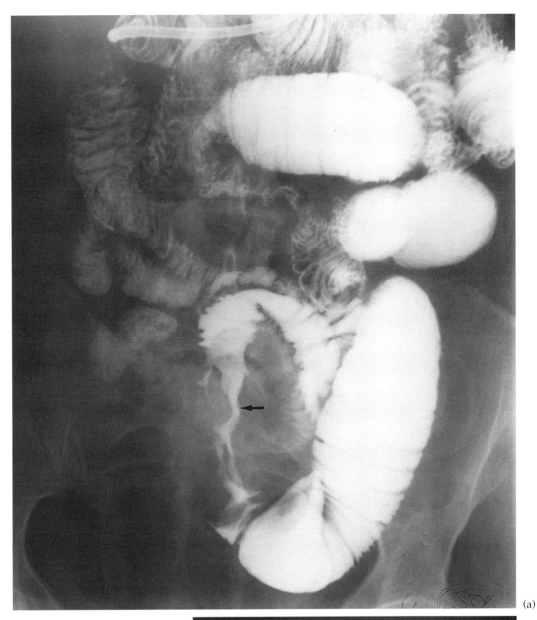

(a)

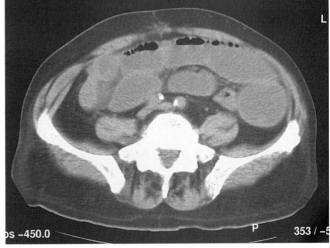

(b)

Fig. 5.50 Small-bowel obstruction secondary to recurrence of colon cancer. (a) This patient had had a previous sigmoid resection for carcinoma; there was a recent history of colicky abdominal pain, distension and weight loss. The SBE shows multiple small-bowel strictures and dilated segments. A grossly irregular lower abdominal stricture is shown (arrow), but with no evidence of ulceration. The differential diagnosis includes Crohn's disease, lymphoma, primary small-bowel carcinoma, radiation enteritis and tuberculosis. (b) In a second similar case, spiral CT shows marked fluid distension with much less marked gaseous distension producing a 'string-of-beads' sign. The obstructing lesion is not seen on this section. This method has the advantages of speed, it may provide information beyond the bowel wall, and it does not require oral contrast or intubation.

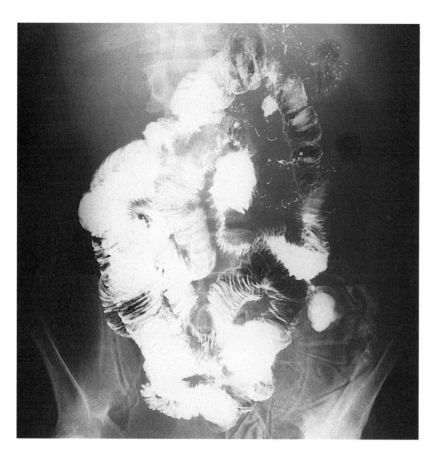

Fig. 5.51 Small-bowel serosal metastases. The elderly male patient had a previous history of gastric carcinoma, with recent pain and distension. There is marked deformity of the small bowel, with segmental loss of distensibility and marked thickening and deformity of the circular fold pattern, in keeping with tumour infiltration.

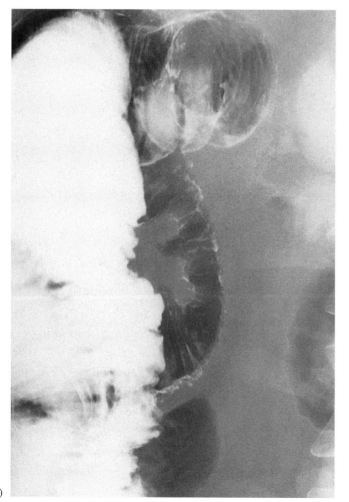

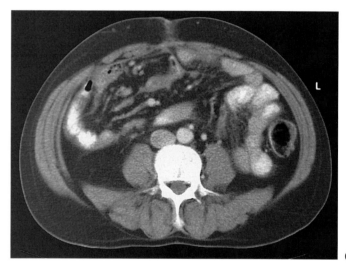

(b)

Fig. 5.52 Small-bowel serosal metastases from colonic carcinoma. This patient had had a previous colonic resection for Dukes B carcinoma, with recent colicky abdominal pain and some distension. (a) The BMFT late film shows a constricted segment of small bowel, with marginal irregularity, suggestive of tumour infiltration. (b) A spiral CECT scan in the same patient shows thickening of a small-bowel loop in the right flank, together with thick linear opacities in the adjacent small-bowel mesentery, in keeping with diffuse lymphatic infiltration.

(a)

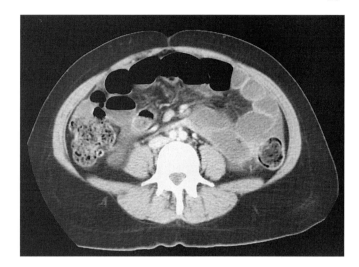

Fig. 5.53 Small-bowel obstruction secondary to ovarian carcinoma. Abdominal pain and distension occurred in this patient with proved ovarian carcinoma. The spiral CT scan shows generalized small-bowel gaseous and fluid distension; some matting of loops is apparent.

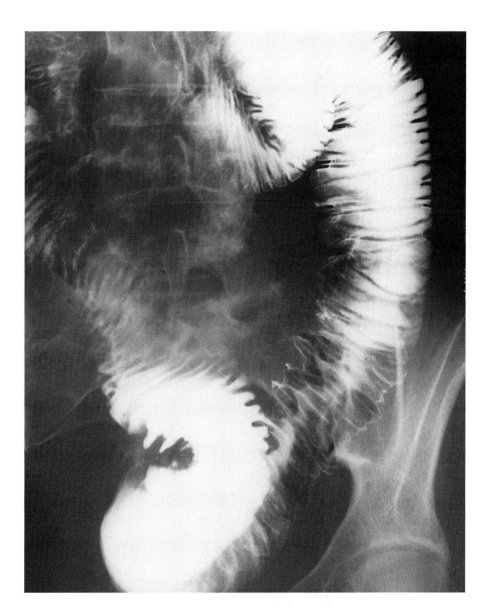

Fig. 5.54 Small-bowel serosal metastases from ovarian carcinoma. A 45-year-old female patient had colicky abdominal pain and distension. The SBE shows small-bowel distension, thickening and deformity of the wall of the small bowel. Surgical confirmation.

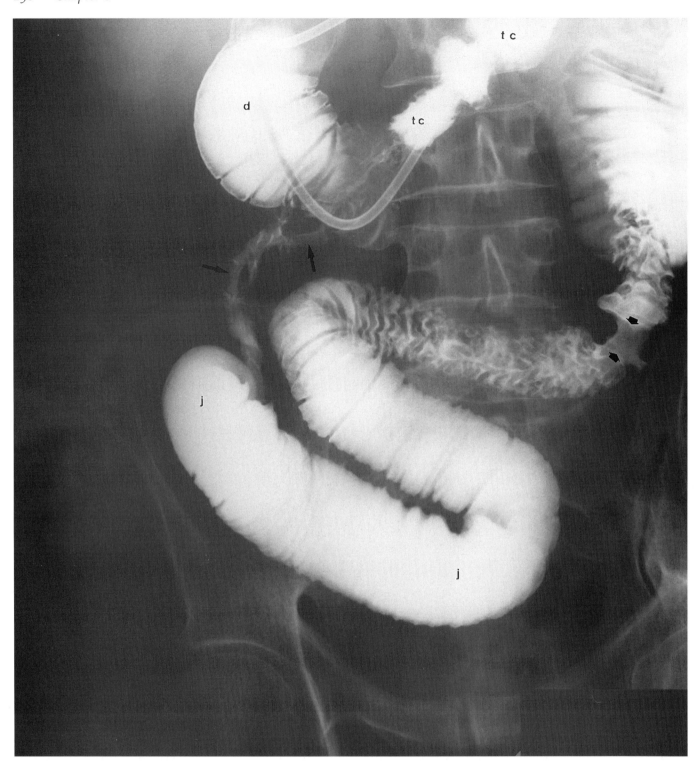

Fig. 5.55 Ischaemic strictures of the small bowel. Two months previously, the patient had had an emergency laparotomy, at which there was very extensive ischaemia of the right hemicolon and most of the small intestine. At that time, a right hemicolectomy and resection of most of the small bowel was performed. Two months later, the SBE shows a very short small bowel, there being a 2 cm partial stricture proximally (arrowheads) and a much longer, tighter ischaemic stricture of the jejunum (arrows) proximal to the jejunocolic anastomosis. In this projection, the transverse colon is superimposed on the distal duodenum. d, duodenum; j, jejunum; tc, transverse colon.

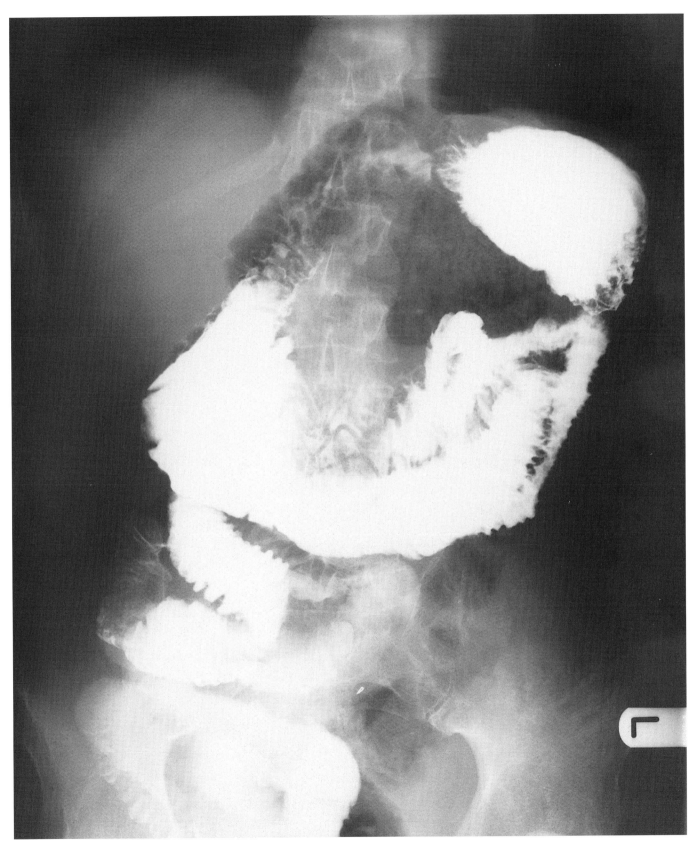

Fig. 5.56 Radiation jejunitis. A male patient presented with a past medical history of radiation to the upper para-aortic nodes for metastatic seminoma. The stomach and first three parts of the duodenum are seen to be distended. There is loss of distensibility of the fourth part of the duodenum and the proximal jejunum, with marked thickening and spiking of the jejunal folds.

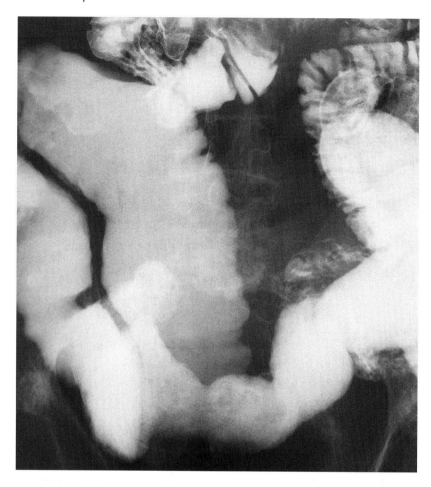

Fig. 5.57 Radiation enteritis. The patient gave a history of radiotherapy 20 years previously, as well as recent abdominal pain, distension and bleeding per rectum. The BMFT shows dilatation of the ileum to 7.5 cm, loss of the circular fold pattern and marginal irregularity. Histological confirmation.

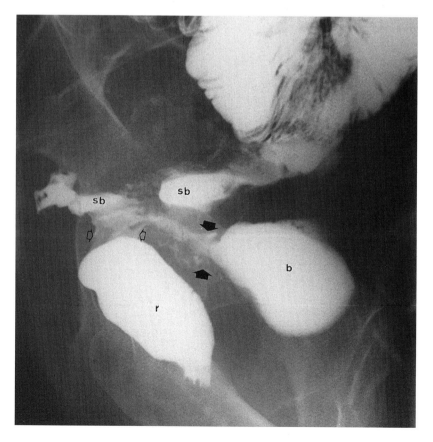

Fig. 5.58 Radiation enteritis with fistulae. A female patient had a past history of radiotherapy for colonic carcinoma. The SBE shows gross deformity of a loop of small bowel (sb) in the pelvis, from which contrast rapidly fills the bladder (b) through a wide fistula (black arrowheads). Through a second wide fistula (open arrowheads), contrast also rapidly fills the rectum (r) from the same small-bowel loop.

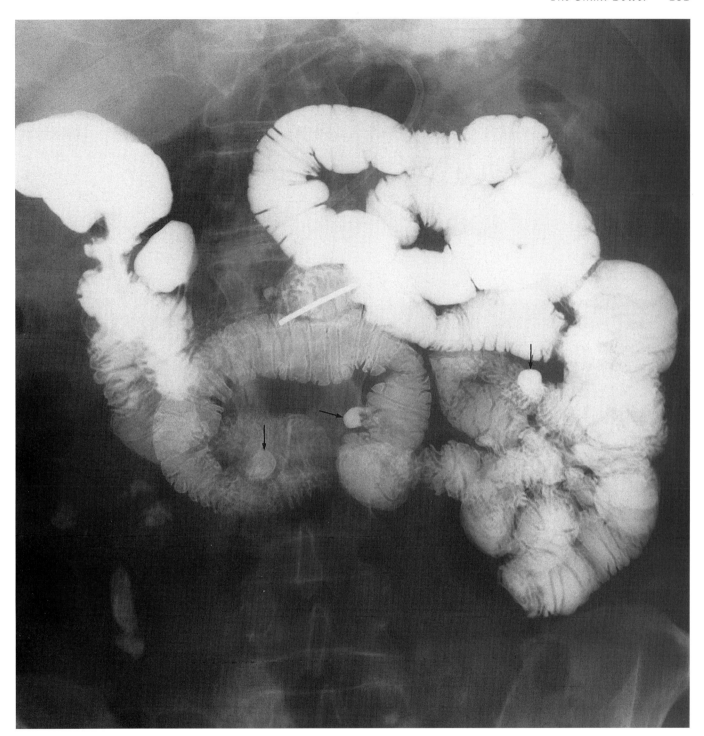

Fig. 5.59 Jejunal diverticula. An SBE in an elderly male patient with diarrhoea revealed a moderately large diverticulum of the second part of the duodenum and several much smaller jejunal diverticula (arrows). No other small-bowel abnormality was demonstrated. The large ovoid calcified opacity in the right lower quadrant was subsequently shown to be a ureteric calculus.

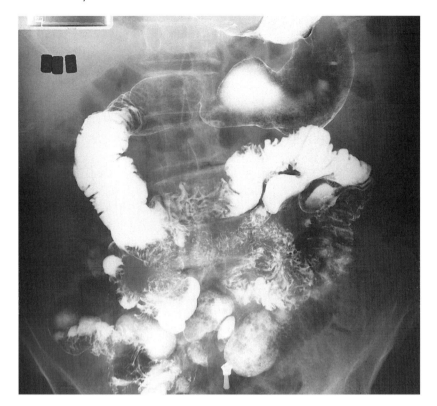

Fig. 5.60 Jejunal diverticula. Dysphagia and anorexia were found in an elderly male patient. Multiple jejunal diverticula were demonstrated in this limited follow-through examination as an incidental finding. The patient has a carcinoma of the distal oesophagus and proximal stomach. Of small-bowel diverticula, 80% occur in the jejunum, 15% in the ileum and 5% in both the jejunum and ileum. The differential diagnosis includes pseudodiverticula in systemic sclerosis.

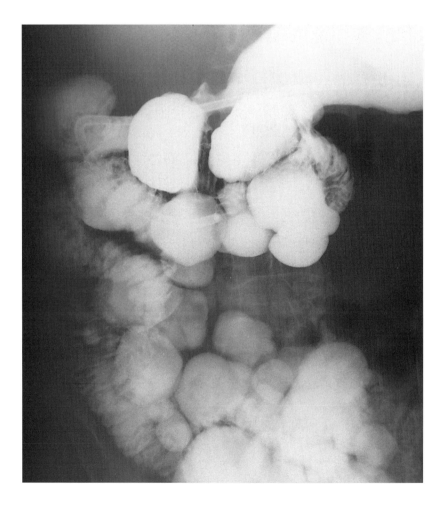

Fig. 5.61 Jejunal diverticulosis. An SBE of a patient with weight loss, steatorrhoea and malabsorption shows numerous large jejunal diverticula.

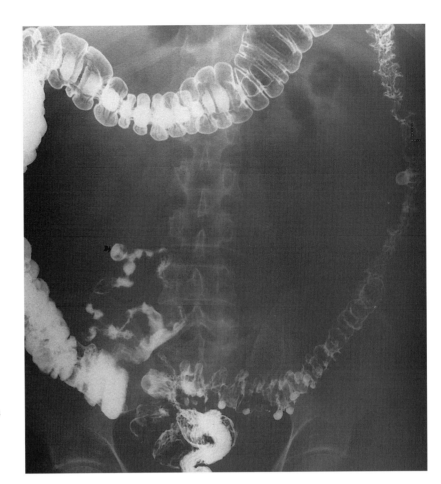

Fig. 5.62 Meckel's diverticulum. This was an incidental finding on a postevacuation barium-enema film. The diverticulum (arrow) represents a persistent remnant of the vitellointestinal duct and it occurs in 2–3% of the population, almost always on the antimesenteric border of the ileum within 2 m of the ileocaecal valve.

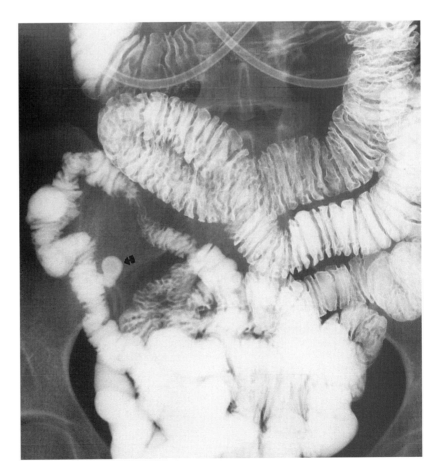

Fig. 5.63 Meckel's diverticulum. An SBE in a 45-year-old female patient with a past history of Crohn's disease. The SBE was normal, apart from the presence of this Meckel's diverticulum (arrow).

(a)

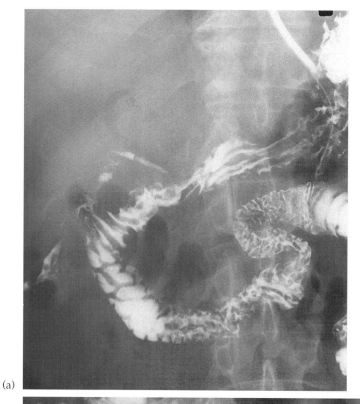

(b)

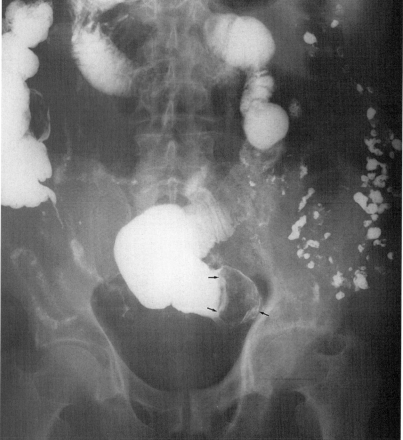

Fig. 5.64 Gallstone ileus. (a) A 90-year-old male patient presented with vomiting and prerenal uraemia. The SBE proximally shows no jejunal lesion, but there is air in the biliary tree and the barium is seen to escape from a fistula in the second part of the duodenum into the gallbladder and also produces partial filling of the cystic duct. (b) A more distal film of the same examination shows jejunal obstruction, with a large intraluminal filling defect (arrows). This represented a large gallstone, which was subsequently removed surgically. The patient also has a barium residue in the colon from a previous examination, there being diverticular disease of the left side. The patient also has Paget's disease of his left hemipelvis.

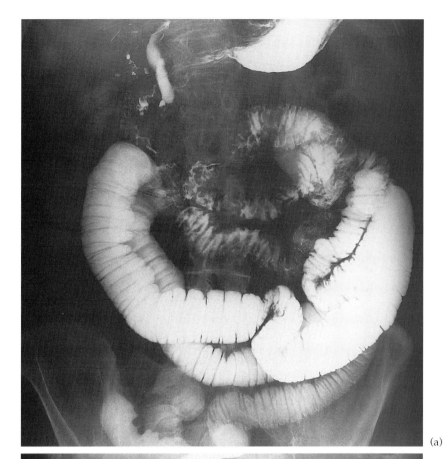

(a)

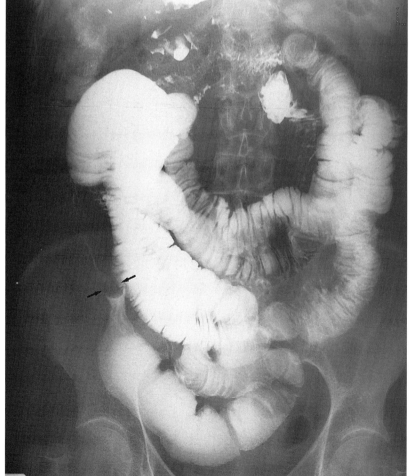

Fig. 5.65 Gallstone ileus. An elderly patient presented with abdominal pain and subacute small-bowel obstruction. (a) The SBE shows generalized dilatation of the small-bowel loops. Contrast is also shown in the biliary tree. (b) A later film of the same examination shows a smooth filling defect in the terminal ileum (arrows). This proved to be a gallstone, which was removed surgically [3, 37]. CT may also be valuable in this diagnosis [38].

(b)

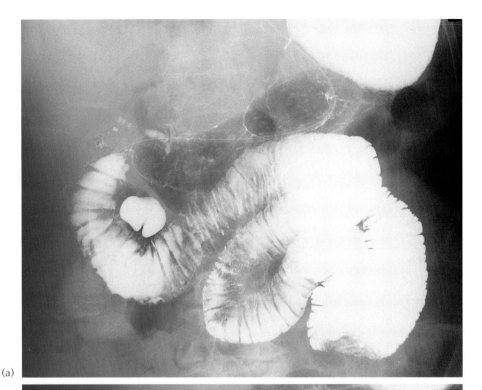

(a)

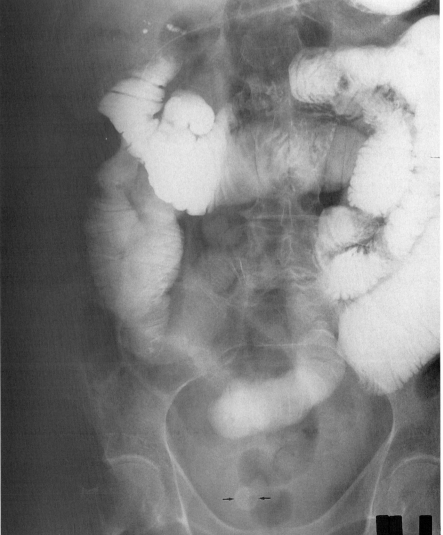

(b)

Fig. 5.66 Gallstone ileus. An elderly female patient had colicky abdominal pain and distension. (a) The SBE shows generalized distension of the small bowel, an incidental duodenal diverticulum and air in the biliary tree. There is also evidence of contrast escaping from the second part of the duodenum via a fistula into the neck of the gallbladder and some contrast is shown in the cystic duct. (b) A slightly later film again shows the above features and there is a calcified opacity in the pelvis, which at operation was shown to be a gallstone. At surgery, the gallstone was much larger than the apparent size depicted by the calcification.

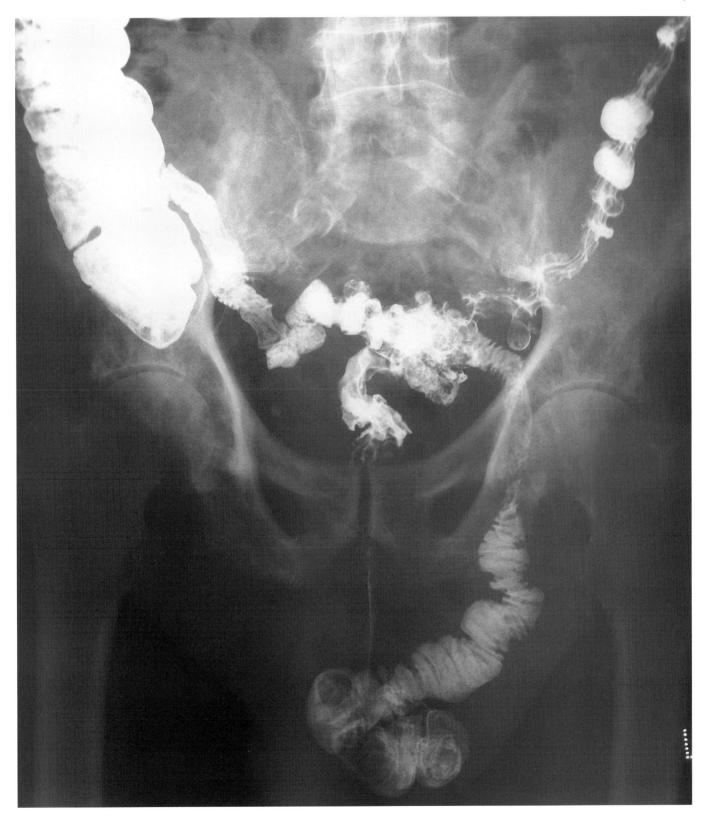

Fig. 5.67 Small bowel contained in a left inguinal hernia. A postevacuation barium-enema film shows a length of contrast-filled small bowel within a left inguinal hernia sac. The patient had no symptoms or signs of small-bowel obstruction. Diverticular disease is shown in the sigmoid colon. The patient also has Paget's disease of the pelvis.

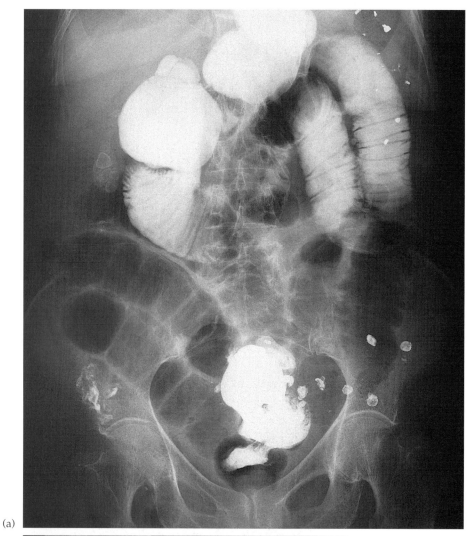

(a)

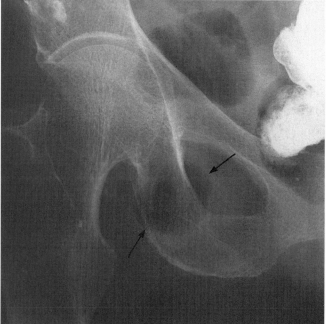

(b)

Fig. 5.68 Small-bowel obstruction due to an incarcerated right femoral hernia. An elderly female patient with subacute small-bowel obstruction was obese and no hernia could be manually palpated. (a) There is generalized small-bowel distension on this Gastrografin follow-through. Multiple gallstones are shown in the gallbladder. An abnormal gas shadow is projected over the right ischiopubic ramus. This is more clearly shown in (b). A diagnosis of obstructed femoral hernia (arrows) was made and, at operation, this was confirmed and found to be of the Richter type. There is a barium residue in the colon from a previous examination.

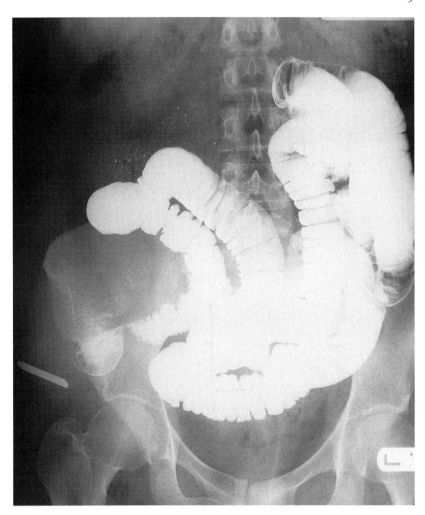

Fig. 5.69 Spigelian hernia. This barium follow through examination shows dilated loops of the small bowel and a Spigelian hernia in the right lower quadrant. A metallic skin marker indicates the position of the palpable mass. (Courtesy of Dr Richard D. Edwards.)

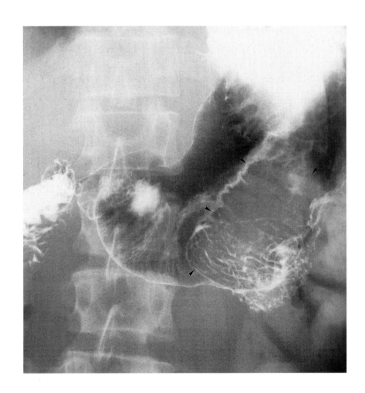

Fig. 5.70 Retrograde intussusception of the efferent limb of gastrojejunostomy into the stomach. This patient had a previous history of gastrojejunostomy and vagotomy, with a recent history of vomiting. On this double-contrast barium meal examination, there is a large constant filling defect occupying the greater-curve aspect of the body and proximal antrum of the stomach (arrowheads). There is evidence of transverse folds corresponding with jejunal mucosa. This finding was confirmed endoscopically [39].

6: The Colon and Rectum

Introduction

The large bowel consists of the caecum, the ascending, transverse, descending and sigmoid (or pelvic) colon and the rectum. The muscular wall of the colon consists of outer longitudinal muscle fibres organized in three narrow longitudinal bands, called taenia coli. The inner circular muscle coat forms a complete layer. The wall is sacculated and the narrower segments between the sacculations are called haustrations. The haustra are less obvious in the sigmoid colon and are sometimes absent in the normal descending colon [1]. The caecum, which may measure up to 9 cm in diameter is normally completely invested with peritoneum, but sometimes is attached by a mesentery, affording considerable mobility and resulting in a predisposition to volvulus. The transverse colon and sigmoid both have mesenteries, whereas the ascending and descending colon are normally partly extraperitoneal. However, these sections may also have a mesocolon, in 26 and 36% of cases, respectively [2]. The junction of the small bowel and the large bowel is marked by the ileocaecal valve, which prevents reflux on barium-enema examinations in more than 50% of cases, but this can be overcome with IV glucagon in most cases. The autonomic nerve plexus of Auerbach is located between the longitudinal and circular muscle layers of the colon and rectum.

The rectum commences at the level of S3, is approximately 12–15 cm in length and ends at the anal canal. Anteriorly, a peritoneal reflection forms the rectovesical pouch in males and the pouch of Douglas in females. The upper third of the rectum is covered with peritoneum laterally and anteriorly, while the middle third is covered with peritoneum only anteriorly. The lower third of the rectum is entirely extraperitoneal. The globular shape of the rectum is modified by three crescentic folds, called the valves of Houston. The muscular wall of the rectum continues into the internal sphincter of the anal canal and the external anal sphincter represents the continuation of the levator ani pelvic-floor muscles. The presacral space is normally less than 1 cm at the fourth sacral segment, as seen on a lateral-view double-contrast barium enema (DCBE) [3]; others accept up to 1.5 cm [1], except in disease and obesity.

The mucosa of the large bowel is normally smooth, as demonstrated by DCBE, but may include innominate grooves, which are multiple, slender, parallel grooves running transversely. In addition, lymphoid follicles, which are contained within the lamina propria, may be visible and, provided these do not exceed 2–3 mm in diameter, can be regarded as normal [4]. The blood supply is provided by the superior mesenteric artery (SMA) and the inferior mesenteric artery (IMA). The caecum, ascending and transverse colon and a variable part of the splenic flexure are supplied by the SMA branches. The remainder of the colon is supplied by the IMA. In the mesenteric border of the colon, a vascular arcade is seen, which gives off long and short branches (vasa recta). The veins follow the course of the arteries. The blood supply to the rectum is provided by the right and left divisions of the superior haemorrhoidal continuation of the IMA. These anastomose with the middle rectal branches of the hypogastric arteries and with the inferior rectal branches of the pudendal arteries. The venous drainage of the rectum is significant, in that, below the dentate line, which marks the squamocolumnar junction, rectal veins drain via the external venous plexus into the internal pudendal veins and ultimately into the systemic circulation of the inferior vena cava. Veins above the dentate line drain via the internal rectal plexus and superior haemorrhoidal veins into the portal system. Consequently, there is a potential porto-systemic anastomosis. The anal canal is sealed by three anal cushions, which are specialized subepithelial venous dilatations [5]. The lymphatic drainage of the large bowel largely follows the course of the chief blood vessels. The lymph nodes are divided into four groups. The epicolic nodes are situated on the wall of the gut, while the paracolic lymph nodes lie on the medial side of the ascending and descending colon, behind the posterior parietal peritoneum. They also lie above and below the transverse colon and sigmoid and between the two layers of each mesocolon. Thirdly, the intermediate lymph nodes are associated with the main branches of the mesenteric vessels and, fourthly, the terminal-group nodes lie along the SMA and IMA trunks.

Plain film radiography

The gas content of the normal colon is extremely variable and multiple fluid levels in the colon, which may be several centimetres in length, can be accepted as normal [6]; almost one in five of normal people also have a caecal fluid level [7]. The diameter of the colon is very variable and there is substantial overlap between normal and abnormal. The generally accepted upper normal limit for the transverse colon is 5.5 cm [8]. The diameter of the caecum should not exceed 9 cm. Plain films are useful in the evaluation of colonic obstruction and, in the UK, the commonest cause of large-bowel obstruction is carcinoma. The site of obstruction and whether or not the ileocaecal valve is competent determine the plain-film appearance. If both small and large bowel are seen to be dilated, the radiographic appearance may be identical to that produced by paralytic ileus. However, the absence of gas in the rectum should suggest a mechanical obstruction. All forms of paralytic ileus can produce gross colonic distension and there are many causes of colonic distension without obstruction. Typical plain-film diagnostic signs may be observed in a volvulus of the sigmoid colon and caecum. Free perforation of the colon or the intraperitoneal part of the rectum may be recognized by the presence of a pneumoperitoneum. However, plain films are less reliable than CT scans. Nevertheless, it is possible to recognize as a little as 1 ml of gas on an erect chest X-ray or a left lateral decubitus abdominal film [9]. The extent of mucosal involvement in acute colitis can usually be predicted from plain films [10]. Plain films are extremely important in the diagnosis of, and assessing the progress of, toxic dilatation, this diagnosis depending on the demonstration of abnormal dilatation and the presence of mucosal islands.

Barium studies

The DCBE is the examination of choice for a routine examination of the large bowel. Success depends on many factors, but a clean colon is a prerequisite for an accurate study. A variety of preparations have been recommended [11]. Unless there is a risk of perforation, barium sulphate suspension, with a density of 75–95% [1] or 100% [4], is the contrast medium of choice. A relatively small volume of barium (for example, 300–600 ml) and a larger volume of gas—normally air—are employed, but CO_2 can be used and is more comfortable [12]. This is being increasingly used. The barium and gas are used to coat and distend, respectively, the large bowel and, by a combination of fluoroscopy and appropriate films, the surface pattern of the whole of the large bowel is examined in detail, the distensibility tested and fistulae noted. An IV smooth-muscle relaxant—0.5–1 mg glucagon or 20 mg hyoscine—is used routinely or whenever

pain or spasm are encountered. Retention of the enema is assisted by the use of a balloon-type self-retaining catheter. This should be necessary only in older patients. The radiation dose can be significantly reduced by using digital equipment.

The examination is contraindicated immediately after biopsy of normal or inflamed rectal mucosa with large biopsy forceps, which is a major cause of rectal perforation [13, 14]. In these circumstances, the enema should be postponed for more than 5 days. However, biopsies of tumours or biopsies with small forceps through flexible endoscopes need not contraindicate an early enema examination. Other contraindications include severe inflammatory bowel disease, toxic dilatation, suspected perforation and peritonitis. Glucagon is contraindicated in patients with phaeochromocytoma and insulinoma. Hyoscine causes blurring of near vision for up to half an hour in one in 10 patients and it causes mouth dryness. There is also a risk of precipitating hypotension in patients on β-blockers. Such patients and also patients with a significant cardiac history should be given IV glucagon if indicated. There is also a risk of precipitating an acute attack of glaucoma in those with early closed-angle glaucoma.

Inaccuracy with DCBE may be due to poor technique, perceptive error or a combination of both [15]. Perceptive errors may be reduced by double reading of the films, as in screening mammography. If systematic double reading by two observers is not practicable, the radiologist should review the films at the time of the examination and separately during the reporting session. A significant cause of difficulty is in patients with marked sigmoid diverticular disease, in whom the DCBE may be supplemented, using 500–700 ml of water or very dilute barium. Thus better sigmoid images can be obtained in 65–75% of patients studied [16].

The DCBE is a very safe technique. A perforation rate, varying between 1/2500 and 1/12500, has been variously reported [17–20] and the mortality in these patients is reported as 13–80%, with a mortality of 40–50% of patients with intraperitoneal perforation. However, if standard enema catheter tips are used, a perforation rate of 1/25000 has been cited [5]. The causes of perforation include excessive inflation of the balloon catheter, particularly in the presence of rectal disease [21]. The perforation rate following colonoscopy has been variously reported as 1/1700 [22] or 1/500 to 1/1000 [23, 24]. The overall complication rate for diagnostic colonoscopy is said to be 0.1–0.2% [25]. Following barium enema, transient bacteraemia has been reported in some studies, although clinical problems have not been recorded [26]. Patients with high-risk cardiac lesions—for example, artificial heart valves—should probably have prophylactic antibiotics [27]. Other complications include water intoxication and detergent colitis. A single-contrast barium enema using 15–20% w/v barium [1] is of limited clinical value. It is not indicated in patients with a history of, or a family history of, polyps or colorectal cancer or for the diagnosis of inflammatory bowel disease in mobile patients. It may be of use in confirming or excluding an obstructing lesion in the frail elderly patient.

Instant enema

This is sometimes of value in assessing inflammatory bowel disease without bowel preparation. Severe disease, including toxic dilatation, should be excluded by a single abdominal plain film. The examination has no value in searching for dysplasia or carcinoma in patients with long-standing colitis, since a completely clean colon is essential in that situation.

Water-soluable contrast studies

If perforation is suspected or an anastomosis is being assessed, the enema examination, which may be limited to the area of interest, should be done with a water-soluble contrast agent—for example, meglumine diatrizoate (Gastrografin), diluted if necessary with water, or Urografin 150.

Double-contrast barium enema or colonscopy?

The relative merits of DCBE and colonoscopy are frequently discussed. Colonoscopy has the great advantage of being able to obtain biopsies, identify angiodysplasia and provide therapeutic intervention, using electrocoagulation or photocoagulation with a laser. However, colonoscopy is incomplete in at least 10% of cases in skilled hands [28]. The DCBE is likely to be quicker, is less expensive, carries a smaller risk and is more complete. Colonoscopy detects small polyps better, even though they may not be clinically significant [29, 30]. Very few lesions of 10 mm or larger are likely to be missed by either technique, provided the highest standards are maintained.

Computerized tomography scanning

The colon and rectum are visible on routine abdominal CT scanning, but, because of faecal content and normal contractility, pathology cannot be confirmed or excluded with a useful degree of confidence. Much more accurate information can be obtained by specific bowel preparation to produce a clean colon and sufficient distension, either by air CT pneumocolon or water [31, 32] introduced per rectum. The oral administration of contrast medium—for example, 2–3% Gastrografin or 2% barium sulphate suspension—produces good opacification of the large bowel, but its distensibility is not reliably tested. Computerized tomography has been used in staging colorectal neoplasms, in inflammatory bowel disease and in staging gynaecological malignancy. The technique lends itself to the assessment of the mural, serosal and mesenteric extent of pathology. However, individual layers cannot be identified as with endoscopic US

[33, 34]. The preoperative staging of colorectal cancer is not widely accepted and staging is normally done surgically. It has been found that CT is of limited value, since it cannot accurately determine the extension of tumour through the wall and therefore cannot distinguish T2 vs. T3 or Dukes A vs. Dukes B categories. The assessment can be improved by using water as an intraluminal contrast. Computerized tomography cannot detect tumour in normal-sized lymph nodes. Early studies suggested that CT was a very good staging procedure, with an overall accuracy of 77–100%. Later studies in less advanced tumours have been less encouraging. Therefore, CT should be used to stage only patients with suspected advanced disease and not routinely [35]. It has an established role in demonstrating liver and lymph-node metastases and lung and pelvic deposits prior to adjuvant chemotherapy [36]. Currently, CT is preferred to MRI because of its ability to rapidly assess all sites of potential disease in the abdomen and pelvis [36]. Also, CT has a key role in the detection of local pelvic and abdominal recurrence of colorectal cancer. Following abdominoperineal resection, CT can detect recurrence in 69–90% [35, 36] and is highly accurate, provided there is invasion of adjacent structures, an enlarging irregular mass or a perineal location. Granulation tissue and fibrous scar tissue cannot be distinguished from tumour purely on the basis of their CT appearance and MRI may provide further information. A baseline CT scan may be of help in distinguishing between postoperative fibrosis and tumour recurrence.

Endoscopic ultrasound

Rectal endosonography may be used to stage rectal carcinoma, five layers of the bowel wall being distinguishable using high-frequency transducers—for example, 10 MHz. A water-filled balloon in the rectum is used as an acoustic window. In colorectal cancer, endoscopic US is highly accurate in determining the T and N stage of disease, with reported accuracy ranging between 75 and 95%, for both T staging and N staging [37–39]. The clinical value of endoscopic US in staging colonic rather than rectal malignancy is less clear. Endoscopic US is emerging as the method of choice in evaluating complex perianal rectal fistulae [40]. Faecal incontinence can be investigated by endoscopic US to confirm or exclude damage to the sphincter. The transducer probe is modified with a rigid tip.

Angiography

This technique may be of value in the diagnosis and sometimes in the treatment of acute bleeding from the large bowel. It is more difficult to demonstrate a source of haemorrhage than in the upper gastrointestinal tract. It is said that active bleeding at a rate of 0.1 ml/min can be detected by radionuclide scanning [41–43]. Selective angiography will not demonstrate bleeding at a rate less than 0.5 ml/min at the time that the contrast is injected. Clearly, if a radionu-clide scan using technetium-labelled red cells or technetium sulphur colloid is negative, arteriography will be futile. Chronic blood loss from the alimentary tract will manifest through a positive faecal occult blood (FOB) test or iron-deficiency anaemia. In these cases, it is important to exclude obvious pathology by colonoscopy or DCBE and, in these circumstances, angiography is most likely to demonstrate angiodysplasia. Despite excellent technique, however, a cause for lower gastrointestinal haemorrhage may not be found [44].

Arteriography may be helpful in investigating patients with chronic abdominal pain and/or weight loss in whom mesenteric ischaemia may be a cause, and lateral flush aortography and selective mesenteric angiography may demonstrate stenotic or occlusive lesions in the SMA and/or IMA.

References

1 Stevenson G.W. (1994) Normal anatomy and techniques of examination of the colon. In: Freeny P.C. & Stevenson G.W. (eds) *Margulis and Burhenne's Alimentary Tract Radiology*, 5th edn. St Louis: Mosby, 692–724.

2 Williams P.L. & Warwick R. (eds) (1980) *Gray's Anatomy*, 36th edn. Philadelphia: W.B. Saunders.

3 Teplick S.K., Stark P., Clark R.E. *et al.* (1978) The retro-rectal space. *Clinical Radiology* **29**, 177–184.

4 Laufer I. (1994) Barium studies. In: Gore R.M., Levine M.S. & Laufer I. (eds) *A Textbook of Gastro-intestinal Radiology*. Philadelphia: W.B. Saunders, 1028–1040.

5 Bartram C.I. (1997) The large bowel. In: Grainger R.G. & Allison D.J. (eds) *Diagnostic Radiology*, 3rd edn. New York: Churchill Livingstone, 1009–1044.

6 Gammill S.L. & Nice C.M. (1972) Air fluid levels: their occurrence in normal patients and their role in the analysis of ileus. *Surgery* **71**, 771–780.

7 Graham D.A. & Johnson F.H. (1966) The incidence of radiographic findings in acute appendicitis compared to two hundred normals. *Military Medicine* **131**, 272–276.

8 Jones H.L. & Chapman M. (1969) Definition of megacolon in colitis. *Gut* **10**, 562–564.

9 Miller R.E. (1973) The technical approach to the acute abdomen. *Seminars in Roentgenology* **8**, 267–269.

10 Hals J. & Young A.C. (1964) Plain abdominal films in colonic disease. *Proceedings of the Royal Society of Medicine* **57**, 893–894.

11 Bartram C.I. (1994) Bowel preparation—principles in practice. *Clinical Radiology* **49**, 365–367.

12 Coblentz C.L., Frost R.A., Molinaro V. *et al.* (1985) A prospective double blind trial to compare pain following barium enema when using carbon dioxide and air for gas contrast. *Radiology* **157**, 35–36.

13 Maglinte D.D.T., Strong R.C., Strate R.W. *et al.* (1982) Barium enema after colorectal biopsies: experimental data. *American Journal of Roentgenology* **139**, 693–697.

14 Harned R.K., Consigny P.M. & Cooper N.B. (1982) Barium enema examination following biopsy of the rectum or colon. *Radiology* **145**, 11–16.

15 Markus J.B., Somers S., O'Malley B.P. & Stevenson G.W. (1990) Double contrast barium enema studies: effect of multiple reading on perception error. *Radiology* **175**, 155–157.

16 Lappas J.C., Maglinte D.D.T. & Copecky K.K. (1988) Diverticular disease: imaging with post double contrast sigmoid flush. *Radiology* **168**, 35–37.

17 Seaman W.B. & Wells J. (1965) Complications of the barium enema. *Gastroenterology* **48**, 728–737.

18 Han S.Y. & Tishler J.M. (1982) Perforation of the colon above the peritoneal reflection during the barium enema examination. *Radiology* **144**, 253–255.

19 Gardener H. & Miller R.E. (1973) Barium peritonitis—a new therapeutic approach. *American Journal of Surgery* **125**, 350–352.

20 Masel H., Masel J.P. & Casey C.V. (1971) A survey of colon examination techniques in Australia and New Zealand with a review of complications. *Australasian Radiology* **15**, 140–144.

21 Nelson J.A., Davis A.U. & Dodds W.J. (1979) Rectal balloons: complications, causes and recommendations. *Investigative Radiology* **14**, 48–54.

22 Cotton P.B. & Williams C.B. (1990) *Practical Gastro-intestinal Endoscopy*, 3rd edn. Oxford: Blackwell Scientific Publications, 160.

23 Gilbert D.A., Hallstrohm A.P., Shaneyfelt S.L. *et al.* (1984) The national ASGE complications of colonoscopy surgery. *Gastrointestinal Endoscopy* **30**, 156 (Abstract).

24 Rogers B.H.G., Silvis S. & Nebel O.T. (1975) Complications of flexible fibreoptic colonoscopy and polypectomy. *Gastrointestinal Endoscopy* **22**, 73–75.

25 Salena B.J. & Hunt R.H. (1997) Lower gastro-intestinal endoscopy. In: Grainger R.G. & Allison D.J. (eds) *Diagnostic Radiology*, 3rd edn. New York: Churchill Livingstone, 1145–1152.

26 Butt J., Hentges D., Pelican G. *et al.* (1978) Bacteraemia during barium enema study. *American Journal of Roentgenology* **130**, 715–718.

27 Dajani A.S., Bisno A.L., Kyung J. *et al.* (1990) Prevention of bacterial endocarditis: recommendations by the American Heart Association. *Journal of the American Medical Association* **264**, 2919–2922.

28 Marshall G.B. & Barthel J.S. (1993) The frequency of total colonoscopy and terminal ileal intubation in the 1990s. *Gastrointestinal Endoscopy* **39**, 518–520.

29 Stryker S.J., Wolff B.E., Culp E.E. *et al.* (1987) Natural history of untreated colonic polyps. *Gastroenterology* **93**, 1009–1013.

30 Atkin W.S., Morson B.C. & Cuzick J. (1992) Long term risk of colorectal cancer after excision of rectosigmoid adenomas. *New England Journal of Medicine* **326**, 658–662.

31 Angelelli G. & Macrani L. (1988) CT of the bowel, use of water to enhance depiction. *Radiology* **169**, 848–849.

32 Gossios K.J., Tsianos E.V. & Contogiannis D.S. (1992) Water as contrast medium for computed tomography study of colonic wall lesions. *Gastro-intestinal Radiology* **17**, 125–128.

33 Wilson S.R. (1992) The gastro-intestinal tract. In: Rumack C.M., Wilson S.R. & Charboneau J.W. (eds) *Diagnostic Ultrasound*. St Louis: Mosby Yearbook, 181–207.

34 Carroll B.R. (1989) Ultrasound of the gastro-intestinal tract. *Radiology* **172**, 605–608.

35 Rankin S.C. (1996) CT in the staging of gastro-intestinal malignancy. In: *Proceedings of the London CT/MRI Course*. Gleneagles, Scotland, 64–68.

36 Husband J. (1997) Pelvic malignancy—the role of CT. In: *Proceedings of the London CT/MRI Course.* Gleneagles, Scotland, 73–83.

37 Tio T., Coene P., van Deldin O. *et al.* (1991) Colorectal carcinoma: pre-operative TNM classification with endosonography. *Radiology* **179**, 165–170.

38 Herzog U., von Fluee M., Tondelli P. *et al.* (1993) How accurate is endorectal ultrasound in the pre-operative staging of rectal cancer? *Diseases of the Colon and Rectum* **36**, 127–134.

39 Scialpi M., Andretta R., Agugiaro S. *et al.* (1993) Rectal carcinoma: pre-operative staging and detection of post-operative local recurrence with transrectal and transvaginal ultrasound. *Abdominal Imaging* **18**, 381–389.

40 McLean A. & Fairclough P. (1996) Endoscopic ultrasound— current applications. *Clinical Radiology* **51**, 83–98.

41 McKuscik K.A., Froelick J., Callaghan J.R. *et al.* (1981) 99m Tc red blood cells for detection of gastro-intestinal bleeding— experience with 80 patients. *American Journal of Roentgenology* **137**, 1113–1118.

42 Alavi A. & Ring E.J. (1981) Localisation of gastro-intestinal bleeding—superiority of 99m Tc sulphur colloid compared with angiography. *American Journal of Roentegenology* **137**, 741–748.

43 Alavi A. (1980) Scintigraphic demonstration of acute gastro-intestinal bleeding. *Gastro-intestinal Radiology* **5**, 205.

44 Keller F.S., Barton R.E. & Rosch J. (1994) Angiographic diagnosis and therapy of gastro-intestinal tract bleeding. In: Freeny P.C. & Stevenson G.W. (eds) *Margulis and Burhenne's Alimentary Tract Radiology,* 5th edn. St Louis: Mosby, 994–1016.

45 Gore R.M., Levine M.S. & Laufer I. (eds) (1994) *A Textbook of Gastro-intestinal Radiology.* Philadelphia: W.B. Saunders.

Suggested further reading

Smith C. (1997) Colo-rectal cancer radiologic diagnosis. In: Gore R.M. (ed.) *Staging Gastrointestinal Malignancy.* Radiologic Clinics of North America, Vol. 35(2). Philadelphia: W.B. Saunders, 439–456.

Thoeni R.F. (1997) Colo-rectal cancer radiologic staging. In: Gore R.M. (ed.) *Staging Gastrointestinal Malignancy.* Radiologic Clinics of North America, Vol. 35(2). Philadelphia: W.B. Saunders, 457–485.

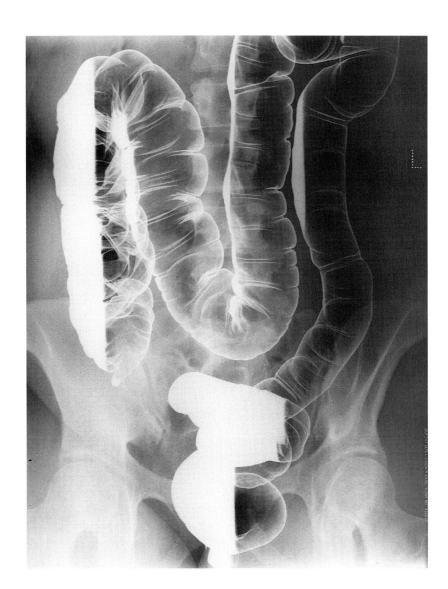

Fig. 6.1 Normal DCBE. Right lateral decubitus film shows normal colonic distensibility with air and mucosal coating with barium. The accuracy depends on thorough bowel preparation. The tortuosity of the large bowel is such that colonoscopy may be incomplete in a significant number of patients, at least 10% even in expert hands [28].

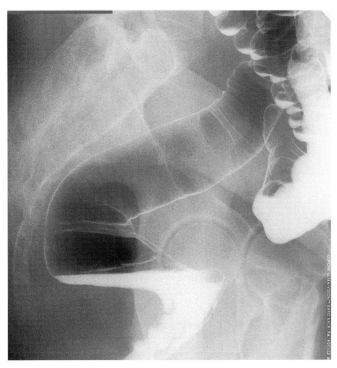

Fig. 6.2 Normal rectum, erect DCBE. The mucosa is smooth, the distensibility is normal, with a presacral space of less than 1 cm.

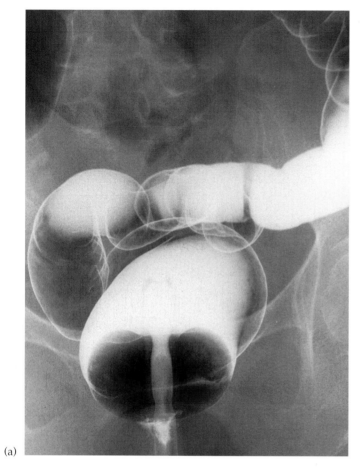

(a)

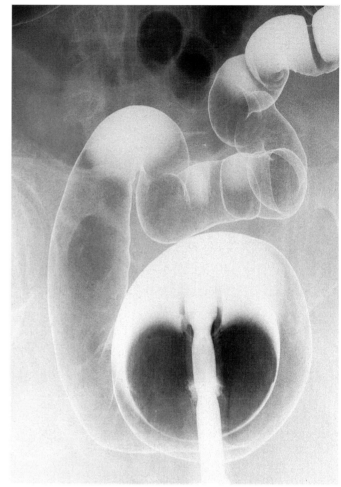

(b)

Fig. 6.3 Normal DCBE. (a) The sigmoid distends normally, but there is a moderate degree of overlapping of segments, partly obscured by the barium pool. (b) The view of the sigmoid is much improved in this prone view with X-ray tube angulation 35° to the patient's feet and most of the barium has been displaced by air in the lower sigmoid region to give a clearer mucosal view.

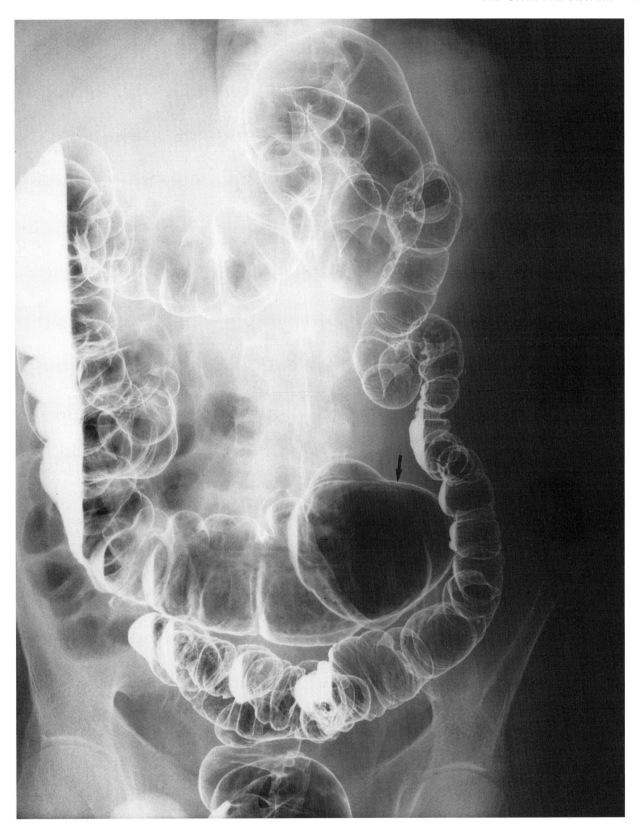

Fig. 6.4 Mobile caecum, normal DCBE. A right lateral decubitus film showing normal gaseous distension of the caecum which is seen to lie in the left iliac fossa (arrow). This is made possible by a substantial caecal mesentery, which allows it to be much more mobile than usual. This predisposes to volvulus of the caecum.

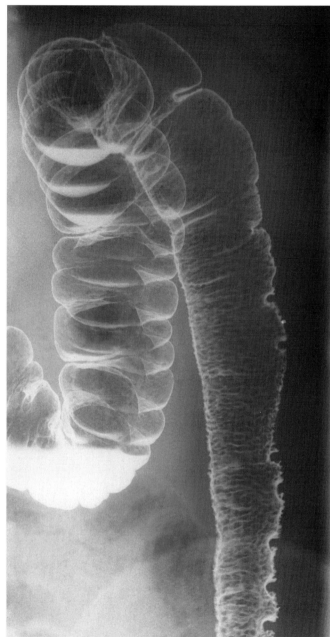

(a)

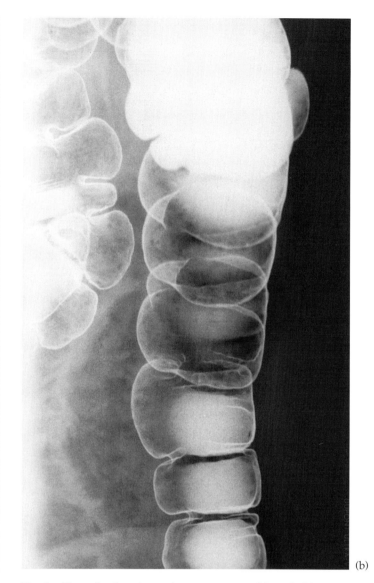

(b)

Fig. 6.5 Normal colon, innominate grooves and lymphoid follicles. (a) The descending colon is momentarily contracted by peristalsis, resulting in the appearance of transverse folds (innominate grooes) and, in addition, very small circular filling defects are visible, corresponding to lymphoid follicles. These can be considered normal if they do not exceed 3 mm in diameter [4]. (b) A few seconds later, the descending colon in the same patient has relaxed and the innominate grooves are no longer visible. The lymphoid follicles are less conspicuous.

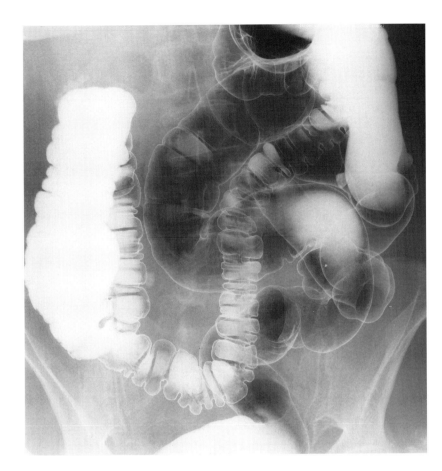

Fig. 6.6 Normal colon, with marked tortuosity. The DCBE shows a normal haustral pattern in the transverse colon, with an almost complete lack of haustral pattern in the descending colon and sigmoid colon, which are seen to be markedly tortuous. A single diverticulum is shown. Multiple calcified gallstones are also visible adjacent to the hepatic flexure.

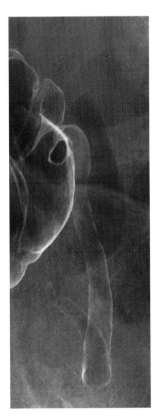

Fig. 6.7 Normal vermiform appendix. The DCBE shows normal filling of the appendix, which is lying in the right iliac fossa. The caecal orifice of the appendix is clearly shown.

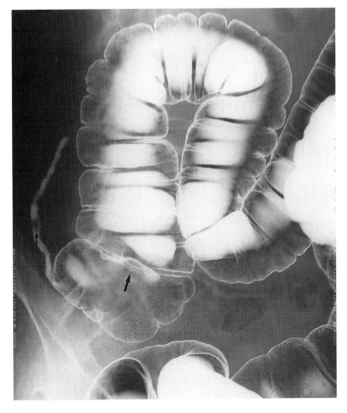

Fig. 6.8 Normal caecum and appendix. The DCBE shows normal mucosal coating of the caecum and filling of the appendix, which lies in a retrocaecal position and contains inspissated faeces (small arrow). The ileocaecal valve is indicated by the larger arrow.

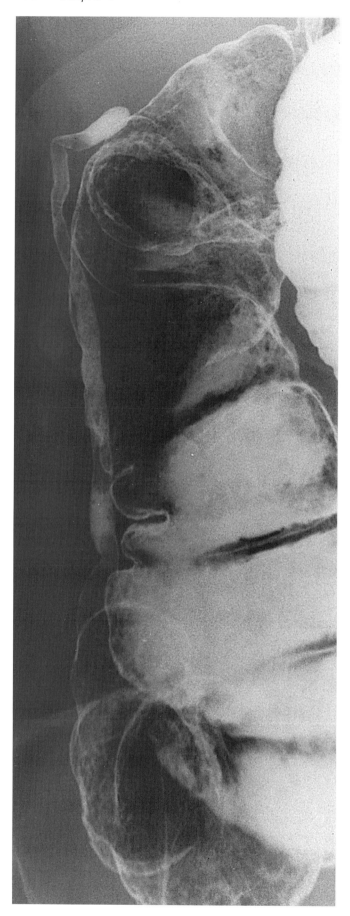

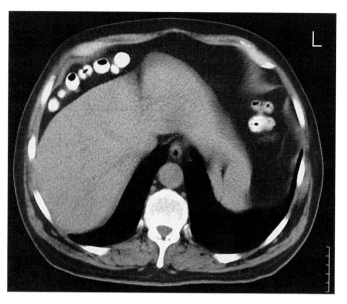

Fig. 6.10 Interposition of the colon between the right hemidiaphragm and the liver. This spiral CT scan shows contrast-filled colon located between the right hemidiaphragm anteriorly and the right lobe of liver as an incidental finding.

Fig. 6.9 Inversion of the pole of the caecum with a very long retrocaecal appendix. These were incidental findings on this DCBE. The appendix is seen to measure 15 cm in length, with its tip adjacent to the hepatic flexure.

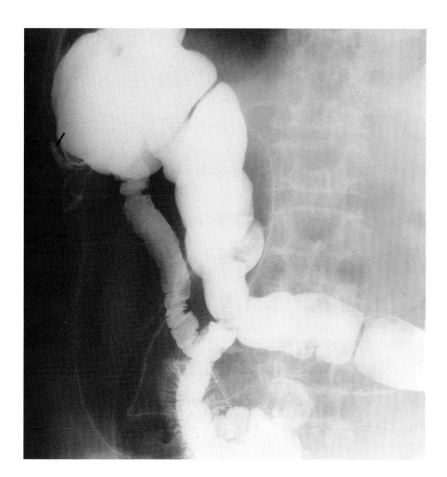

Fig. 6.11 Congenital malrotation of the colon. In this middle-aged male patient, the caecum is seen to be located at a high level under the right hemidiaphragm. The appendix is indicated by the arrow. In addition, a long redundant loop of sigmoid colon is also located in the right side of the abdomen and is superimposed on the transverse colon and terminal ileum in this projection.

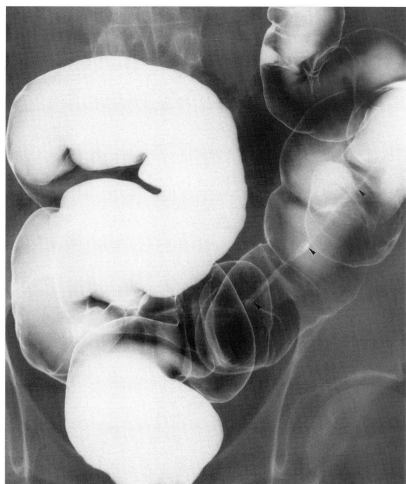

Fig. 6.12 Band of mucus artefact in the sigmoid colon. A long linear opacity is projected within the sigmoid colon (arrowheads). This is the result of barium mixing with adherent mucus. It should not be confused with the stalk of a pedunculated polyp.

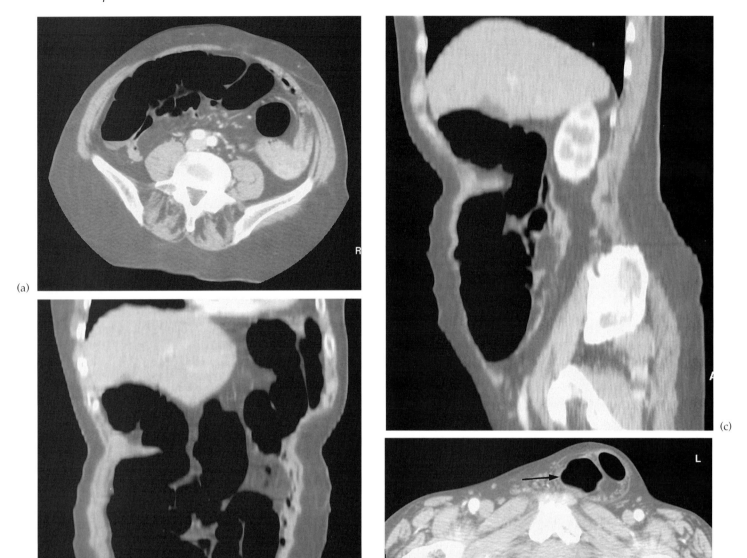

Fig. 6.13 (a–c) Normal large bowel, CT pneumocolon. (a) After bowel preparation, the colon is distended with air or CO_2 with a rectal catheter and a volume acquisition with IV contrast enhancement is obtained. The whole of the large bowel may be examined with a single breath-hold. (b) A coronal reconstruction of the same examination shows gaseous distension of the normal colon. Although only a single coronal section is illustrated, the whole of the large bowel may be inspected using the multiplanar reconstruction method. (c) Sagittal reconstruction of the same examination through the abdomen in the plane of the hepatic flexure, ascending colon and caecum. The right lobe of the liver and the right kidney are clearly shown. (Five millimetre collimation, pitch 1.4, 3 mm reconstruction.) **(d) CT pneumocolon complicated by extraluminal air.** This elderly male patient, with a moderately large sliding colonic hernia (large arrow), had a previously failed barium enema and colonoscopy. The spiral CECT was complicated by perirectal, extraperitoneal accumulation of air (arrowheads). The patient was completely asymptomatic during the procedure and for 5 days follow-up without any treatment. Small arrow, rectal wall.

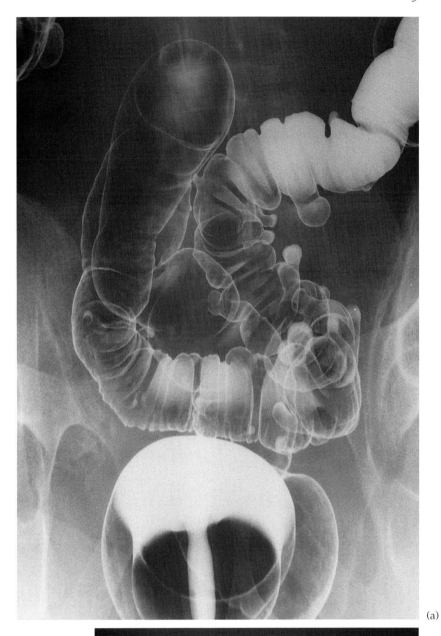

(a)

(b)

Fig. 6.14 **Diverticular disease of the colon.** (a) This 35° prone angled view of the rectosigmoid region shows satisfactory separation of the convoluted sigmoid, in which there are multiple diverticula. There is no evidence of stricture and no other abnormality is visible. (b) CT pneumocolon: rectal insufflation of air, IV hyoscine 20 mg and spiral CECT shows uncomplicated diverticular disease in the sigmoid region.

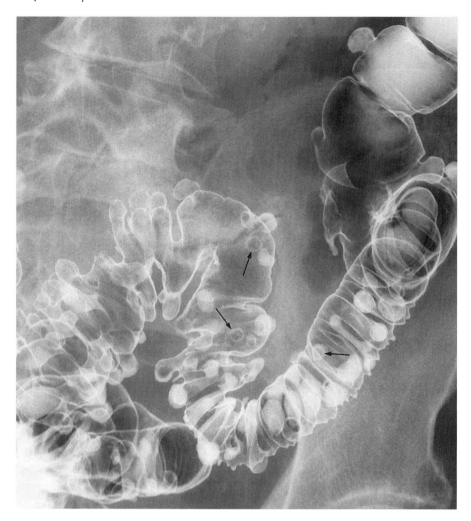

Fig. 6.15 Diverticular disease of the colon. This DCBE shows numerous diverticula in the sigmoid colon, many of which are seen in profile and some are shown as ring shadows *en face* (arrows). These may be difficult to distinguish from polyps.

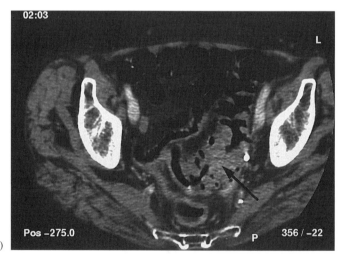

(a)

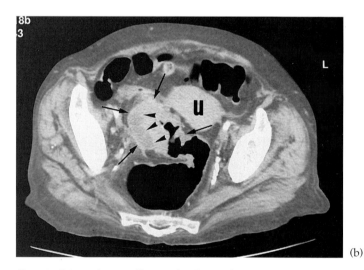

(b)

Fig. 6.16 Diverticular disease of the colon. (a) This spiral CT scan through the pelvis shows the typical sawtoothed deformity of the sigmoid colon with pockets of gas within the diverticula. The marked muscular hypertrophy of the wall of the bowel, which is a prominent feature of diverticular disease, is indicated by the arrow. There was no bowel preparation. (b) Sigmoid diverticulitis with a small pericolic abscess (CT pneumocolon). The sigmoid lumen is irregularly contracted and the wall is markedly swollen (arrows) within which there is an area of reduced attenuation in keeping with a small abscess (arrowheads). u, uterus.

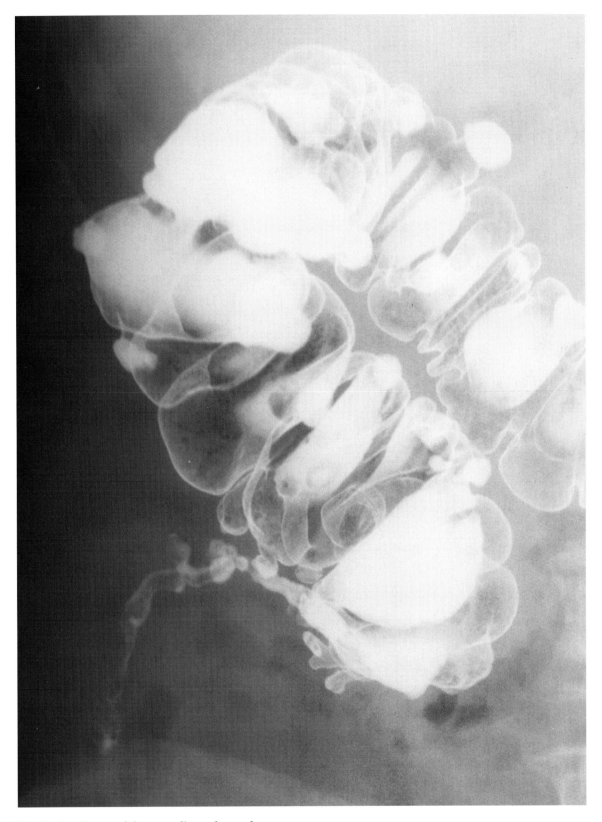

Fig. 6.17 Diverticular disease of the ascending colon and appendix. The DCBE shows multiple diverticula affecting the caecum and ascending colon, which are less frequent than left-sided diverticula. Diverticula of the appendix are very rare.

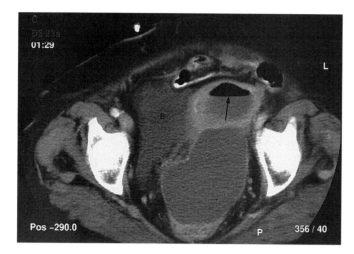

Fig. 6.18 Colonic diverticular disease complicated by pelvic abscess. A 76-year-old female patient was known to have diverticular disease with lower abdominal pain, pyrexia and a high white-cell count. A spiral CT scan of the pelvis shows a huge pelvic abscess containing gas and a fluid level, indicated by the arrow. B, bladder.

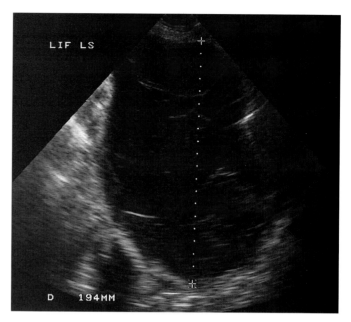

Fig. 6.19 Sigmoid diverticular disease complicated by pelvic abscess. This ultrasound scan shows a huge abscess in the left iliac fossa measuring 19 cm in anteroposterior diameter. Some echoes are visible within it. The patient had a white-cell count of 17 000. A 10 F drainage catheter was inserted percutaneously and 1500 ml of frank pus were drained.

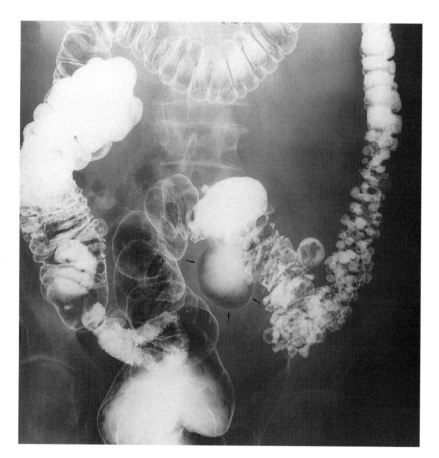

Fig. 6.20 Colonic diverticular disease complicated by giant cyst. A DCBE in this male shows gross diverticular disease affecting the pelvic and lower descending colon, with a 5.5 cm cystic dilatation arising from the inferior aspect of the mid-sigmoid region (arrows).

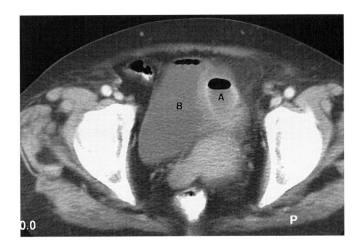

Fig. 6.21 Sigmoid diverticular disease complicated by pericolic abscess and colovesical fistula. A spiral CT scan through the lower pelvis shows air within the bladder (B). The left lateral wall of the bladder is compressed and displaced by the pelvic abscess, which is also seen to contain gas (A).

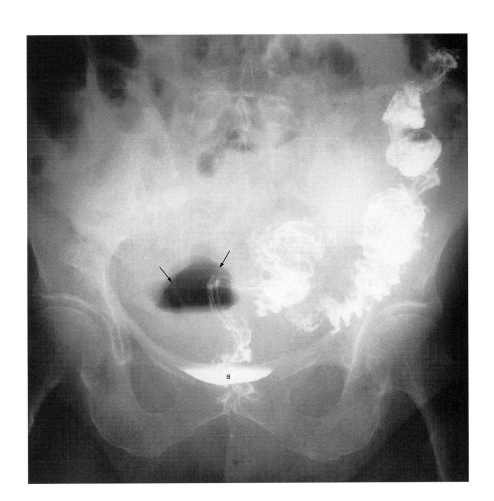

Fig. 6.22 Diverticular disease complicated by colovesical fistula. A postevacuation film shows a residue of barium in the colon and rectum. On this erect view, a pool of contrast is shown in the base of the bladder (B). In addition, the bladder contains a considerable volume of air (arrows).

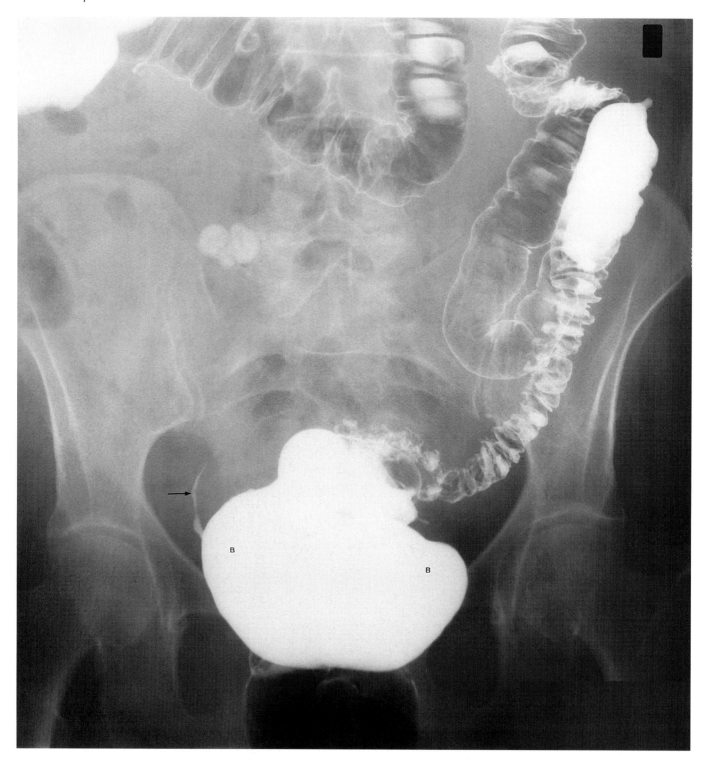

Fig. 6.23 Diverticular disease complicated by colovesical fistula.
A DCBE in this patient with altered bowel habit shows fairly
extensive diverticular disease in the left side of the colon. A large
volume of contrast has entered the bladder (B) and some contrast
has refluxed into the right ureter (arrow).

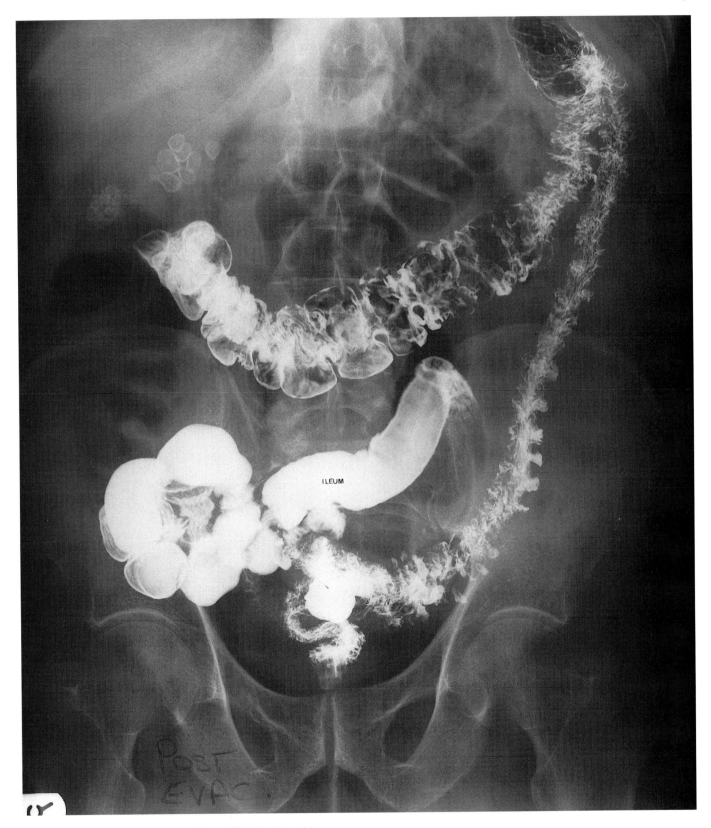

ILEUM

Fig. 6.24 Diverticular disease complicated by ileosigmoid fistula. Postevacuation film in a 65-year-old male patient with mucus and blood per rectum. There is diverticular disease in the sigmoid colon. Barium is seen to fill the small bowel before it has reached the caecum. Multiple calcified gallstones are also visible.

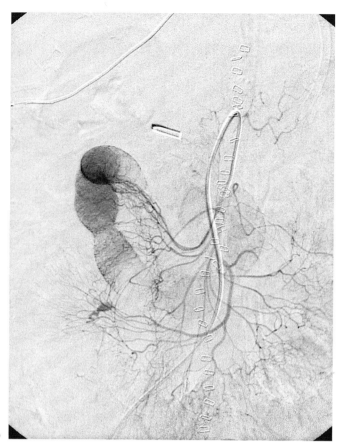

(a)

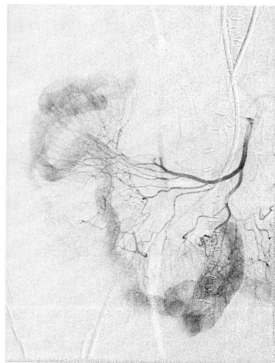

(b)

Fig. 6.25 Diverticular disease complicated by haemorrhage.
(a) This selective superior mesenteric angiogram, performed after right hemicolectomy, shows an area of extravasation in the right lower quadrant. This was due to a bleeding diverticulum supplied by the middle colic artery. (b) Superimposed vessels may make visualization of the bleeding point difficult. A selective ileocolic angiogram shows no extravasation. (Courtesy of Dr Richard D. Edwards.)

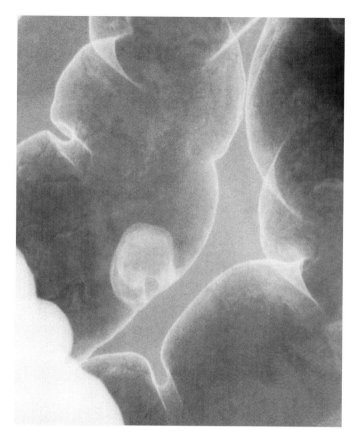

Fig. 6.26 Polypoid adenoma. A sessile polypoid filling defect is shown on this DCBE. The detection of polyps depends on thorough preparation and careful technique.

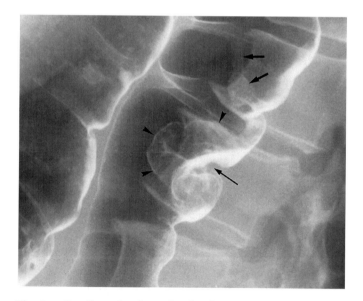

Fig. 6.27 Sessile and pedunculated polyps. A DCBE in this 68-year-old female patient (same patient as in Fig. 6.26) shows a broad-based slightly lobulated mass measuring 3 cm in diameter (arrowheads). The long arrow indicates indrawing of the base of the polyp, a feature which is suggestive of, but not diagnostic of, malignancy. In addition, there is an adjacent smaller polypoid lesion suspended by a short pedicle (short arrows). Histology of the resected sessile polyp indicated a villotubular adenoma, with moderate dedifferentiation of epithelium, but with no evidence of invasion. Histology of the pedunculated lesion showed no features of malignancy.

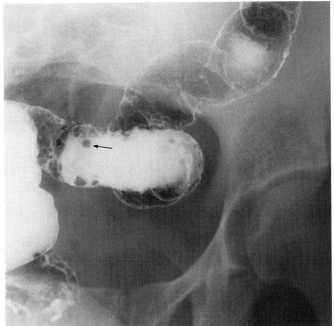

(a)

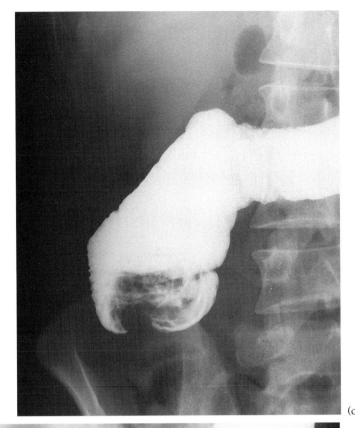

(c)

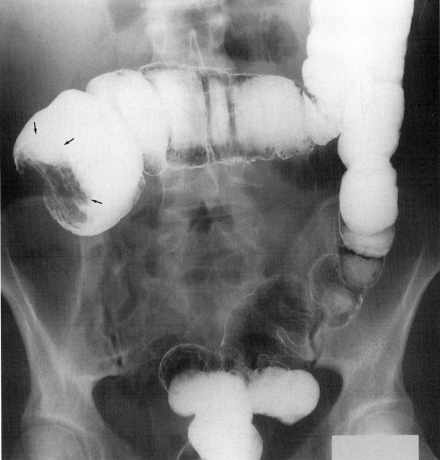

(b)

Fig. 6.28 Familial polyposis coli complicated by carcinoma, complicated by intussusception. (a) The DCBE of the sigmoid colon shows numerous small rounded filling defects (arrow). Endoscopic confirmation of polyposis. (b) In the same patient, there is a large filling defect at the hepatic flexure (arrows). (c) Ten minutes later, the intussusception at the hepatic flexure was at least partly reduced, with a residual large filling defect in the ascending colon. At surgery, this was found to be a carcinoma complicating polyposis coli.

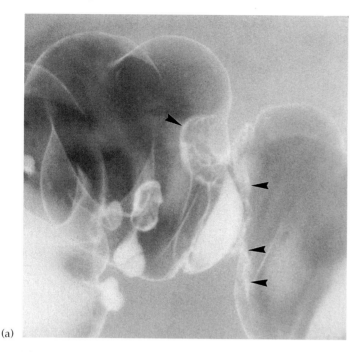

(a)

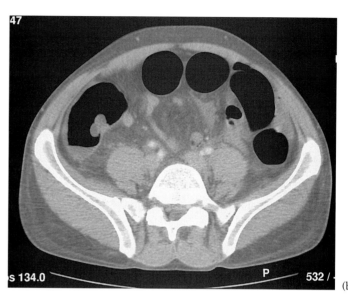

(b)

Fig. 6.29 Colonic carcinoma, early disease. (a) The DCBE in this patient with a short history of rectal bleeding shows a broad-based 2 cm polyp in the right side of the transverse colon. There is persistent deformity of the mucosa to the left of the main lesion, which is seen to extend inferiorly (arrowheads).

Endoscopic confirmation of malignancy. (b) A CT pneumocolon in a 45-year-old male patient with iron-deficiency anaemia shows a 2.5 cm sessile polypoid lesion in the medial wall of the ascending colon. The success of this method depends on thorough bowel preparation, adequate bowel distension by air insufflation, fine collimation, reconstruction of overlapping slices and adequate breath-holding for the volume acquisition of data.

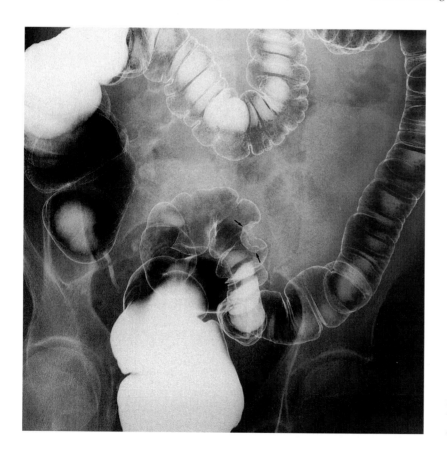

Fig. 6.30 Colonic carcinoma. A DCBE in a 70-year-old male patient with iron-deficiency anaemia shows a 2.5 cm diameter sessile polypoid lesion (arrows) arising from the mesenteric aspect of the mid-sigmoid colon, with conspicuous indrawing of the base of the lesion. Malignancy was confirmed and the lesion was treated by anterior colonic resection.

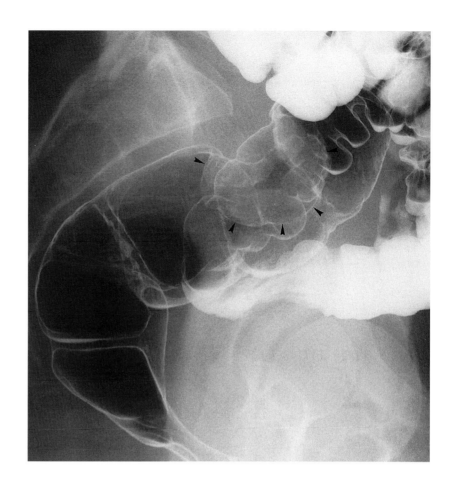

Fig. 6.31 Carcinoma of the rectosigmoid junction. A DCBE lateral view of the rectum and lower sigmoid shows a constant 5.5 cm diameter filling defect (arrowheads) arising from the posterior wall of the rectosigmoid junction. Carcinoma was confirmed histologically.

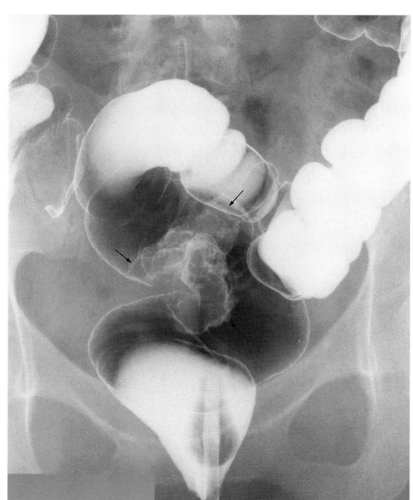

Fig. 6.32 Rectal carcinoma. The DCBE in this patient with a short history of rectal bleeding shows an irregular eccentric mass lesion arising from the middle third of the rectum (arrows). The appearance is typical of carcinoma with obvious mucosal destruction.

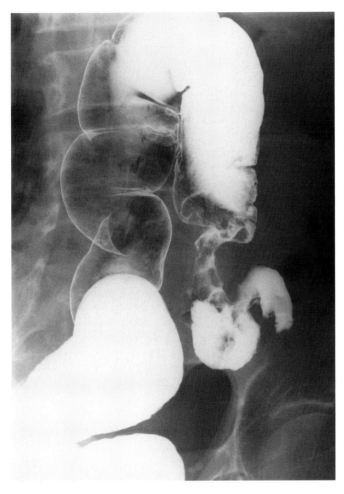

Fig. 6.33 Sigmoid carcinoma. A DCBE of a 59-year-old male patient with recent alteration in bowel habit. There is an annular stricture resembling an apple core, with shouldered margins, in the mid-sigmoid colon, the appearance being characteristic of carcinoma. There is no evidence of diverticular disease.

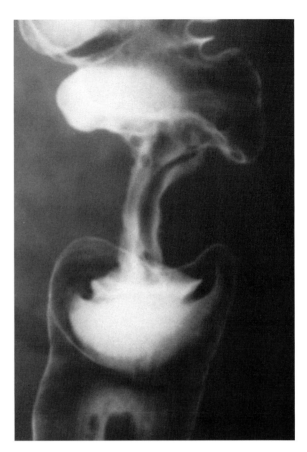

Fig. 6.34 Carcinoma of the descending colon. A DCBE in a 63-year-old male patient with colicky abdominal pain. An annular carcinoma with shouldered margins is clearly visible in the proximal descending colon. Histological confirmation.

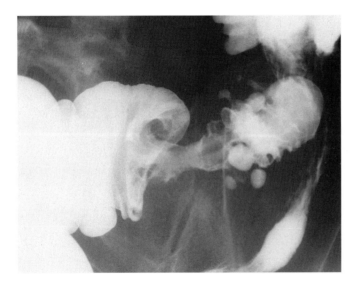

Fig. 6.35 Coexistent carcinoma and diverticular disease. The DCBE shows an irregular stricture with a shouldered margin at its distal end in a patient who also has sigmoid diverticular disease. Carcinoma is clearly not a complication of diverticular disease, but they frequently coexist. The differential diagnosis of sigmoid strictures may be difficult, but the appearance of this lesion makes malignancy almost certain. Histological confirmation.

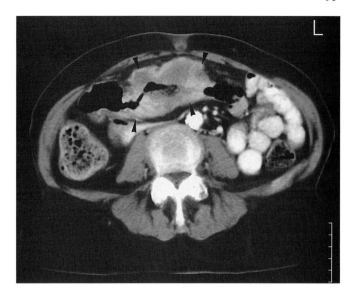

Fig. 6.36 Carcinoma of the transverse colon. A 74-year-old female patient presented with a palpable central abdominal mass. A spiral CT scan with contrast enhancement shows a long irregular stricture of the transverse colon, with marked thickening of the bowel wall. A fat plane between the posterior surface of the lesion and the duodenum is preserved (arrowheads).

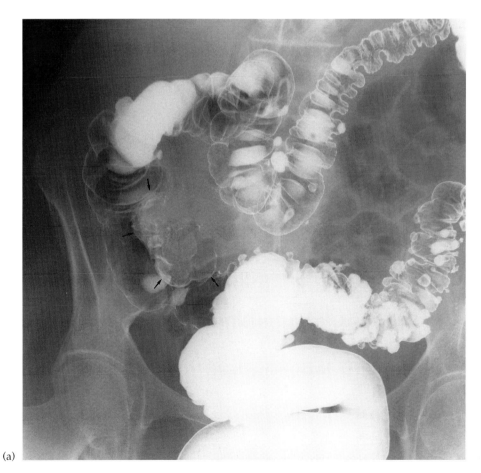

(a)

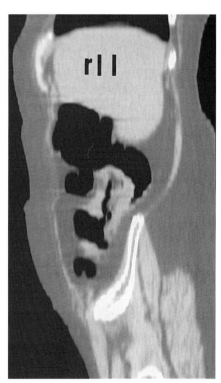

(b)

Fig. 6.37 (a) Carcinoma of the caecum. The DCBE of this patient with altered bowel habit and anaemia shows extensive diverticular disease, particularly in the sigmoid region. In addition, there is a large eccentric exophytic mass lesion arising from the medial wall of the caecum (arrows). **(b) Carcinoma of the ascending colon.** A sagittal multiplanar reconstruction (MPR) of a spiral CT pneumocolon with IV contrast shows an apple-core lesion in the ascending colon of a 67-year-old female patient with iron-deficiency anaemia and altered bowel habit. rll, right lobe of the liver.

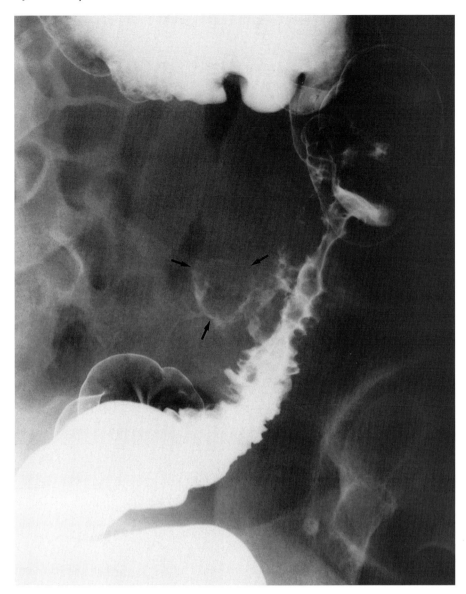

Fig. 6.38 Sigmoid carcinoma complicated by pericolic abscess. The DCBE shows a long, very irregular, ulcerated stricture of the sigmoid colon. There is extensive leakage of contrast from the stricture into an irregular cavity on the mesenteric side of the colon (arrows). Colonoscopy of this lesion suggested Crohn's disease, but the biopsy indicated carcinoma.

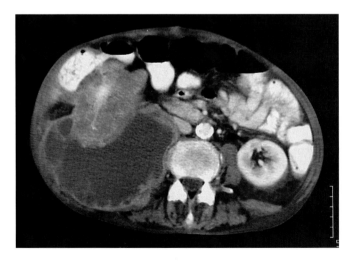

Fig. 6.39 Carcinoma of the ascending colon complicated by retrocolic abscess. A spiral CT scan in a 72-year-old male patient with pain and fullness in his right flank, pyrexia, raised white-cell count and anaemia. There is marked thickening of the wall of the ascending colon, which is displaced forwards by a large irregular fluid-filled cavity, which partly surrounds it posteriorly. Some of the sections showed pockets of gas within this lesion. Pus was removed by percutaneous drainage. Colonic carcinoma was confirmed at autopsy. (Courtesy of Dr F.G. Adams.)

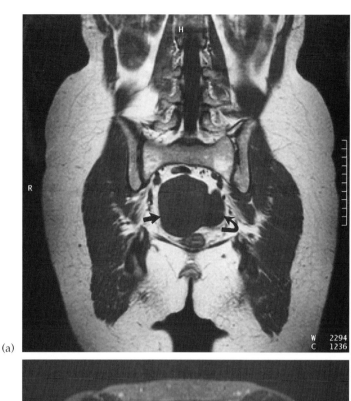

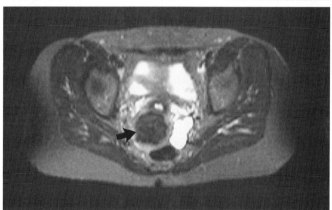

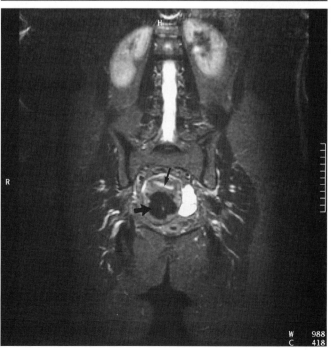

(a)

(b)

(c)

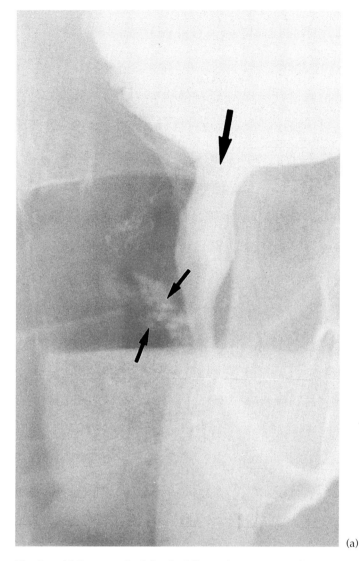

(a)

Fig. 6.41 (a) Rectourethral fistula. Micturating cystogram in a 74-year-old male patient, who had had an anterior resection for a locally advanced rectal carcinoma. During voiding, contrast is shown in the bladder neck (large arrow). Contrast is seen to escape from a fistula arising in the posterior urethra (small arrows).

Fig. 6.40 Pelvic mass in a patient with previous colonic carcinoma. (a) A coronal T_1 SE MRI scan of pelvis shows a 6 cm intermediate signal mass (arrow) posterior to the bladder with a left-sided 4 cm mass (curved arrow) of low signal. (b) An axial T_2 FSE shows the larger mass (arrow) to have low signal and the smaller mass to have a high signal. (c) A coronal STIR shows the larger low-signal mass lying in the wall of the uterus (small arrow, endometrial stripe), in keeping with uterine fibroids, while the smaller mass (thick arrow) is in keeping with an ovarian cystic mass (surgical confirmation). (Courtesy of Dr J. Graeme Houston.)

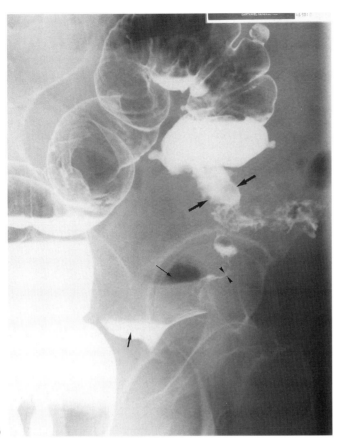

(b)

Fig. 6.41 *Continued.* **(b) Sigmoid carcinoma with colovesical fistula.** An elderly female patient presented to the urology department with urinary-tract symptoms. Cystoscopy revealed tumour in the wall of the bladder, the biopsy of which indicated adenocarcinoma. This erect lateral DCBE shows a constant irregular stricture of the sigmoid colon (large arrows), from which the contrast is seen to escape via a fistula (arrowheads) into the bladder, forming a pool of barium (short arrow). Air (thin arrow) is seen above a fluid level of urine in the bladder.

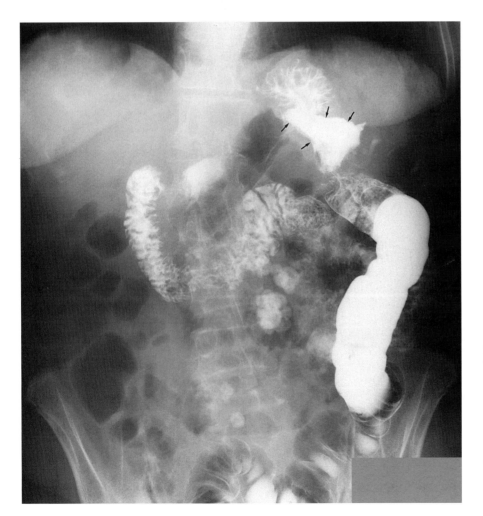

Fig. 6.42 **Colonic carcinoma complicated by gastrocolic fistula.** This DCBE shows a grossly deformed splenic flexure of the colon, which includes a huge ulcer (arrows), which has produced a fistula into the fundus of the stomach. All of the contrast in the stomach, duodenum and jejunum has followed this route. Other causes of gastrocolic fistula include gastric carcinoma, pancreatic carcinoma, Crohn's disease and peptic ulceration.

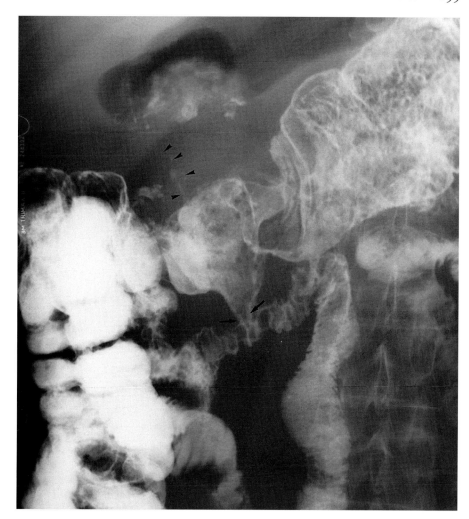

Fig. 6.43 Colonic carcinoma complicated by enterocolic fistula and duodenocolic fistula. This patient had altered bowel habit, diarrhoea and recent rectal bleeding. A postevacuation barium-enema film shows barium in the large bowel, with an annular stricture in the transverse colon close to the hepatic flexure. Contrast was seen to have reached a loop of small bowel via a fistula arising in the tumour (arrows). A second fistula arising from the superior aspect of the tumour drained contrast into the duodenum (arrowheads).

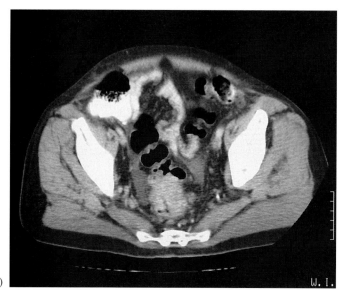

(a)

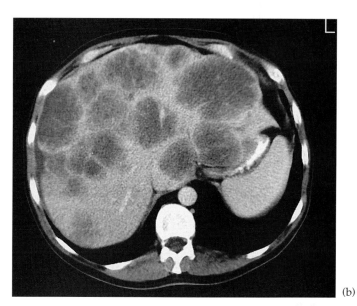

(b)

Fig. 6.44 Rectal carcinoma with metastatic liver disease.
(a) There is an irregular mass lesion within the rectum. Internal iliac lymph nodes are visible and these are about the upper limit of normal. (b) The liver is markedly enlarged and is extensively replaced by numerous low-attenuation metastatic deposits. The patient also had metastatic lung disease.

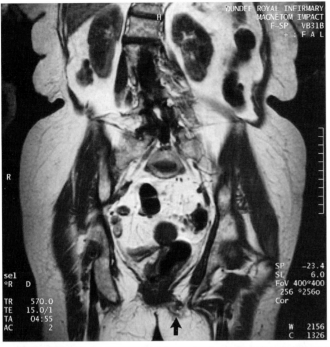

(a)

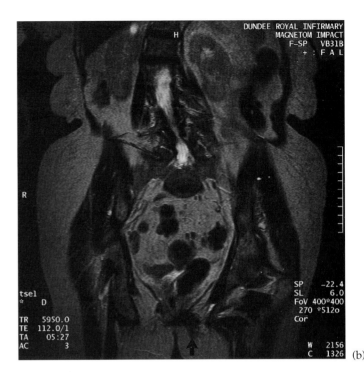

(b)

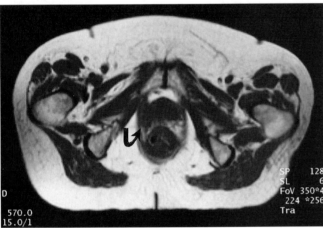

(c)

Fig. 6.45 Staging rectal carcinoma. A 79-year-old male patient with rectal carcinoma was scanned. (a) A coronal T_1 SE MRI scan of the pelvis and (b) a coronal T_2 FSE show a low-signal rectal mass on the T_1-weighted image and an intermediate signal on the T_2-weighted image, with lateral extension into the left ischiorectal fossa (arrows). (c) Right periprostatic spread (curved arrow) indicating T3 rectal carcinoma. (Courtesy of Dr Graeme Houston.)

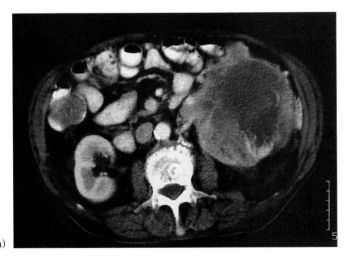

(a)

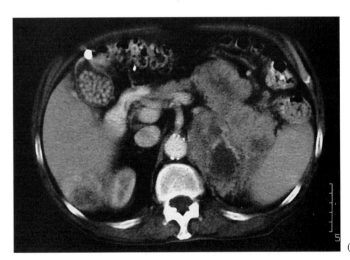

(b)

Fig. 6.46 Carcinoma of the caecum with primary renal carcinoma. (a) There is a constant filling defect in the caecum, which was shown to be primary carcinoma. There is also a much larger solid mass lesion arising from the left kidney, which was a separate primary renal cancer. (b) This shows the primary renal lesion on the left side, together with a metastatic deposit posteriorly in the liver. Numerous gallbladder calculi are also visible.

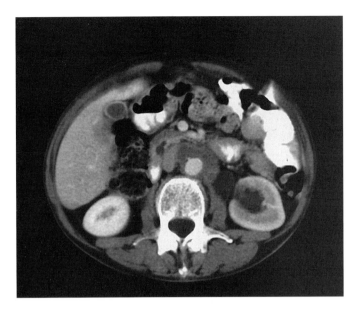

Fig. 6.47 Metastatic colon cancer. There is retroperitoneal lymphadenopathy in this contrast-enhanced spiral CT scan in a 66-year-old female patient, who previously had had a colonic resection for carcinoma. She had recent back pain and weight loss.

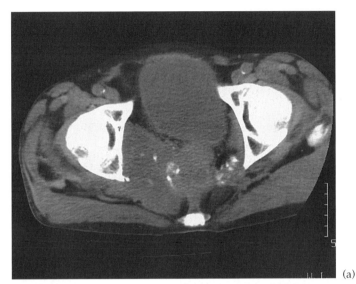

(a)

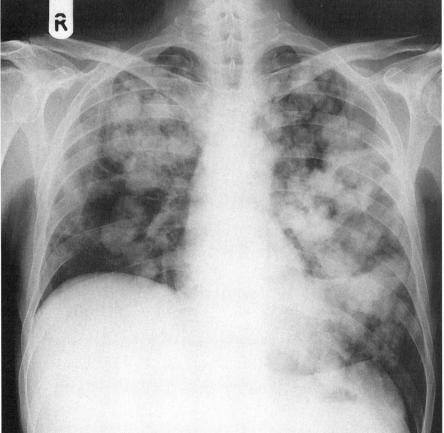

Fig. 6.48 Recurrent rectal carcinoma with pulmonary metastases. This patient had had a surgical resection of rectal carcinoma 1 year previously, and now has recent pelvic pain, weight loss, breathlessness and ankle oedema. (a) A solid mass lesion is shown centrally between the bladder and the sacrum and this is seen to extend laterally on both sides to the side wall of the pelvis. This extensive local recurrence shows patchy calcification, which is typical of mucin-secreting adenocarcinoma. (b) A posteroanterior chest X-ray in the same patient shows numerous pulmonary metastases.

(b)

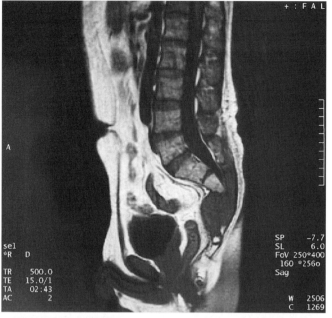

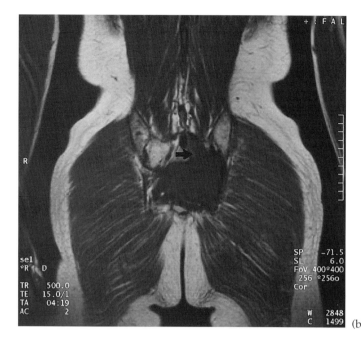

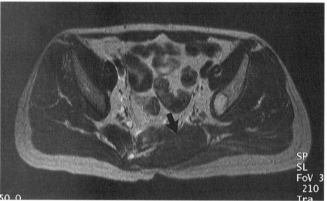

Fig. 6.49 Recurrent rectal carcinoma. This 42-year-old male patient had had a previous anterior resection of rectal carcinoma. (a) A sagittal and (b) a coronal T_1 SE of the pelvis show low-signal sacral recurrence extending superiorly to involve the left ala of the sacrum (arrow). (c) An axial T_2 FSE shows a left sacral mass extending into the piriformis muscle (arrow). (Courtesy of Dr Graeme Houston.)

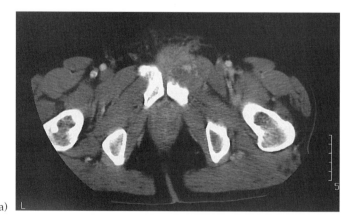

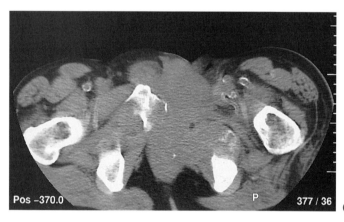

Fig. 6.50 Recurrent rectal carcinoma. (a) A spiral CT scan of the pelvis in a patient with previous anterior resection of rectal carcinoma shows an irregular mass lesion in the left pubic area, with an irregular anterior margin, in keeping with infiltration of the subcutaneous fat. The lesion is seen to extend posteriorly, with destruction of the body of the pubis on the left side. (b) The same patient 18 months later shows more extensive bone destruction and extensive soft-tissue tumour infiltration.

The Colon and Rectum 203

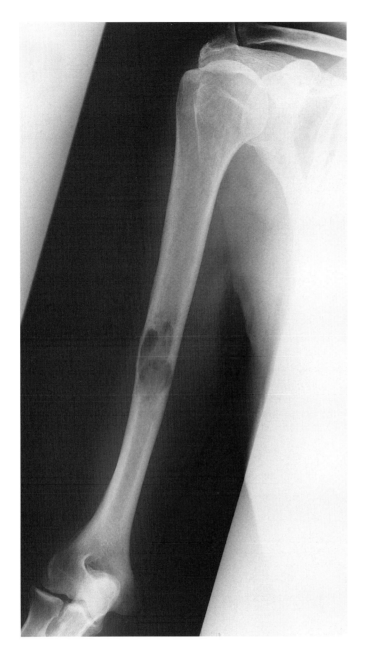

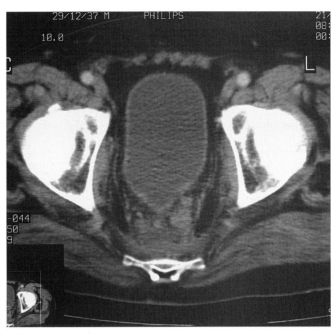

Fig. 6.52 Recurrent rectal carcinoma. Spiral CT scan in a patient with previous abdominoperineal excision of the rectum. A lobulated mass lesion is visible in the presacral space. There was biopsy confirmation of carcinoma. The distinction between postoperative scar tissue and recurrent tumour may be impossible on the basis of a single CT scan and sequential studies and biopsy may be required.

Fig. 6.51 Bone metastasis from colonic carcinoma. A 63-year-old male patient with a history of colonic resection for adenocarcinoma had a 3-week history of pain and tenderness in his right arm. An AP view of the humerus shows an extensive osteolytic lesion involving the middle third of the humerus. Of patients with metastatic bone disease, 1% have a colorectal primary.

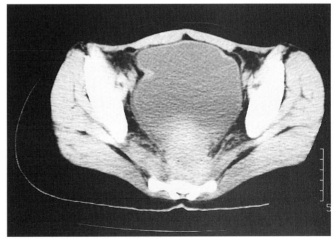

Fig. 6.53 Recurrent rectal carcinoma. A 24-year-old female patient presented with a past history of abdominoperineal excision of rectum and constant pelvic pain. The spiral CT scan shows a solid presacral mass lesion extending laterally on the right side into the piriformis muscle.

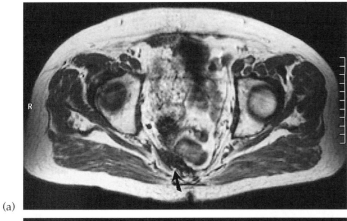

(a)

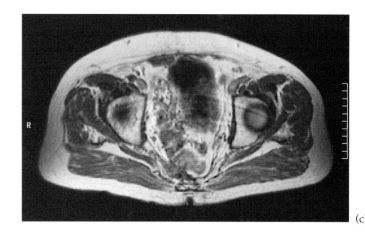

(c)

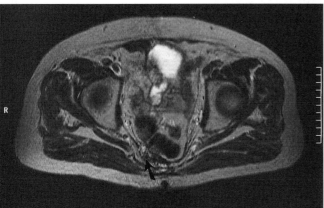

(b)

Fig. 6.54 Postsurgical change in rectal carcinoma. This 54-year-old male patient had a previous anterior resection of rectal carcinoma. (a) An axial T_1 SE of the pelvis and (b) a T_2 FSE show a right presacral 3 cm × 2 cm mass (arrows). (c) An axial T_1 SE with post gadolinium enhancement (0.1 mmol/kg) shows no significant enhancement, in keeping with postinflammatory change (biopsy confirmation). (Courtesy of Dr J. Graeme Houston.)

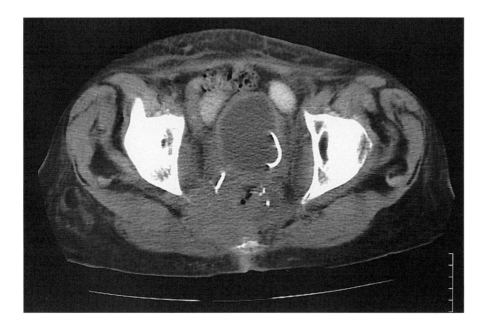

Fig. 6.55 Recurrent anal carcinoma. This patient had low back pain and previous abdominoperineal excision of the anus and rectum for anal carcinoma. The spiral CT scan shows an extensive presacral soft-tissue mass extending into the piriformis muscle on the right, as well as the bladder wall. Bilateral ureteric stents are shown.

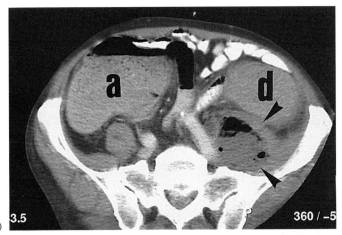

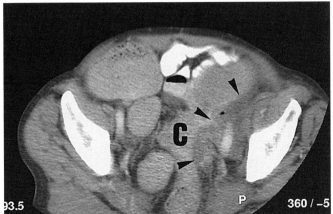

Fig. 6.56 Recurrent sigmoid carcinoma; large bowel obstruction and psoas abscess. The patient gave a history of painful abdominal distension 2 years after sigmoid colectomy for cancer. (a) The spiral CECT shows obstructed ascending (a) and descending (d) colon. The left psoas muscle is expanded and extensive gas formation (arrowheads) was visible on multiple sections. (b) At a lower level in the pelvis, there is a left-sided solid mass lesion (arrowheads) deforming the pelvic colon (c). On other sections the left ureter was obstructed producing hydronephrosis.

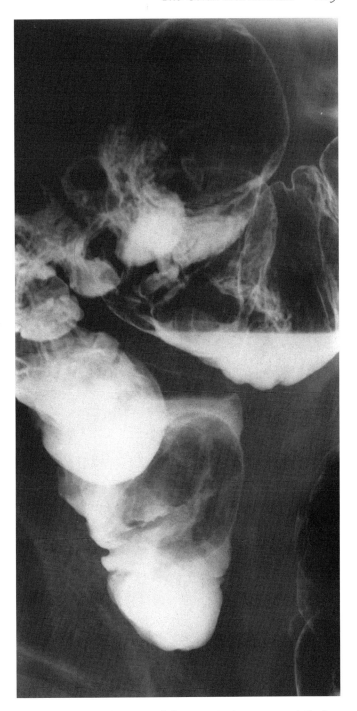

Fig. 6.57 Carcinoid tumour of the caecum. A constant, relatively smooth filling defect is shown in the caecum on this single-contrast barium enema (SCBE). Biopsy of this lesion indicated carcinoid tumour.

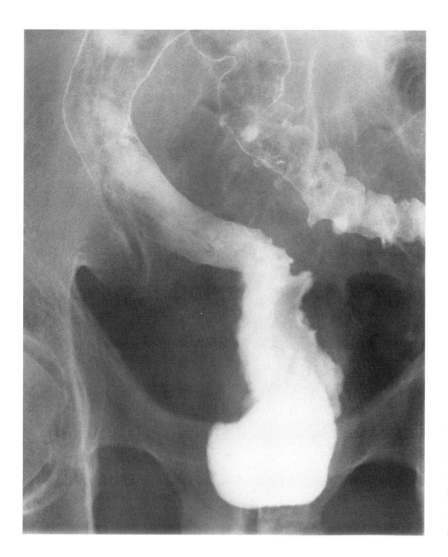

Fig. 6.58 Lymphoma of the rectum. An 80-year-old retired anaesthetist had a history of altered bowel habit and rectal bleeding. The wall of the rectum shows extensive irregularity and there is considerable loss of distensibility. The changes are non-specific and biopsy indicated lymphoma. Diverticular disease is present in the sigmoid colon.

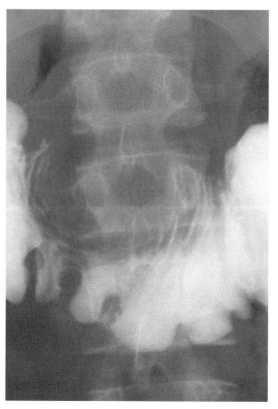

Fig. 6.59 Secondary involvement of the colon by paraganglionoma. This 55-year-old male patient had intermittent abdominal pain and a palpable epigastric mass. A large eccentric filling defect is seen to affect the transverse colon, sparing the inferior margin. There is no shouldered margin and no evidence of mucosal destruction. This was due to a paraganglionoma arising in the transverse mesocolon.

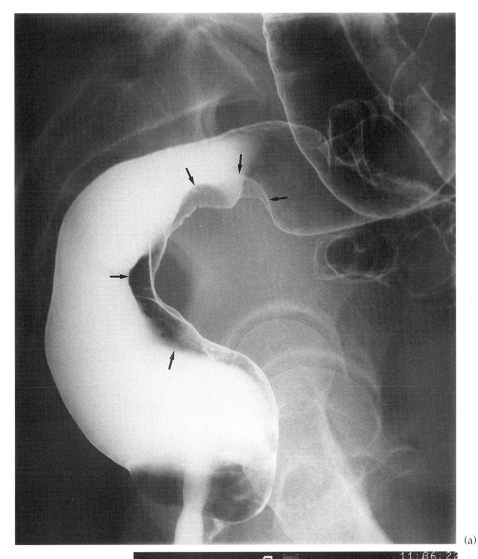

(a)

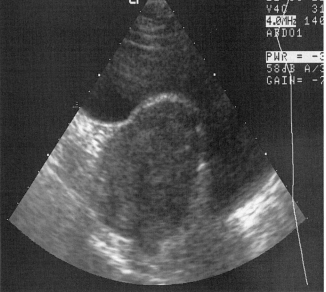

Fig. 6.60 Secondary involvement of the rectum by gynaecological malignancy. Colonoscopy in this patient revealed some deformity of the anterior wall of the rectum, but the mucosa was normal. (a) The lateral-view DCBE shows a very extensive lobulated filling defect (arrows) affecting the anterior wall of the rectum and distal sigmoid, but with no evidence of mucosal involvement. (b) An ultrasound of the same patient shows a large, solid, pelvic mass lesion, apparently contiguous with the uterus. The appearance is non-specific. At laparotomy, the pelvis was found to be 'frozen', resulting from stage 3 ovarian carcinoma (poorly differentiated on biopsy).

(b)

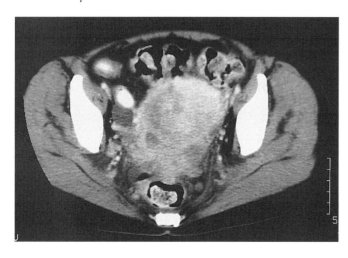

Fig. 6.61 Extension of carcinoma of the cervix into the rectum.
The spiral CT scan shows a large pelvic mass of uneven
attenuation extending through the anterior wall of the rectum.
The mass proved to be stage 3B carcinoma of the cervix.

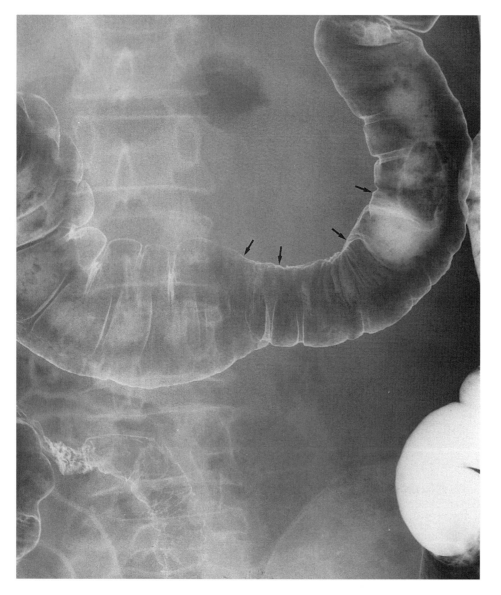

**Fig. 6.62 Extrinsic compression of
the transverse colon by pancreatic
pseudocyst.** A DCBE in this male
patient with a palpable abdominal
mass shows slight loss of
distensibility of the left side of the
transverse colon and a moderate
impression on its superior aspect
(arrows). A CT scan in this patient
indicated a large pancreatic
pseudocyst.

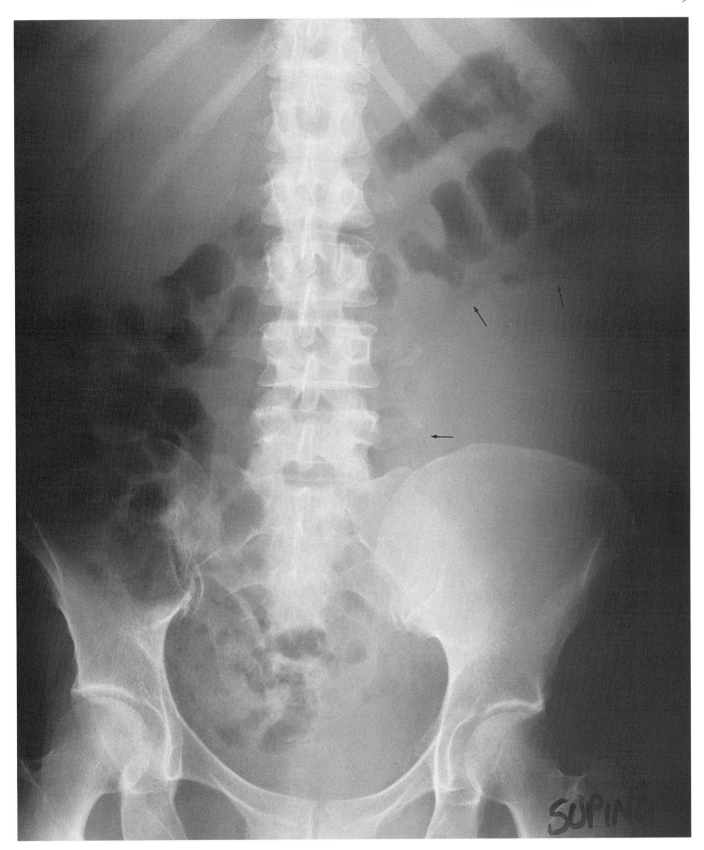

Fig. 6.63 Displacement of the descending colon by retroperitoneal haematoma. A 35-year-old female patient sustained a blunt abdominal injury in a road traffic accident. This plain abdominal film shows evidence of a large soft-tissue swelling in the left flank and left iliac fossa, with marked medial displacement of the gas shadow of the descending colon (arrows). Fractures of the left fourth and fifth lumbar transverse processes are also shown.

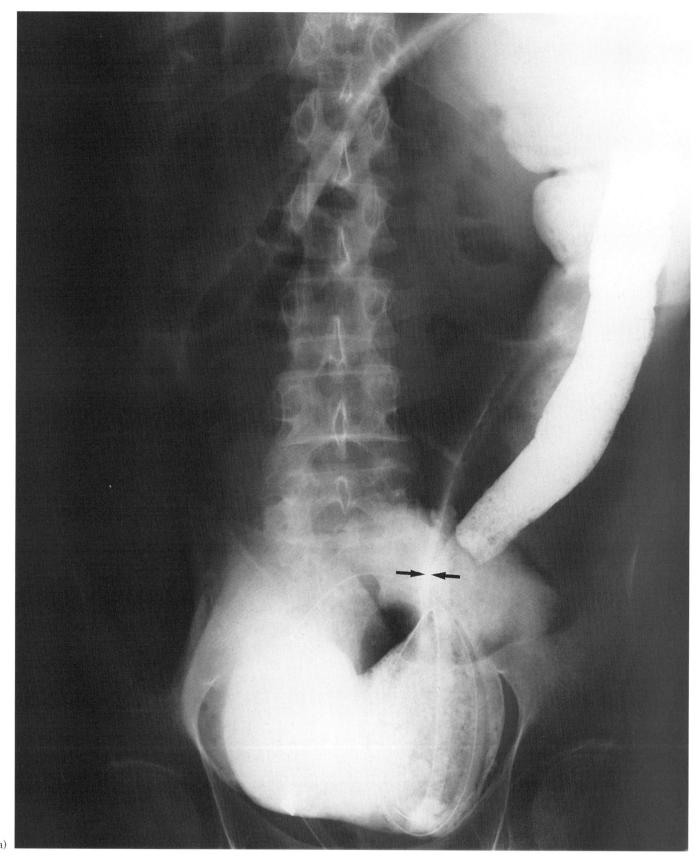

(a)

Fig. 6.64 Sigmoid volvulus. An elderly male patient with progressive abdominal distension was given oral Gastrografin and this is seen to fill the descending colon. (a) This film was obtained after a Gastrografin enema, in which there is partial filling of one limb of the massively distended sigmoid loop with contrast. The positive signs of sigmoid volvulus in this case are the left flank overlap sign, inferior convergence on the left (arrows), an air/fluid ratio greater than 2/1 and an ahaustral margin to the distended sigmoid loop.

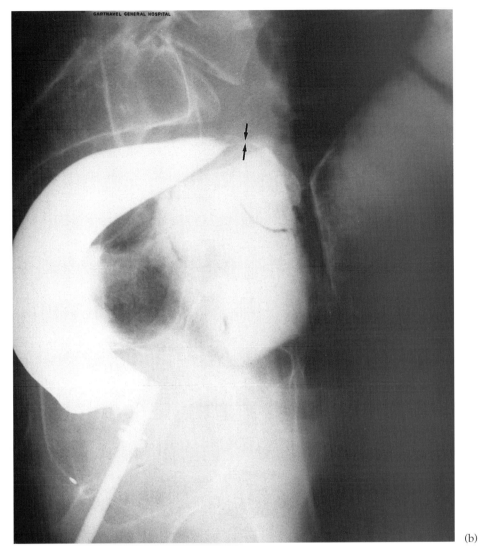

(b)

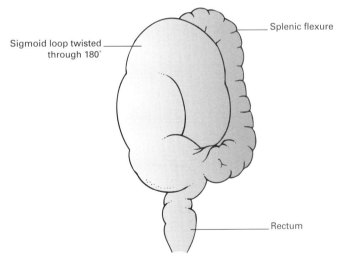

Splenic flexure

Sigmoid loop twisted
through 180°

Rectum

(c)

Fig. 6.64 *Continued.* (b) The lateral view of the rectum shows the typical bird-beak sign at the level of the twisted mesentery (arrows). (c) Diagram of a sigmoid volvulus. (Redrawn from [45] with permission.)

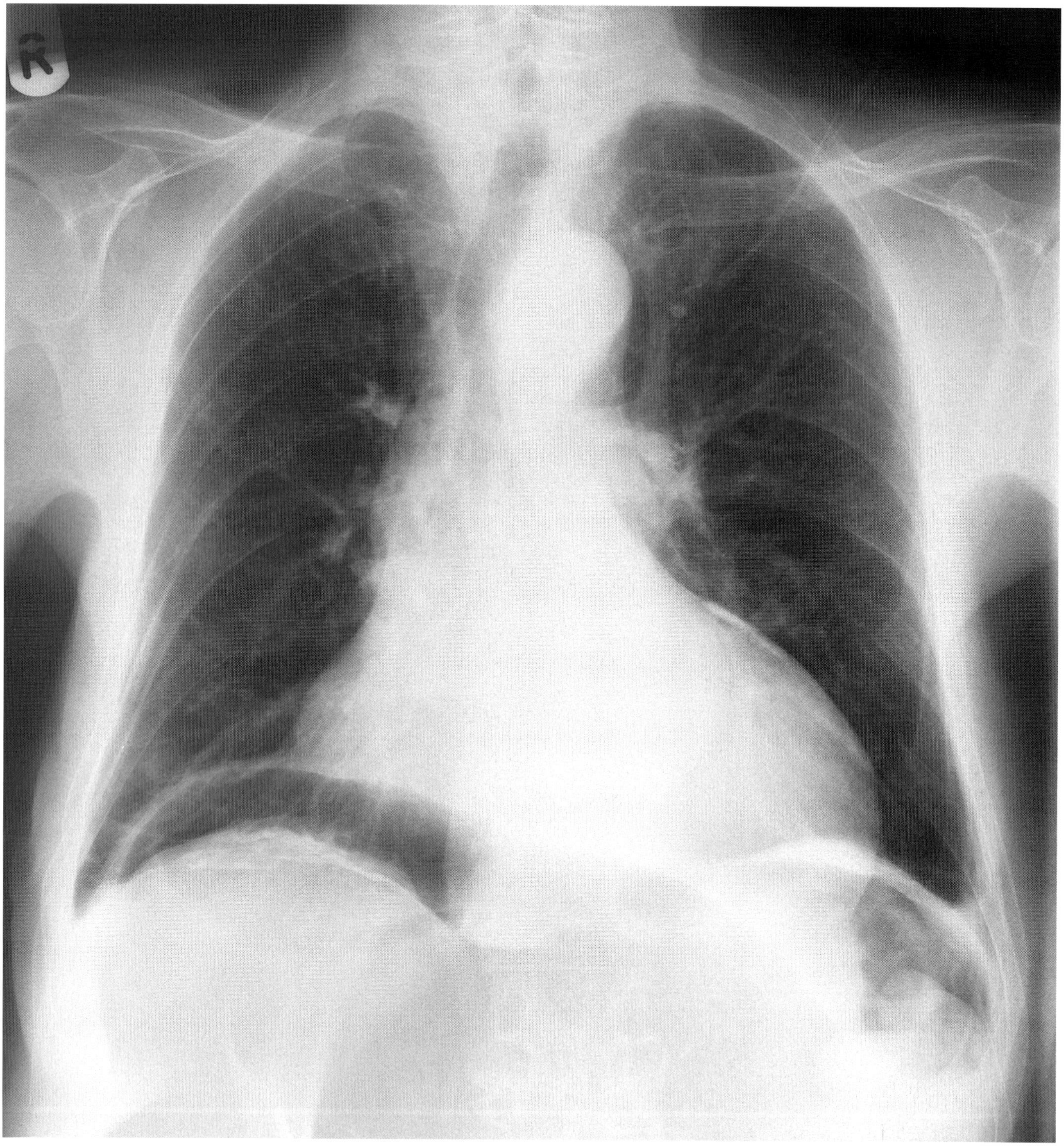

Fig. 6.65 Sigmoid volvulus. In another patient with sigmoid volvulus, the apex of the massively distended sigmoid loop is seen to be interposed between the diaphragm and the liver. This should not be confused with a pneumoperitoneum. In addition, the patient has bilateral pleural calcification as a result of previous exposure to asbestos.

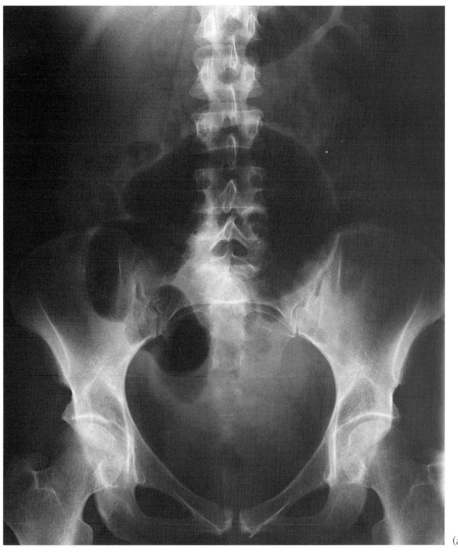

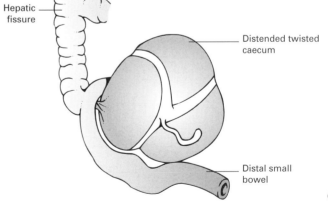

Fig. 6.66 Volvulus of the right hemicolon. A middle-aged female patient presented with central abdominal pain and distension. (a) A plain supine X-ray shows a large central abdominal gas shadow, with a slightly distended gas-filled small bowel in the right iliac fossa. A volvulus of the caecum was confirmed at operation 2 h later. (b) Diagram of a caecal volvulus showing the relationship between the twisted, obstructed caecum, the normal colon beyond the obstruction, and the distal small bowel. (Redrawn from [45] with permission.)

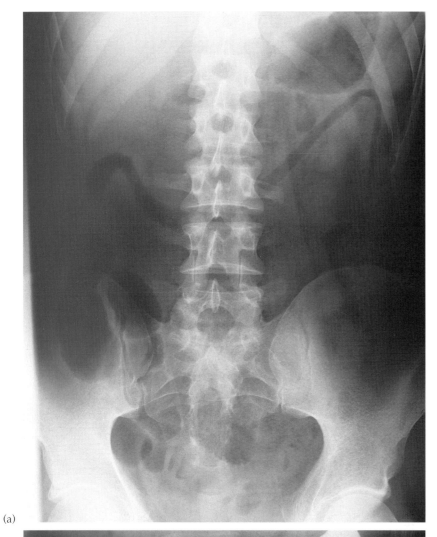

(a)

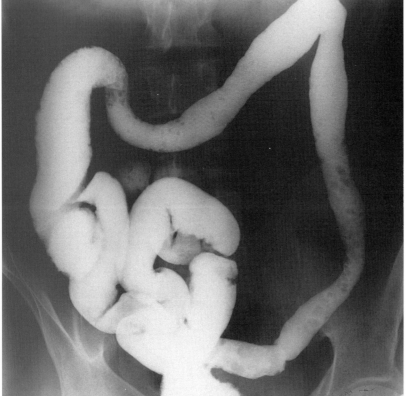

(b)

Fig. 6.67 Ulcerative colitis (advanced). (a) The plain film shows a grossly contracted, ribbon-like, colonic gas shadow, which is shortened, completely lacking in a haustral pattern and irregular in outline. (b) A SCBE on the same patient also shows a grossly contracted colon with no haustration, but with multiple filling defects. These pseudopolyps are due to islands of inflamed mucosa in an otherwise denuded bowel wall.

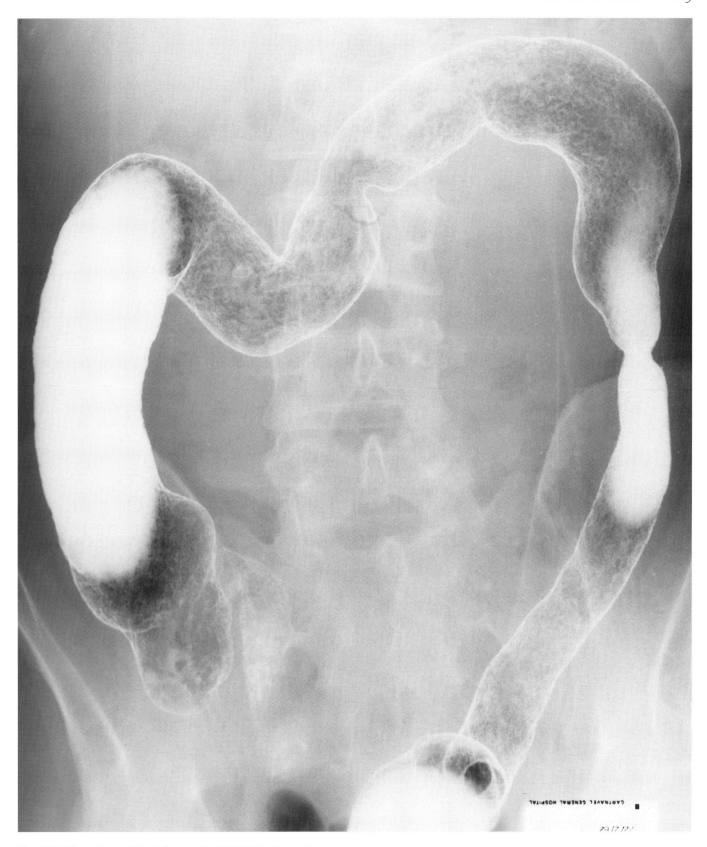

Fig. 6.68 Ulcerative colitis (advanced). A DCBE in this patient
with histologically proved ulcerative colitis shows a generalized
reduction in distensibility, complete loss of haustration and
diffuse mucosal granularity.

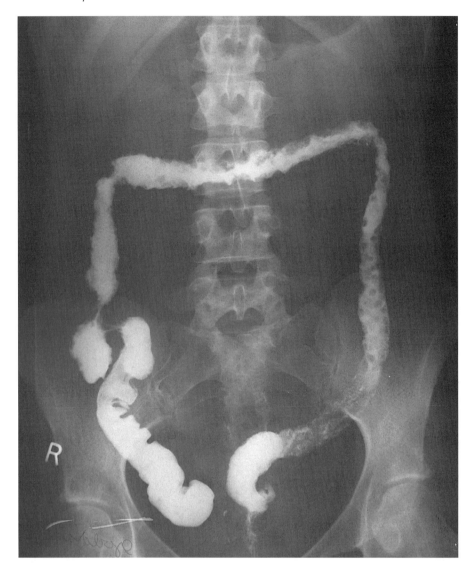

Fig. 6.69 Ulcerative colitis (advanced).
The patient had a long history of
diarrhoea, rectal bleeding, weight loss and
anaemia. This postevacuation DCBE film
shows a shortened contracted colon with
widespread pseudopolyp formation.
There is also a stricture at the hepatic
flexure, which was inflammatory.
Malignancy cannot be excluded without
histology.

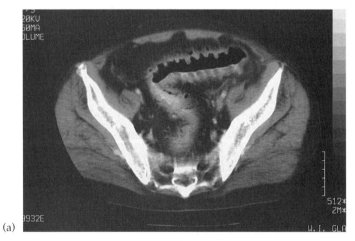

(a)

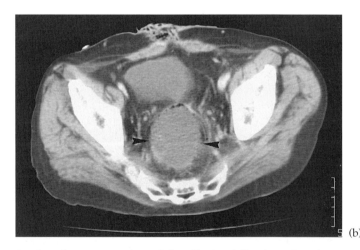

(b)

**Fig. 6.70 Ulcerative colitis complicated by a postoperative
pelvic abscess.** (a) A CT scan through the pelvis shows marked
thickening of the wall of the sigmoid colon, due to oedema, and
there is also pseudopolyp formation. Histology indicated
inflammatory bowel disease without granulomata. (b) The patient
developed a postoperative pelvic collection following subtotal
colectomy and oversewing of the rectum. The white-cell count
was 23 000. A relatively well-defined abscess cavity is shown
posterior to the bladder (arrowheads). Gas bubbles are visible in
the abscess anteriorly.

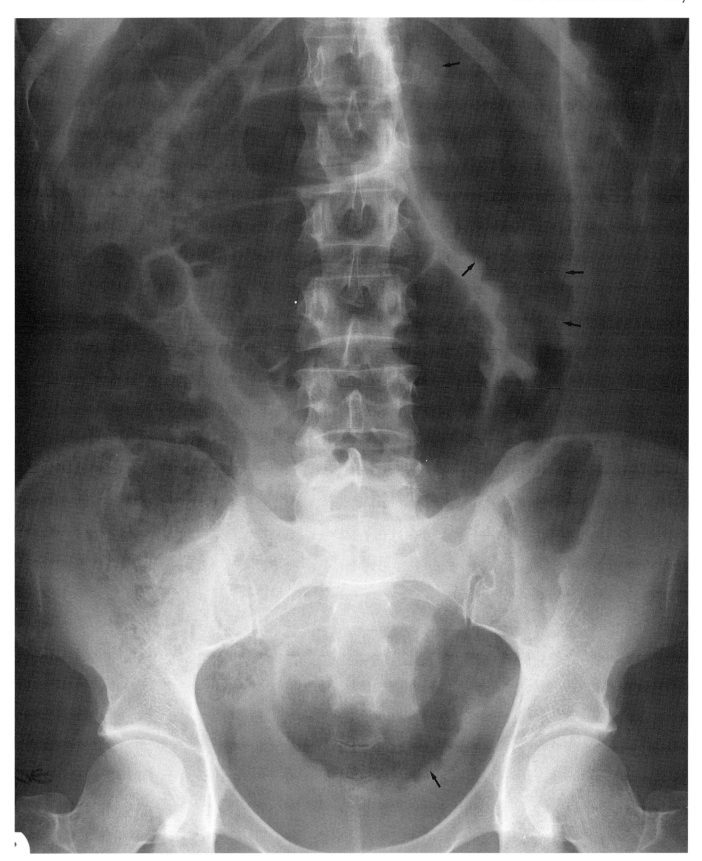

Fig. 6.71 Toxic dilatatation complicating ulcerative colitis. A plain X-ray of a patient with acute exacerbation of ulcerative colitis characterized by worsening diarrhoea, abdominal distension and anaemia. This X-ray shows marked colonic distension—the transverse colon measuring 9 cm. In addition, there are widespread islands of oedematous mucosa (arrows), which together indicate toxic dilation. The mortality associated with this complication is at least 20%.

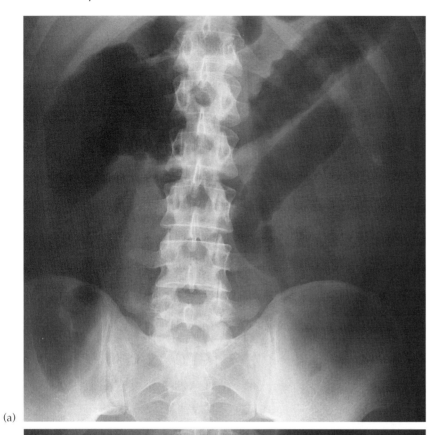

(a)

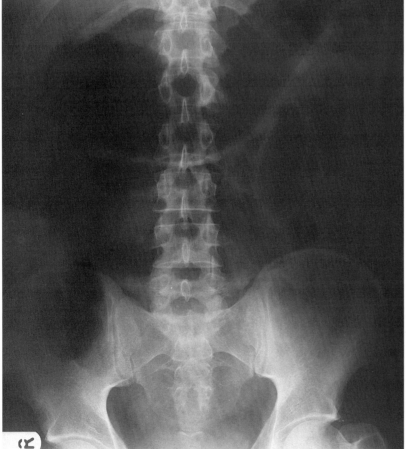

(b)

Fig. 6.72 Toxic dilatation complicating ulcerative colitis. This 36-year-old male patient had worsening diarrhoea and rectal bleeding. (a) The film shows gross mucosal swelling affecting the transverse colon, which, to the right of the midline, is distended. The descending colon is featureless and filled with fluid. (b) A second abdominal film taken 24 h after (a) shows progression of toxic dilatation in the transverse colon. The upper limit of normal is 5.5 cm.

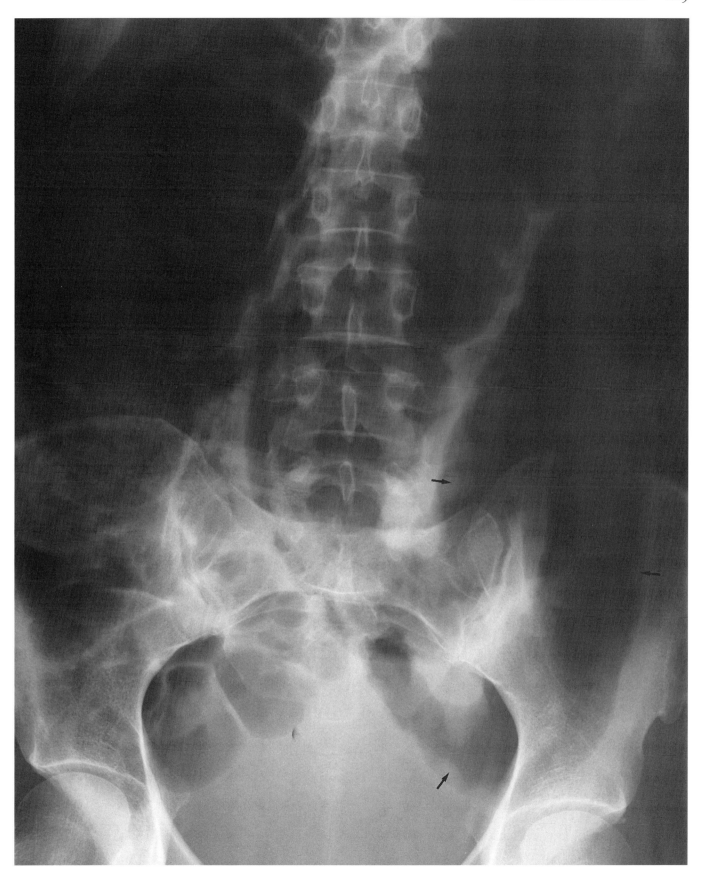

Fig. 6.73 Toxic dilatation complicating ulcerative colitis. A third patient showed gross gaseous colonic distension where the transverse colon measures 10 cm in diameter, and is associated with widespread islands of oedematous mucosa (arrows).

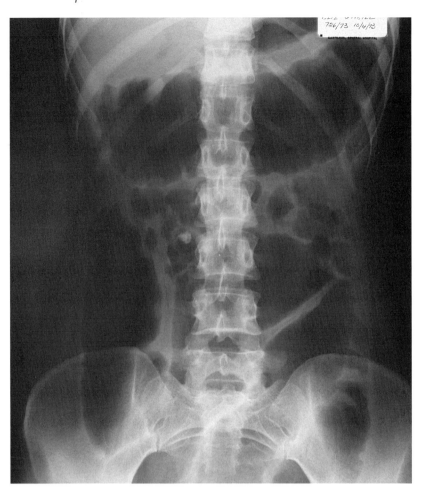

Fig. 6.74 Toxic dilatation complicating ulcerative colitis. This middle-aged female patient had a 2-year history of periodic diarrhoea and rectal bleeding, recent abdominal distension and hypotension. The plain abdominal film shows marked gaseous distension of the transverse colon to 8 cm, together with widespread islands of oedematous mucosa, including the ascending colon. There is also evidence of oedema of the properitoneal fat line.

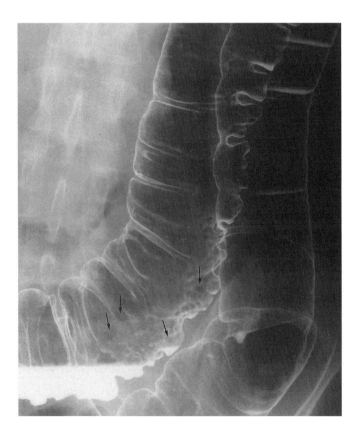

Fig. 6.75 Crohn's disease of the colon. The DCBE shows multiple aphthoid ulcers (arrows), chiefly affecting the inferior margin of the transverse colon, with asymmetrical loss of the haustral pattern in this part of the large bowel.

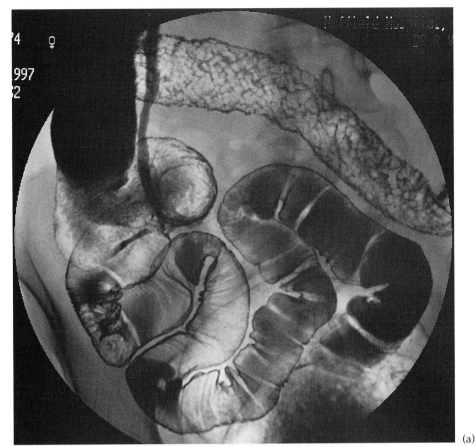

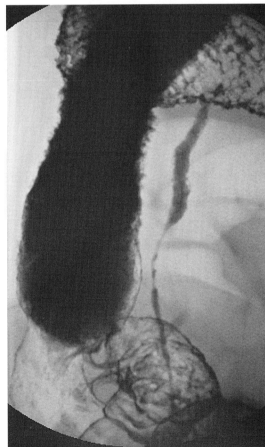

Fig. 6.76 Crohn's disease of the colon and appendix. (a) This DCBE of a 17-year-old girl with several months' history of diarrhoea, weight loss and iron-deficiency anaemia shows complete loss of the haustral pattern, generalized reduced distensibility and a very widespread cobblestone pattern, resulting from mucosal oedema interspersed by longitudinal and transverse ulcers. The appendix is similarly affected. The terminal ileum is conspicuously normal. (b) A spot view with magnification shows the inflammatory changes in the ascending colon and appendix in more detail.

(a)

(b)

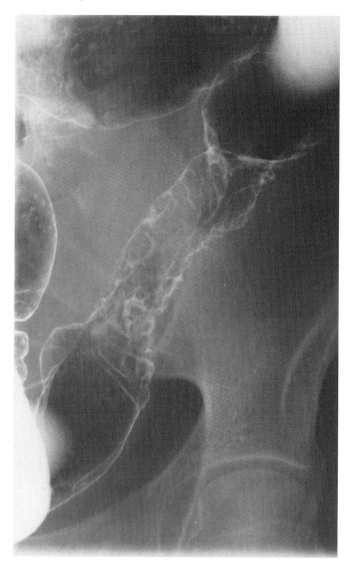

Fig. 6.77 Crohn's disease of the colon. Part of a DCBE showing an 8 cm long stricture of the sigmoid colon, with mucosal nodularity and ulceration. Positive histology for Crohn's disease.

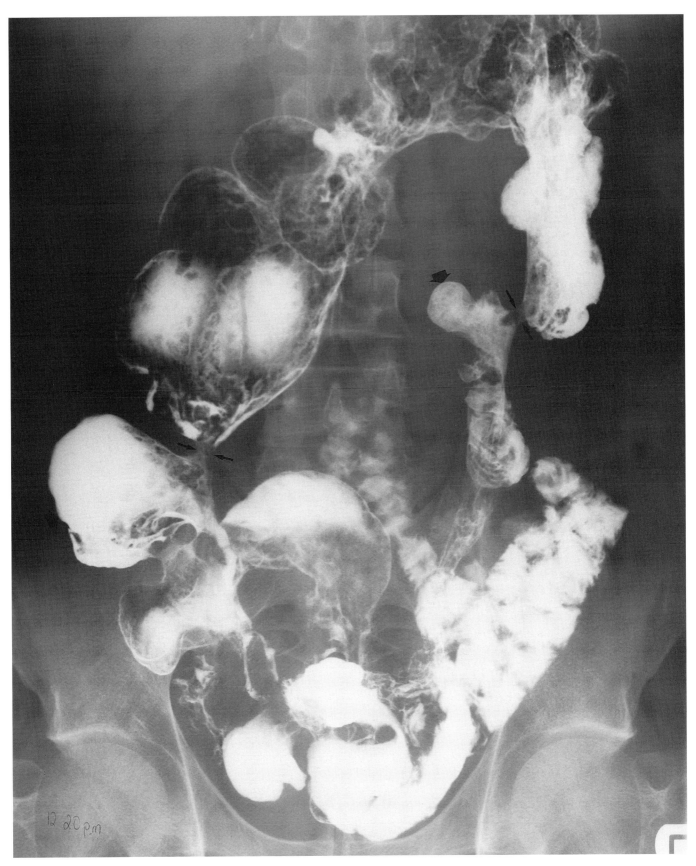

Fig. 6.78 Crohn's disease of the colon and distal small bowel.
This late barium-meal follow-through film shows deformity, dilatation and some stricture formation affecting the distal small bowel. In addition, the large bowel is grossly abnormal, with multiple eccentric strictures (arrows) and intervening sacculations or pseudodiverticula (arrowhead). Aphthoid ulcers are also visible.

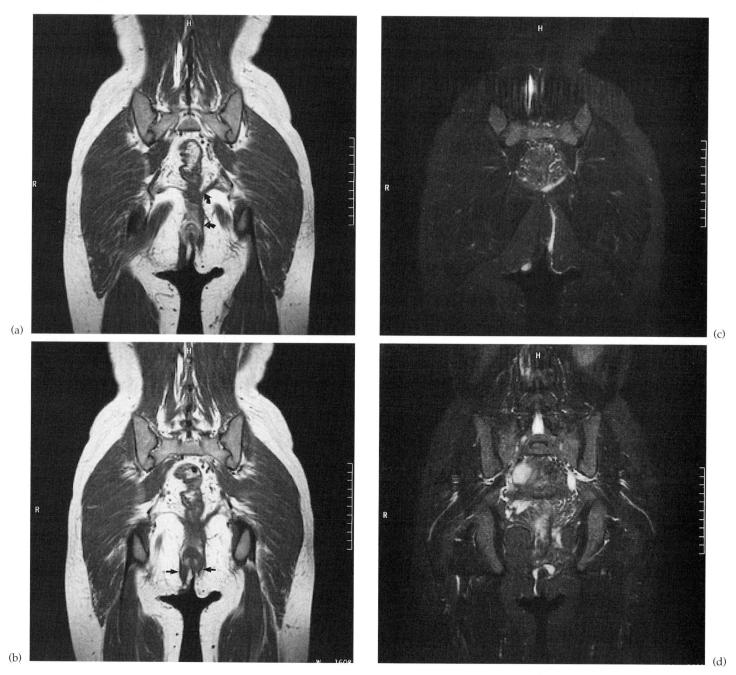

Fig. 6.79 Perianal fistulae. This 33-year-old female patient had Crohn's disease and recurrent perianal fistulae. (a and b) Coronal T_1 SE of the pelvis show low signal confined to the ischiorectal fossa (straight arrows) and high, extending above the levator ani (curved arrows). Fistulous tracks are also seen, which are better demonstrated on coronal STIR (c and d) as high-signal tracks. (Courtesy of Dr J. Graeme Houston.)

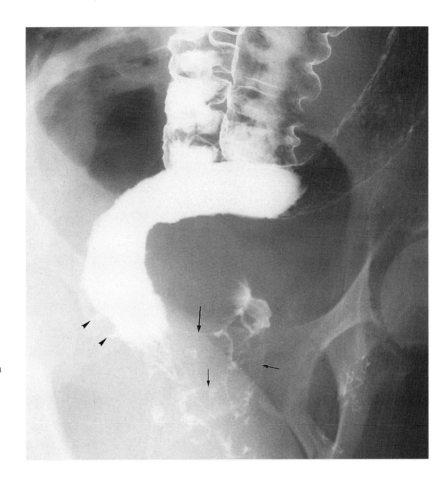

Fig. 6.80 Crohn's disease complicated by complex rectovaginal fistulae. The DCBE shows a grossly contracted and ulcerated rectum and distal sigmoid colon. Several penetrating rectal ulcers are visible (arrowheads). In addition, there are multiple interconnecting fistulae linking the lower rectum and anal canal with the vagina (arrows).

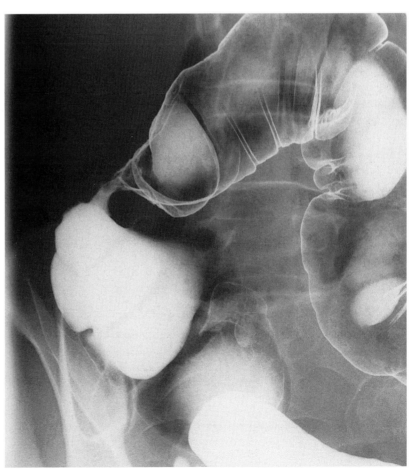

Fig. 6.81 Colonic Crohn's disease complicated by localized stricture. A recent colonoscopy of a female patient with a 2-year history of colonic Crohn's disease (positive biopsy) suggested a stricture involving the caecum. The DCBE shows a tight, eccentric, slightly irregular stricture proximal to the hepatic flexure.

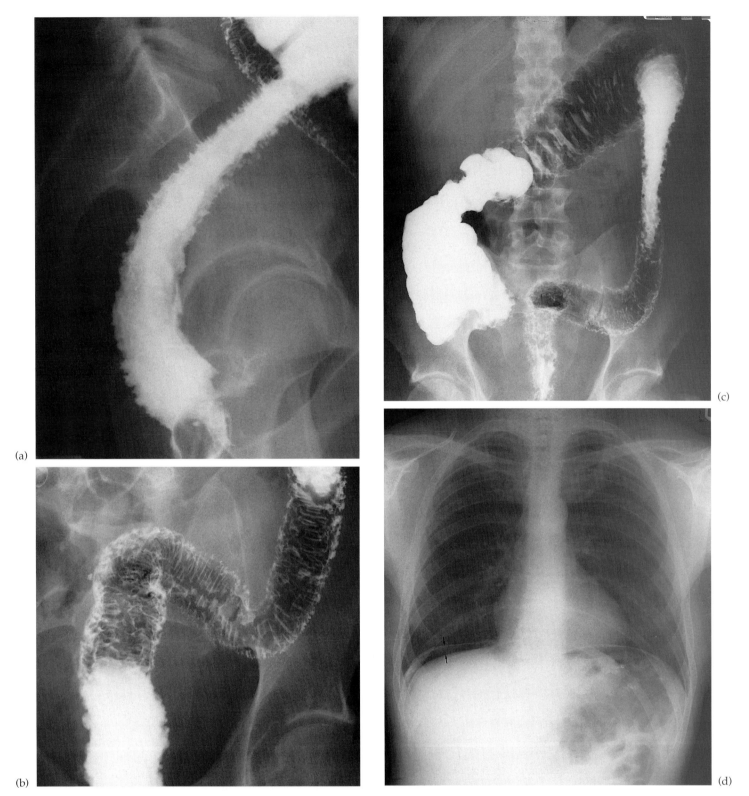

Fig. 6.82 Colonic Crohn's disease complicated by perforation.
(a) A 55-year-old male patient had severe diarrhoea, abdominal pain, weight loss, rectal bleeding and anaemia. A lateral single-contrast view of the rectum shows marked loss of distensibility and very widespread penetrating ulceration. (b) An AP view of the sigmoid colon in the same patient shows florid inflammatory changes also, including conspicuous transverse ulceration. (c) Postevacuation film shows changes of inflammatory bowel disease affecting the whole of the large bowel. There is no evidence of perforation. (d) Having commenced on prednisolone, the patient attended for a small-bowel enema 9 days later, to assess any possible small-bowel involvement. There had been no clinical deterioration in the patient's condition and, in particular, he was still ambulant. Preliminary fluoroscopy demonstrated gas under both diaphragms (arrows). Inflammatory changes are visible on the gas shadow of the splenic flexure. At operation, colonic perforation was confirmed, but there was no evidence of barium in the peritoneal cavity.

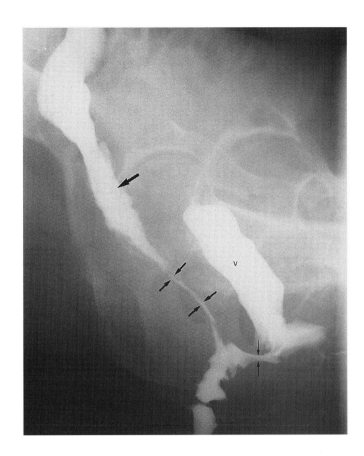

Fig. 6.83 Rectal Crohn's disease complicated by anovaginal fistula. A limited water-soluble contrast enema shows a contracted ulcerated rectum (large arrow), with stricture formation involving the distal rectum (smaller arrows). The contrast is seen to fill the vagina (v) via a very low fistula (thin arrows) connecting the anal canal with the posterior margin of the vagina.

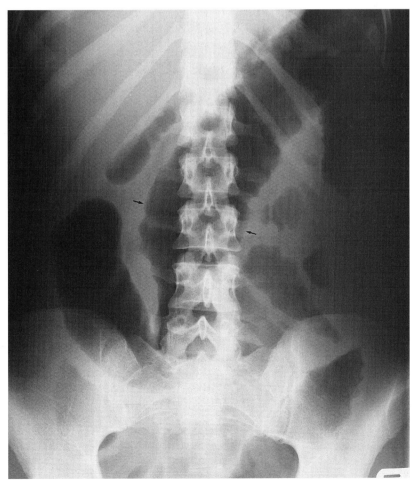

Fig. 6.84 Crohn's disease complicated by toxic dilatation. A plain film was taken of this 23-year-old female patient with rapid deterioration in her general condition, diarrhoea, abdominal distension and rectal bleeding. It shows generalized dilatation of the transverse colon (8 cm between arrows). In addition, there is marginal irregularity, 'thumbprinting', in keeping with diffuse inflammatory change. Toxic dilatation was confirmed at operation. At this stage, it is impossible to distinguish Crohn's disease from non-specific ulcerative colitis on plain films.

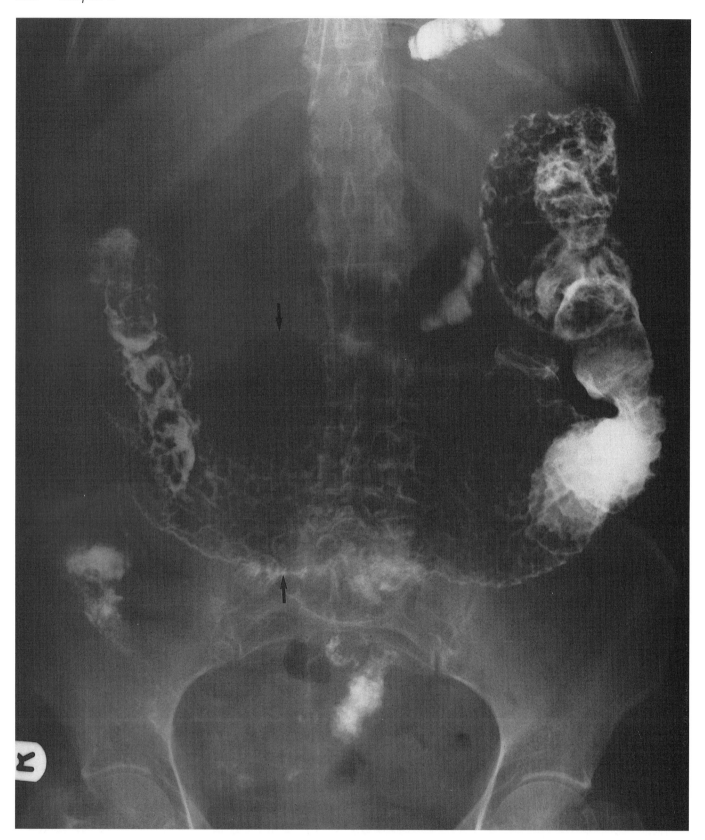

Fig. 6.85 Pseudomembranous colitis complicated by toxic dilatation. A 60-year-old female patient had had a right hemicolectomy for colon cancer 10 days previously, at which time the remainder of the large bowel was normal. A difficult postoperative period was characterized by considerable abdominal distension. Her management included antibiotic therapy. A late film of barium-meal follow-through shows marked dilatation of the transverse colon (11.5 cm between arrows) and the mucosa has a grossly abnormal reticular or cobblestone pattern. There was endoscopic evidence of pseudomembranous colitis.

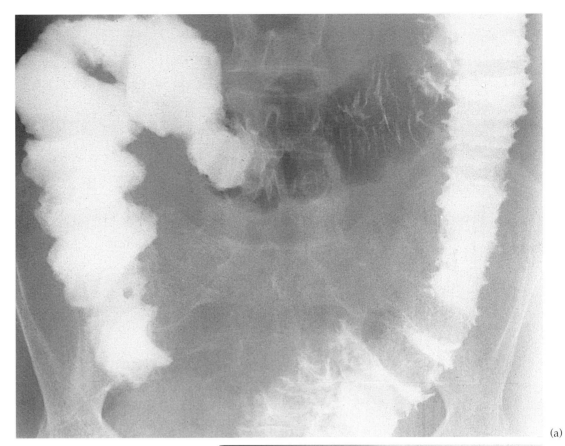

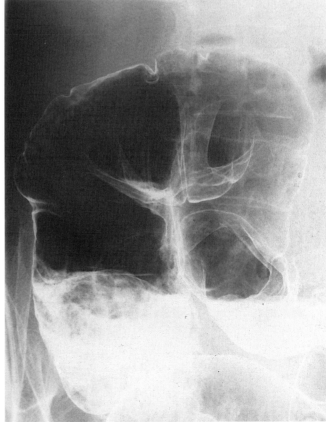

Fig. 6.86 Fat encrustation of the colon. (a) A barium enema in a female patient with known coeliac disease shows a grossly abnormal mucosal coating, which is due to encrustation with fat, resulting from small-bowel malabsorption. (b) A repeat examination 3 months later shows a normal colonic mucosa, the patient having been on a gluten-free diet for 2 months. This condition should not be confused with inflammatory bowel disease.

(a)

(b)

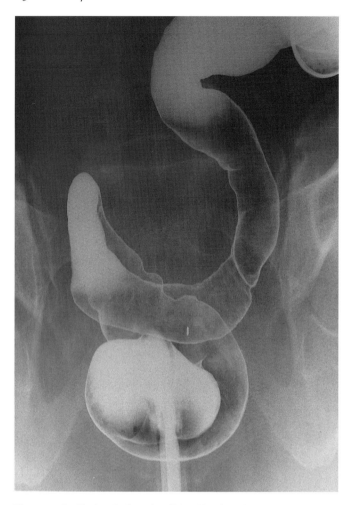

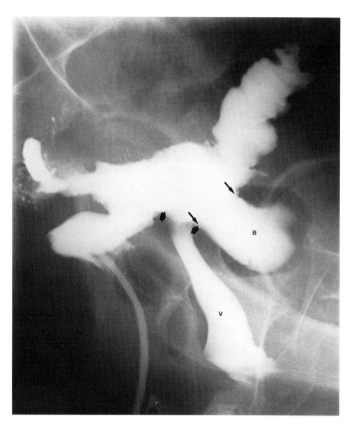

Fig. 6.87 Radiation-induced colitis. This female patient with a past history of carcinoma of the cervix was treated by radiotherapy 2 years previously. She was known to have radiation cystitis. In the past month, she developed rectal bleeding, with both fresh and altered blood. The DCBE shows a moderate reduced distensibility of the upper rectum and lower half of the sigmoid colon, the mucosa having a very fine granular texture. The biopsy was consistent with radiation colitis.

Fig. 6.88 Radiation colitis complicated by fistulae. This female patient had a history of radiotherapy for colorectal carcinoma. The single-contrast water-soluble study via a rectal catheter shows contraction and deformity of the rectum, with a large fistula (arrowheads) into the vagina (V) and an even larger fistula (arrows) into the bladder (B).

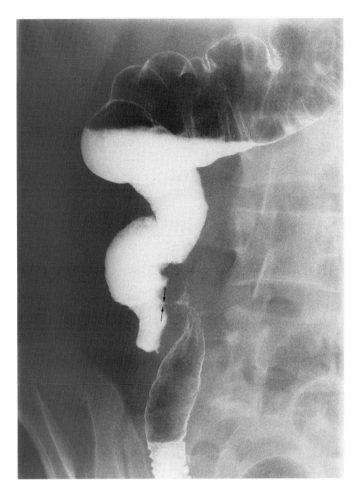

Fig. 6.89 Colonic tuberculosis. An 18-year-old male patient presented with a cold abscess affecting his wrist and subsequently developed diarrhoea. The DCBE erect view shows contraction of the ascending colon and, in particular, the caecum. The ileocaecal valve is irregularly contracted (arrows) and the distal 2 cm of the terminal ileum is irregular in outline, with at least one short sinus track. Acid-fast bacilli were isolated from the cold abscess and from the colon.

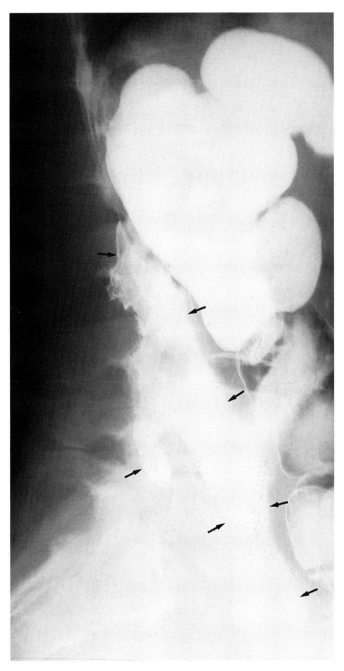

Fig. 6.90 Retrocolic abscess complicating xanthogranulomatous pyelonephritis. This female patient had had a left nephrectomy for xanthogranulomatous pyelonephritis. The lateral view of the descending colon shows a very extensive retrocolic collection of contrast (arrows) filling a large cavity, which communicates with the lumen at the splenic flexure. This was surgically drained, resulting in several cutaneous fistulae, which eventually healed spontaneously.

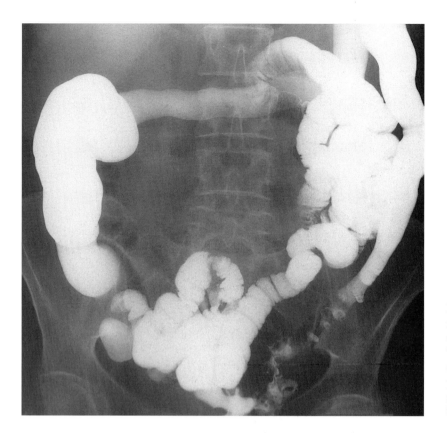

Fig. 6.91 Amoebic dysentery. A 65-year-old female patient had a history of three proved episodes of amoebic dysentery over several years. This SCBE shows generalized contraction of the colon, with virtually complete loss of the haustral pattern. The appearance is indistinguishable from non-specific ulcerative colitis radiologically. Sigmoid diverticula are also visible.

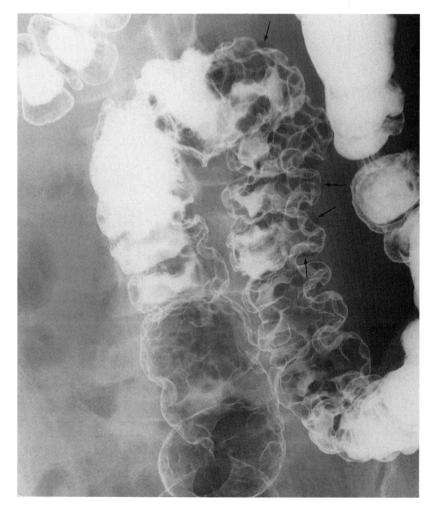

Fig. 6.92 Pneumatosis cystoides coli. This 54-year-old male patient had a history of chronic obstructive airway disease and recent mucous discharge per rectum. The DCBE shows multiple gas-filled intramural filling defects in the sigmoid colon (arrows). Although these are visible on DCBE, they may be more obvious on a CT scan. A subserous location is more frequent than in the submucosa.

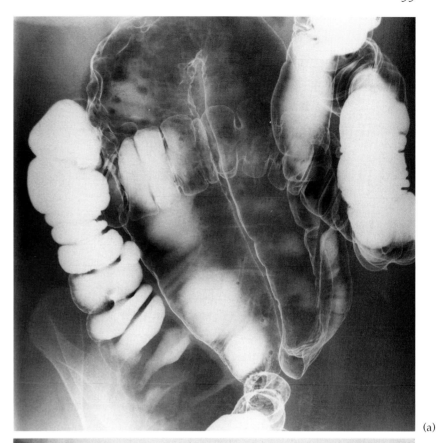

(a)

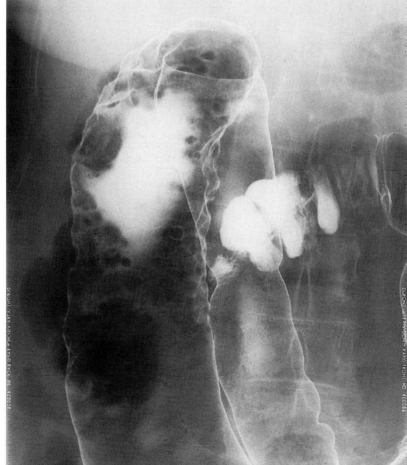

(b)

Fig. 6.93 Pneumatosis cystoides coli in a patient with a history of recurrent sigmoid volvulus. (a) Multiple radiolucent filling defects are shown in the region of the apex of the redundant sigmoid loop. These gas-filled cysts are more obvious in (b). Although no volvulus was present at the time of the examination, the length of the sigmoid loop and the apparent narrowness of the base of the sigmoid mesocolon predispose to recurrent twisting and obstruction. Volvulus is a recognized predisposing factor to pneumatosis, together with obstructive airways disease, cystic fibrosis, artificial ventilation and intestinal ischaemia.

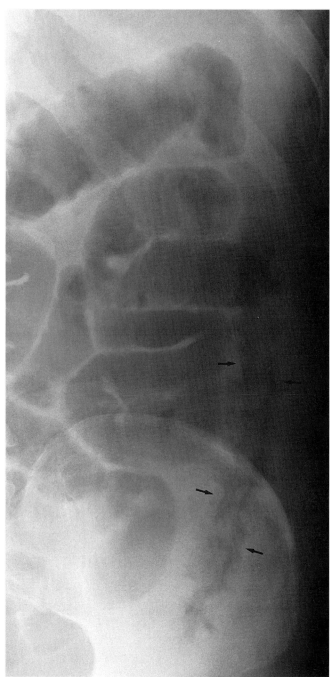

(a)

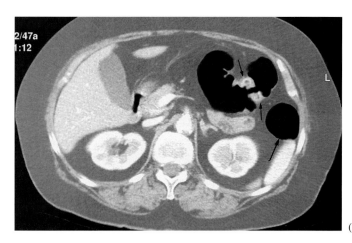

(b)

Fig. 6.94 (a) Ischaemic colitis. The plain supine abdominal film of an elderly male patient with acute onset of rectal bleeding shows a grossly abnormal gas pattern in the descending colon, with a very prominent widespread pattern of thumbprinting (arrows). This is typical of, but not diagnostic of, ischaemic colitis. The splenic flexure is also involved, but less obviously so. In addition, there is non-specific mild gaseous distension of the small-bowel loops. **(b) Colonic stricture resulting from ischaemia.** A CT pneumocolon in an elderly female patient with a short history of abdominal pain shows a short annular stricture of the transverse colon close to the splenic flexure (short arrows). This was thought to be due to carcinoma. At laparotomy no mass was palpable, but an intraoperative colonoscopy was performed via the transverse colon and the stricture was visualized. The bowel resection revealed a short stricture, the pathology of which was consistent with a post-ischaemic stenosis. Large arrow, normal descending colon.

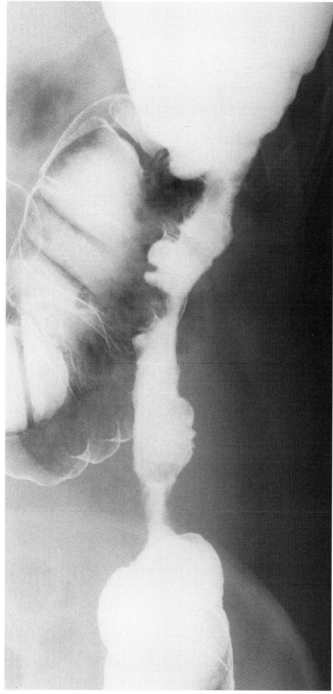

(a)

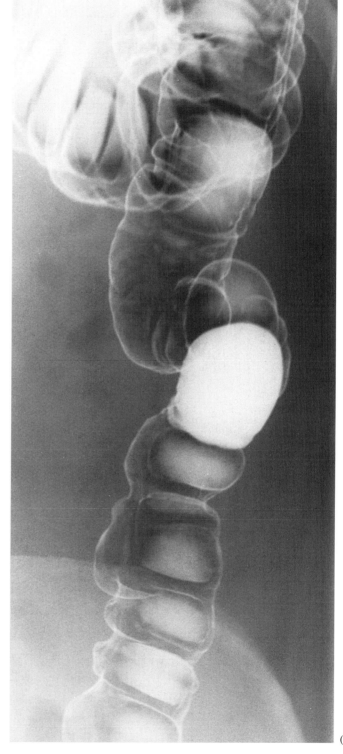

(b)

Fig. 6.95 Ischaemic colitis. Double-contrast barium enemas of a 44-year-old female patient with a sudden onset of severe abdominal pain and rectal bleeding. (a) The first DCBE shows a 12 cm segment of proximal descending colon which is persistently contracted and irregular in outline, but without any definite evidence of ulceration. The location close to the splenic flexure is typical of ischaemia, which represents a watershed between the middle colic territory of the superior mesenteric artery and the left colic territory of the inferior mesenteric artery. (b) A DCBE in the same patient 8 weeks later shows virtually complete reversal of the ischaemic change, with more or less normal distensibility and no mucosal lesion.

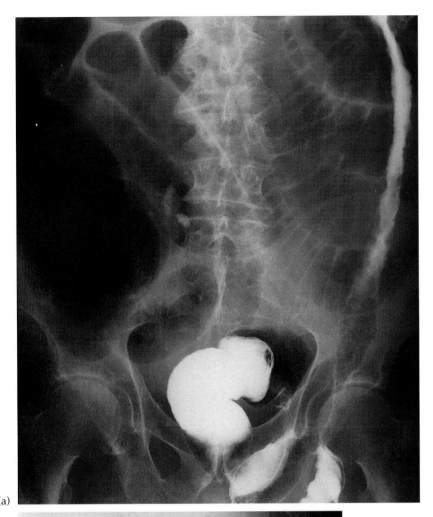

(a)

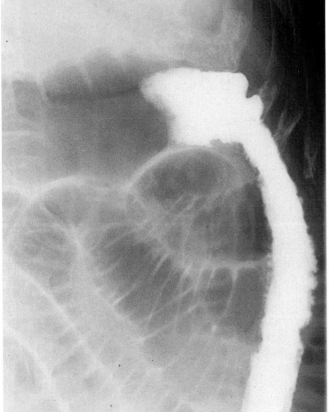

(b)

Fig. 6.96 Colonic obstruction secondary to ischaemic colitis.
An elderly male patient presented with progressive abdominal
distension and obstructive bowel sounds. (a) A limited
Gastrografin enema shows gross gaseous distension proximal to
the splenic flexure. There is also massive dilatation of multiple
small-bowel loops because of patency of the ileocaecal valve.
Gastrografin is shown in the rectum and within a left inguinal
hernia containing sigmoid colon, which was unobstructed. The
whole of the descending colon is grossly contracted and irregular
in outline. (b) The Gastrografin is seen to flow retrogradely
beyond the splenic flexure into the transverse colon, without any
tight stricture being demonstrated. At operation, the same day,
severe chronic ischaemic colitis limited to the descending colon
was confirmed, but associated with massive colonic obstruction
proximal to this. There was no evidence of ischaemia affecting the
small bowel or right hemicolon. The patient died postoperatively.

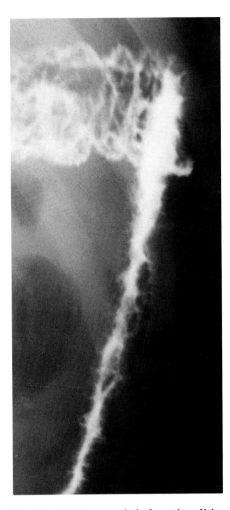

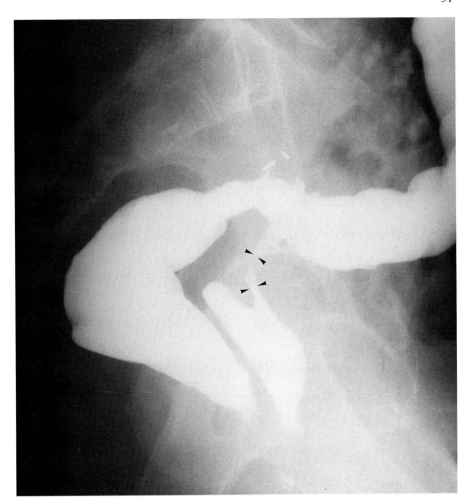

Fig. 6.97 Post-traumatic ischaemic colitis.
A 25-year-old male patient sustained severe abdominal injuries from multiple stab wounds, with extensive trauma to the small bowel and mesentery, resulting in extensive sepsis. A limited barium study of the large bowel approximately 4 weeks after the injury shows gross contraction of the upper descending colon, with marked marginal irregularity, in keeping with ischaemia.

Fig. 6.98 Rectovaginal fistula (postoperative). The patient had had a recent sigmoid colectomy for carcinoma and discharged faeces per vaginam. A lateral view of this single-contrast study shows a fistula (arrowheads) at the level of the colorectal anastomosis marked by the surgical clips. Contrast is seen to drain into the vagina.

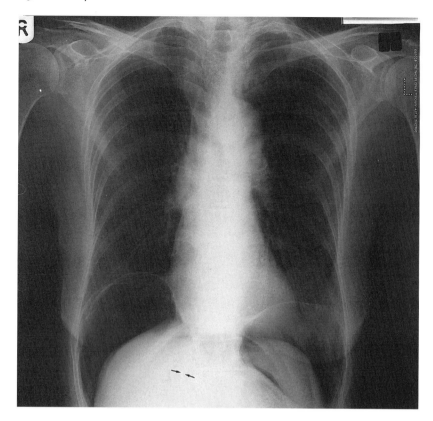

Fig. 6.99 Colonic perforation during colonoscopy. This patient developed sudden abdominal pain during colonoscopy. The erect AP chest X-ray shows a large volume of free air in the peritoneal cavity, the air collecting under both hemidiaphragms. Part of the falciform ligament is also outlined by air (arrows).

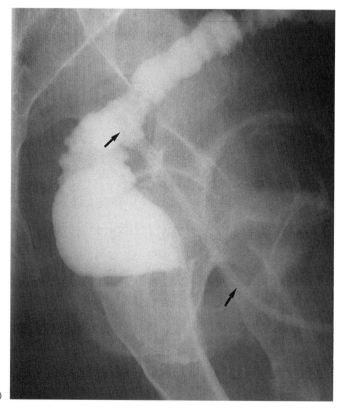

(a)

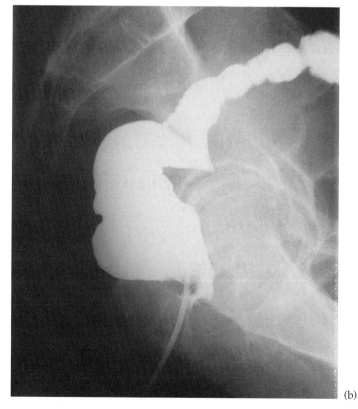

(b)

Fig. 6.100 Rectovesical fistula complicating transurethral prostatectomy. (a) Urografin 150 is introduced via the urethral catheter (arrows). It is apparent that the catheter has crossed a rectovesical fistula, since only the rectum and sigmoid colon are seen to fill with contrast. (b) The SCBE 4 months later shows angular deformity of the anterior wall of the rectum at the site of the previous fistula, but there is no evidence of any persistent connection.

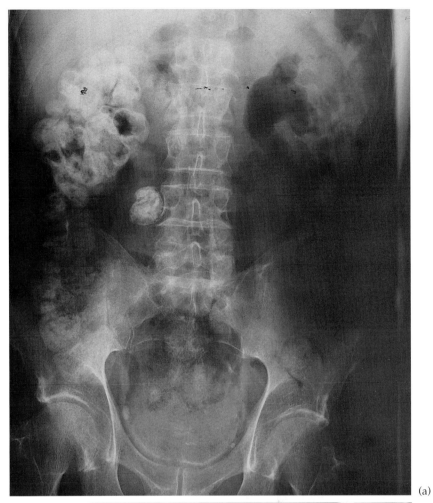

(a)

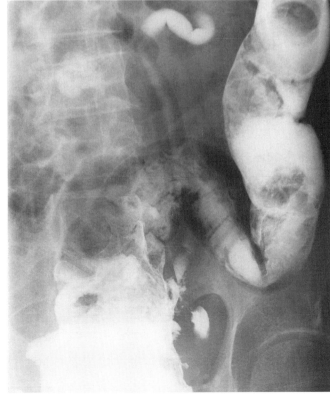

Fig. 6.101 Ureterocolic fistula complicating anterior resection of the colon. (a) The moderately distended collecting system of the left kidney is almost completely outlined by gas. (b) An instant enema with water-soluble contrast shows a connection between the distal colon and the left ureter, which is seen to fill with contrast. Contrast is also seen to escape laterally into a small cavity.

(b)

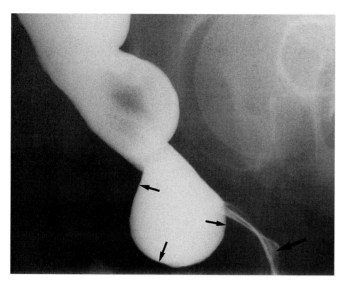

Fig. 6.102 Posterior rectocele. A dynamic proctogram shows a well-defined posterior bulge in the lower rectum (small arrows), which is seen to form when the patient strains. The position of the anal canal is indicated by the large arrow.

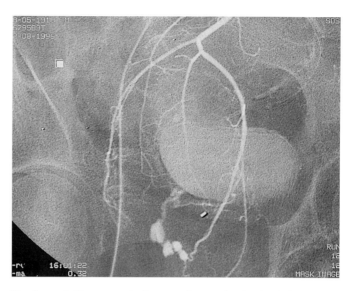

Fig. 6.104 Solitary rectal ulcer syndrome. A selective inferior mesenteric arteriogram shows extravasation from a branch of the superior rectal artery due to a solitary rectal ulcer. (Courtesy of Dr Richard D. Edwards.)

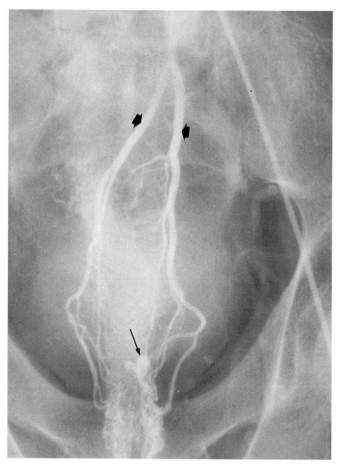

Fig. 6.103 Internal haemorrhoid. A 25-year-old male patient had rectal bleeding, anaemia and a previous haemorrhoidectomy. Recent investigations, including endoscopy and DCBE, were negative. The inferior mesenteric angiogram shows normal filling of the left and right divisions of the superior haemorrhoidal artery (arrowheads). However, there is a contrast-filled varicose vessel (arrow) in the distal rectum, indicating a recurrent haemorrhoid.

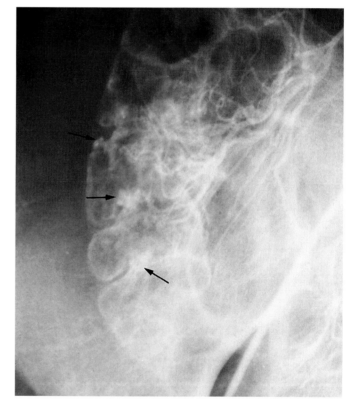

Fig. 6.105 Angiodysplasia of the caecum. A 20-year-old female patient with a long history of rectal bleeding had a normal colonoscopy, DCBE, gastrointestinal endoscopy and double-contrast barium meal. Superior mesenteric angiography shows multiple small dysplastic vessels in the wall of the caecum (arrows).

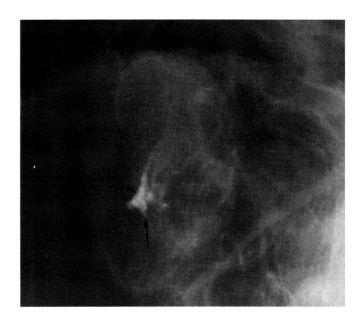

Fig. 6.106 Angiodysplasia of the caecum. A 75-year-old retired medical practitioner with rectal bleeding had a negative previous investigation. Superior mesenteric angiography shows dysplastic vessels in the wall of the caecum (arrows).

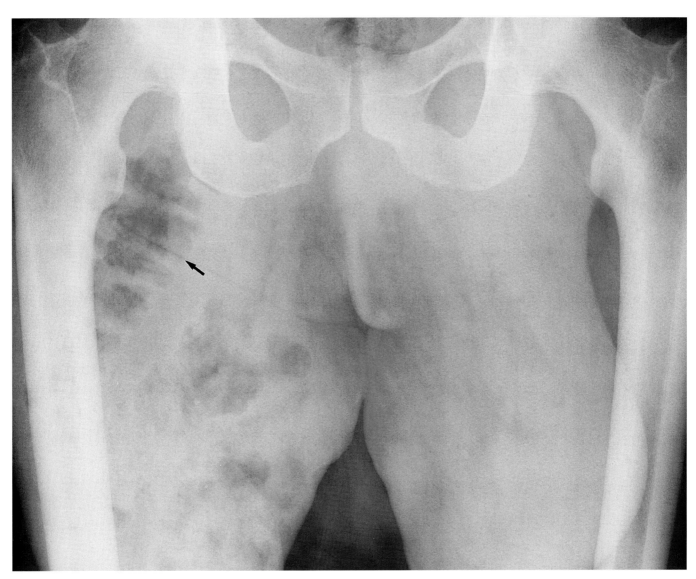

Fig. 6.107 Bilateral inguinal herniae. This patient was referred from a medical ward for ultrasound of the testes. A plain X-ray of the lower pelvis and upper thigh shows a huge bilateral scrotal swelling, with obvious gas shadows on the right side, with a well-developed haustral pattern (arrow), indicating large bowel.

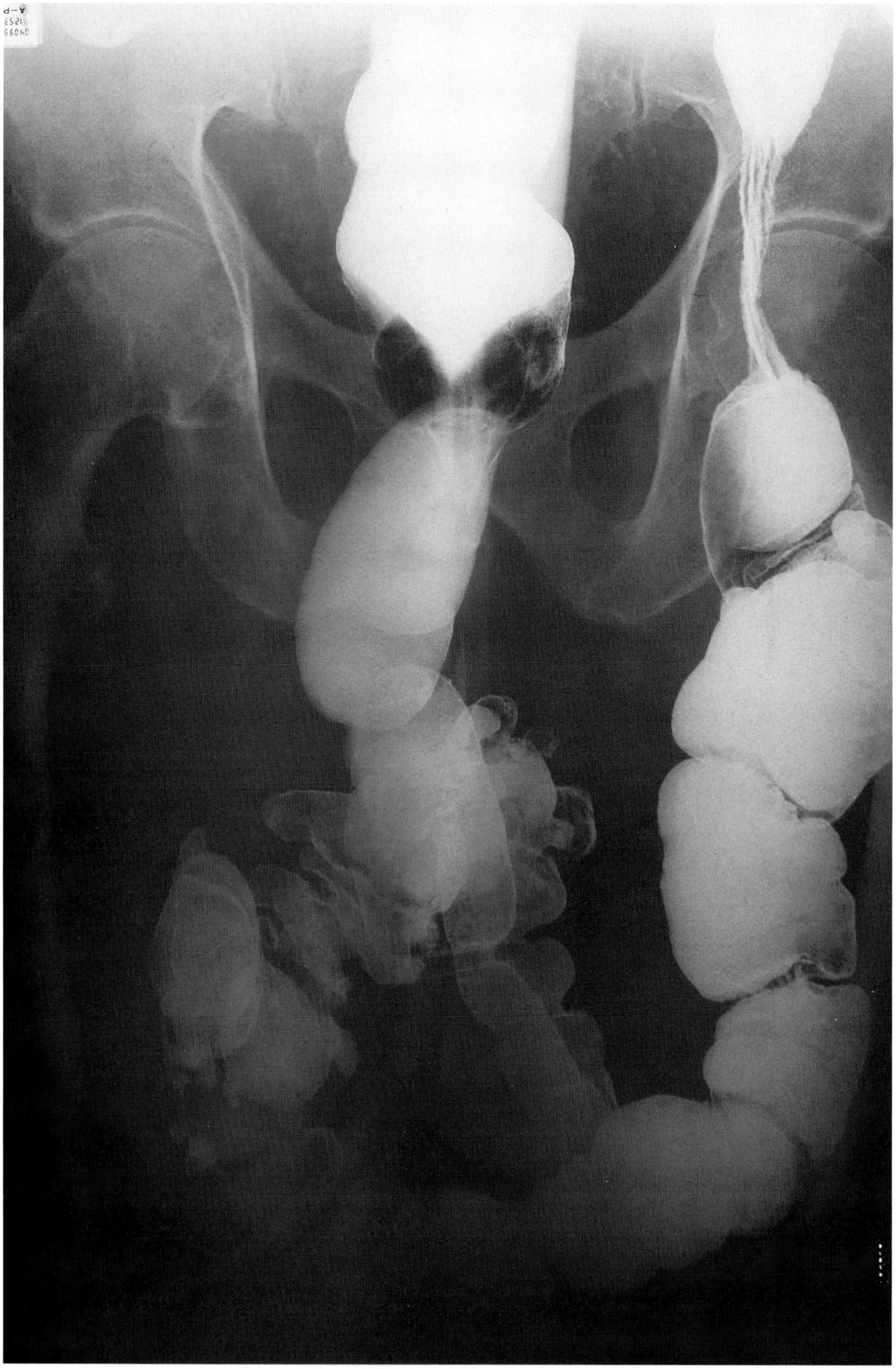

Fig. 6.108 Left inguinal hernia containing colon. An AP view of
the lower pelvis and thigh shows a huge left-sided inguinal
hernia containing a substantial portion of the large bowel, which
is seen to be affected by diverticular disease. The neck of the
hernia sac is very wide, there being no evidence of intestinal
obstruction.

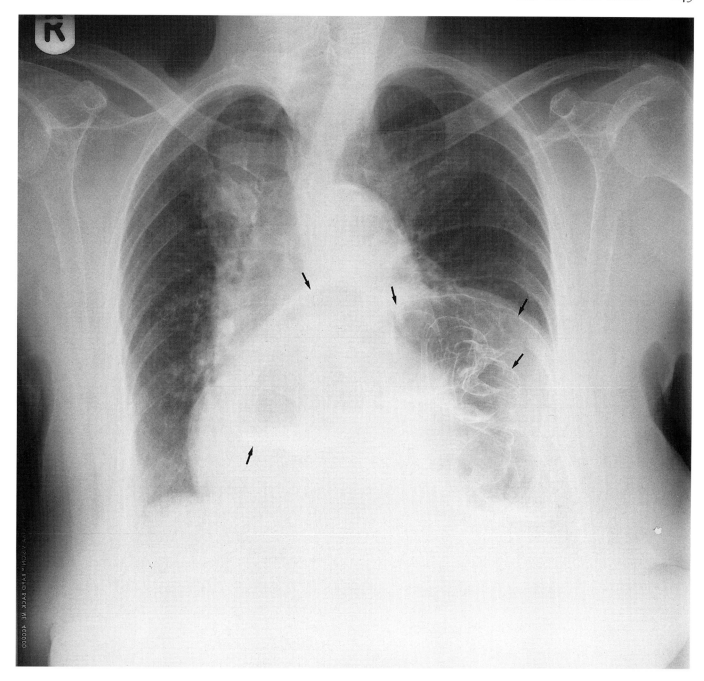

Fig. 6.109 Morgagni hernia. A chest X-ray in an elderly patient immediately after a DCBE shows a large diaphragmatic hernia containing a substantial portion of the large bowel (arrows). On the lateral projections, the colon was seen to reach the chest via an anterior defect in the diaphragm.

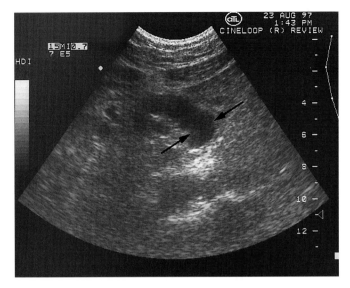

Fig. 6.110 Acute appendicitis. A 43-year-old male patient presented with several hours' history of epigastric pain moving into his right iliac fossa. This was associated with marked tenderness and guarding, pyrexia and a white-cell count of 16 000. Graduated-compression US shows a constant low-attenuation tubular structure in the right iliac fossa, consistent with a swollen appendix, which measures 15 mm in diameter between the arrows. The upper limit of normal is 6 mm. The swollen appendix may be distinguished from fluid-filled small bowel by its lack of peristalsis. The diagnosis was confirmed surgically within the hour.

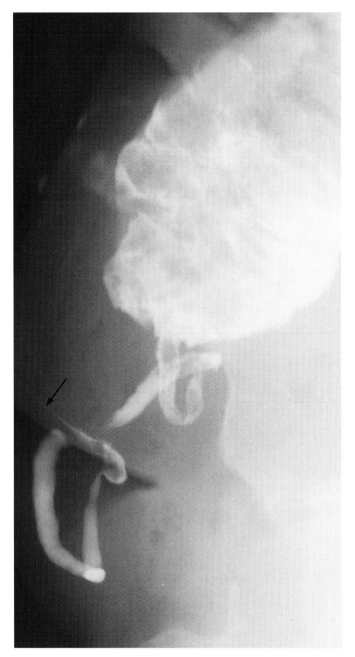

Fig. 6.111 External fistula of the appendix. An elderly female patient developed a small subcutaneous abscess in her right iliac fossa, which quickly discharged pus. After the discharge had continued, a sinogram with water-soluble contrast was performed and this was seen to fill the appendix and caecum. This was treated conservatively and after 5 months it had completely dried up. Arrow, sinogram catheter.

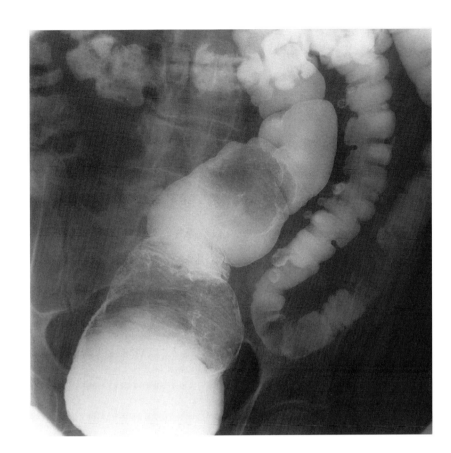

Fig. 6.112 Acquired megarectum. A 73-year-old male patient presented with diarrhoea and a palpable right-sided abdominal mass. A limited single-contrast enema shows impaction of faeces in a markedly distended rectum and distal sigmoid colon. The proximal sigmoid colon is normal apart from diverticular disease.

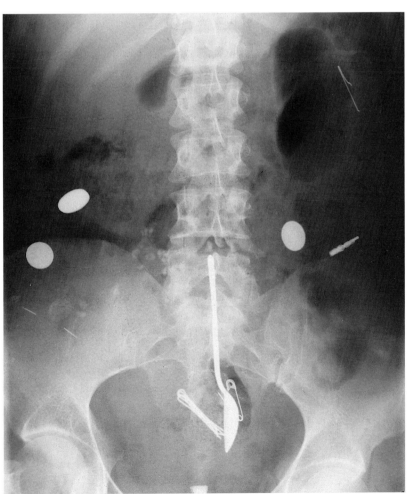

Fig. 6.113 Opaque foreign bodies. A plain abdominal X-ray in a psychiatric patient who has ingested numerous radio-opaque foreign bodies.

7: The Liver

Anatomy

The basic structural unit of the liver is the acinus, which is that portion of liver parenchyma which receives blood from a single portal venule and hepatic arteriole and delivers its bile into a single small duct in the same portal tract. The single acinus lies between two hepatic venules, into which its blood drains [1]. The liver is the largest abdominal organ, the volume of which varies between 1350 and 1500 ml. It is wedge-shaped and lies mostly in the right upper quadrant, extending medially into the epigastrium, and sometimes encroaches on the left upper quadrant. Peritoneum covers most of the hepatic surface, excluding the fossae for the gallbladder and inferior vena cava (IVC) and the bare area where the liver is in direct contact posteriorly with the diaphragm. It is related anteriorly to the anterior abdominal wall and diaphragm. Posterior relations include the right kidney, the right adrenal gland and the IVC, which in its upper portion is surrounded by liver. The duodenum, gallbladder and colon are inferior relations. The dual blood supply is provided by the hepatic artery, arising from the coeliac axis and contributing up to one-quarter of the blood flow, and the portal vein (PV), which contributes 75–80%. These vessels, together with the bile duct, traverse the hepatoduodenal ligament (the lower part of the lesser omentum) to enter the liver at its hilum (porta hepatis). In the porta hepatis, the artery and vein divide to supply the right and left lobes. In the same way, the right and left bile-duct tributaries meet at the hilum to form the common hepatic duct. In the hilum, the orientation of the artery, vein and bile duct is constant, with the PV lying posteriorly, the common hepatic duct lying anteriorly and laterally and the hepatic artery in front and to the left of the PV. The venous drainage from the liver is largely via the three main hepatic veins, namely the middle HV, dividing the liver into the right and left lobes, the right HV, which divides the right lobe into the anterior and posterior segments, and the left HV, which divides the left lobe into the medial and lateral segments. A more detailed subdivision of these segments was devised by Couinaud and has become generally accepted [2]. Each of the four segments is divided by an imaginary transverse line through the right and left PV into anterior and posterior subsegments. These are numbered in anticlockwise fashion from the IVC, the caudate lobe being segment one. This segment should be considered separately, for its blood supply and drainage are independent of the PV division and of the three main hepatic veins. It is located between the PV and the IVC and is supplied by vessels from both the left and right branches of the PV and hepatic artery. Its draining veins flow directly into the IVC.

Plain film radiography

Marginal definition of the liver is dependent on its borders being defined by gas or fat, and these are not constantly present. The superior contour, however, is usually well defined by the air in the right lung base with the intervening right hemidiaphragm, provided that there is no pathology in the lung base, pleura or subphrenic space. Inferior margin definition is unreliable and, in particular, the lower border of the left lobe is only rarely visible on a normal plain film [3]. Inevitably, the assessment of hepatomegaly on plain films is generally inaccurate. However, diffuse enlargement of the right lobe will raise the right hemidiaphragm, and there is likely to be downward displacement of the right kidney and of the hepatic flexure of the colon. There will be a shift in stomach gas to the left and possibly downwards by an enlarged left lobe. Plain films are of value in detecting calcification, either in surrounding structures or as a result of pathology within the liver, or both. Gas within the liver is never a normal finding, but this may be a manifestation of pathology in the biliary tree, the portal veins or surrounding structures—for example, subphrenic or subhepatic abscesses or emphysematous cholecystitis.

Ultrasound

The liver can normally be accessed easily by a subcostal or intercostal approach and this can be a source of much valuable information. High-resolution, real-time scanning with transducers from 3 to 5 MHz in multiple scanning planes makes ultrasound a valuable imaging tool, particularly as a first line of radiological investigation. It is relatively inexpensive and involves no ionizing radiation. In addition, ultrasound equipment is relatively mobile, being readily transported to the very sick or injured patient in the intensive-care unit. It is also extremely useful in guiding needle biopsies. The parenchymal echoes are grey and of uniform intensity, interspersed only by the PV branches and HV tributaries. Like CT and MRI, ultrasound produces tomographic images—that is, images of slices of tissue. The PV, hepatic artery and bile duct can be demonstrated within the lesser omentum and the PV followed into the liver hilum, where it divides into right and left branches, the right branch further dividing into anterior and posterior divisions. The left PV curves anteriorly and to the left before dividing into superior and inferior divisions. The left, middle and right hepatic veins can be readily visualized as they converge towards the IVC. Within the substance of the liver, normal-sized bile ducts are too small to be seen, except under favourable conditions, when the right and left main ducts may be seen, measuring a few millimetres in diameter.

Assessment of liver size tends to be subjective, a volumetric assessment being difficult and time-consuming, and it has failed to gain routine acceptance. In practice, we measure the sagittal diameter in the midclavicular line. This is useful in assessing change in liver size, but gives little guide to the liver volume [4]. In practice, a sagittal diameter of less than 13 cm is considered normal and 13–15.5 cm equivocal; if the sagittal diameter is greater than 15.5 cm, hepatomegaly can be diagnosed with an accuracy of 87% [5].

Intraoperative ultrasound has a useful role in certain situations. Direct contact with the surface of the liver (through the visceral peritoneum) means that the resolution can be substantially improved by increasing the frequency of the probe—for example, 7 MHz. This can be of value in planning segmental resections and also in excluding liver metastatic disease prior to major colorectal surgery [6].

Liver computerized tomography

The CT attenuation of normal liver is 50–70 Hounsfield units (HU) usually, but may vary between 40 and 80 HU without contrast enhancement [7]. The attenuation of pancreas, kidneys and spleen is normally less than liver, which is usually 7–8 HU greater than spleen. Within the unenhanced liver, PV branches and hepatic veins are seen as low-attenuation, linear, branching structures. Gas in the biliary tree or in the portal venous system is readily detected by CT, the latter having a more peripheral distribution, and this may extend to within 2 cm of the capsule.

When IV contrast is given, hepatic artery enhancement begins about 20 s after the start of the injection, but this can be timed exactly on some modern scanners by a bolus-tracking device. At about 70 s, PV enhancement is optimal. Scanning should normally be avoided during the equilibrium phase at greater than 120 s, since focal hepatic lesions tend to become isodense with normal liver. Normal bile-duct tributaries may be visible within the liver, with attenuating values close to that of water—that is, 0 HU. The liver size on CT is normally not greater than 15 cm in craniocaudal diameter [7]. In the investigation of diffuse and focal liver pathology, CT has an established role. The advent of spiral (helical) scanning has been a major advance in this organ [8]. Dynamic incremental scanning is too prolonged to image the liver during both the arterial and portal venous enhancement phases, 1.5–3 min being required to image the whole liver. Spiral CT refers to volume acquisition of image data by rotating the X-ray tube and detectors continuously around the patient, producing a continuous exposure and, at the same time, moving the patient at a constant speed through the scanner. The resultant field of exposure forms a helix or spiral. The very brief scanning time makes it possible to scan the whole organ, once during the arterial phase and once during the portal venous phase. Other benefits of spiral CT include an increased throughput of patients and a reduction in the contrast-medium usage, since a 25% lower iodine dose can be employed compared with incremental CT [9] and, in thin patients, a reduction of iodine dose up to 40% is feasible. Further benefits include a potential for improved multiplanar display and three-dimensional reconstructions. In addition, partial volume averaging is minimized and respiratory misregistration can be eliminated. Portal-vein phase enhancement is optimized in the protocols for incremental CT, because most metastases show reduced vascularity compared with normal liver when imaged during this phase. However, some lesions can become homogeneous in attenuation during the portal venous phase—for example, some primary hepatic neoplasms and some metastases. Consequently, some lesions are more likely to be detected during the arterial phase. Recent studies of patients with hepatoma and a variety of metastases exhibiting increased vascularity have demonstrated an 8–13% increase in lesion detection with dual-phase helical CT, compared with the PV-phase imaging alone [10–13]. When dual-phase CT has been compared with dynamic MR, arterial-phase MR has been shown to be slightly better in finding hepatic lesions [14, 15]. Spiral CT, however, was significantly better for delayed-phase imaging (greater than 3 min) [15]. Three-dimensional reconstructions can be useful in more exact localization of liver tumours prior to surgery.

COMPUTERIZED TOMOGRAPHY ARTERIAL PORTOGRAPHY

Computerized tomography arterial portography (CTAP) is the most sensitive preoperative method of investigating liver masses and it involves the catheter injection of contrast into the superior mesenteric artery (SMA) or splenic artery in order to densely opacify the liver parenchyma via the PV. Since liver tumours are very largely nourished by the hepatic artery, they are therefore seen as low-attenuation lesions, in sharp contrast to the densely opacified normal parenchyma [3]. A suitable protocol would be 150ml of dilute contrast—for example, 140–150mg iodine/ml injected at a rate of 3 ml/s into the SMA. Spiral scanning commences 30–50s after the start of the contrast injection. This produces twice the concentration of dye in the liver compared with an IV infusion [7]. Up to 62% of small metastases may remain undetected by routine CT; less than 20% remain undetected by CTAP [7].

IODIZED OIL COMPUTERIZED TOMOGRAPHY

Iodized oil CT has been proposed as a useful preoperative method to assess vascular tumours—for example, hepatoma. Intra-arterial injection of Lipiodol into the hepatic artery is taken up by normal liver, but is cleared in approximately 7 days, whereas it is taken up and retained by neoplasms. About 10ml of Lipiodol emulsion is injected, followed 7–10 days later by the CT scan. In one series, the procedure was found to be unhelpful [16] and, in a further series, the technique was found to be an insensitive method of detecting small hepatocellular carcinomata in advanced cirrhotic livers, but was slightly superior to ultrasound, CT and angiography [17].

Magnetic resonance imaging

The development of the clinical use of MRI in the abdomen has been relatively slow compared with other clinical applications—for example, in musculoskeletal or CNS imaging. However, with modern equipment and protocols, it is now possible to produce high-quality images of the liver [18]. The main limiting factor in image quality is movement artefact. This can be due either to peristalsis, vascular pulsation or breathing. Compression bands are of benefit in diminishing the amount of abdominal movement, bowel movement can be reduced by IV hyoscine, and respiratory and vascular pulsation artefacts can be reduced by flow-compensation/gradient-moment nulling techniques. With modern equipment also, it may be possible to obtain 12 sections through the liver in a single 18s breath-hold. Metastases greater than 1 cm can be readily identified, but, at the present time, CTAP is the most sensitive test. However, MRI is likely to continue to improve, particularly with the availability for routine clinical use of liver-specific MRI contrast agents—for example, superparamagnetic iron oxide. At the present time, the characterization of small lesions is the greatest challenge in liver MRI [18]. Magnetic resonance imaging has the additional advantages of readily available sagittal and coronal reconstruction, as well as transverse axial sections. There is, of course, no exposure to ionizing radiation. However, for the desperately ill or seriously injured patient, MRI is not currently appropriate. Other contraindications include the presence of ferromagnetic implants.

Angiography

ARTERIOGRAPHY

Major advances in cross-sectional imaging have resulted in contraction of the role of arteriography in this territory. Angiography may provide useful information in the diagnosis of primary tumours, haemangiomata and arteriovenous malformations, as well as focal nodular hyperplasia and metastatic liver disease [3]. While the information provided may not be specific, in the context of the results of other imaging modalities the diagnosis may be confirmed by arteriography. In addition, catheter access to the hepatic arterial tree may facilitate the means of effective therapy—for example, hepatic artery embolization. Liver pathology or trauma, resulting in haemorrhage into the liver parenchyma, under the capsule, into the peritoneal cavity or retroperitoneally or even into the biliary tree, may require arteriography for precise diagnosis and localization of a bleeding point.

PORTAL VENOGRAPHY

Demonstration of the portal venous system may be useful in the diagnosis of portal hypertension and may also be of great value in assessing the surgical resectability of biliary-tract tumours and pancreatic cancer. Contrast medium can be delivered to the portal venous system by *direct* puncture—for example, percutaneous splenoportography—or alternatively by a transjugular approach via a hepatic vein, through which the left or right portal veins may be punctured and catheterized as a precursor to transjugular intrahepatic portosystemic shunting (TIPSS). Transhepatic portography [19] is a further direct method, in which the PV is punctured via a percutaneous transhepatic approach through an intercostal space. The patient's coagulation status needs to be satisfactory. The commonly performed *indirect* method of portal venography consists of injecting contrast medium into the coeliac artery, SMA or even the inferior mesenteric artery, which will ultimately deliver contrast into the portal system. This indirect method has been so improved by the advent of digital-subtraction angiography (DSA) that direct methods are used only where therapeutic or sampling techniques are being employed [3].

References

1 Mowat A., MacSween R.N.M., Percy-Robb I.W. *et al.* (1993) Liver, biliary tract and pancreas. In: MacSween R.N.M. & Whaley K. (eds) *Muir's Textbook of Pathology*, 13th edn. London: Arnold, 741.
2 Cosgrove D.O. (1993) Liver anatomy. In: Cosgrove D.O., Meire H. & Dewbury K. (eds) *Clinical Ultrasound*. Edinburgh: Churchill Livingstone, 227–242.

3 Adam A., Bydder G.M., Urbain J.-L.C. *et al.* (1997) The liver. In: Grainger R.G. & Allison D.J. (eds) *Diagnostic Radiology*, 3rd edn. New York: Churchill Livingstone, 1156.

4 Cosgrove D.O. (1994) Ultrasound in surgery of the liver and biliary tract. In: Blumgart L.H. (ed.) *Surgery of the Liver and Biliary Tract*. Edinburgh: Churchill Livingstone, 189–219.

5 Dahnert W. (1996) *Radiology Review Manual*, 3rd edn. Baltimore: Williams & Wilkins, 485.

6 Plant G.R. (1993) Intra-operative ultrasound. In: Cosgrove D.O., Meire H. & Dewbury K. (eds) *Clinical Ultrasound*. Edinburgh: Churchill Livingstone, 243–250.

7 Burgener F.A. & Kormano M. (1996) *Differential Diagnosis in Computed Tomography*. Stuttgart: Thieme Medical Publishers, 248.

8 Brink J.A., McFarland E.G. & Heiken J.P. (1997) Helical/spiral computed body tomography. *Clinical Radiology* **52**, 489–503.

9 Brink J.A., Heiken J.P., Forman H.P. *et al.* (1995) Hepatic spiral CT, reduction of dose of intravenous contrast material. *Radiology* **197**, 83–88.

10 Bonaldi V.M., Bret P.M., Reinhold C. *et al.* (1995) Helical CT of the liver: value of an early hepatic arterial phase. *Radiology* **197**, 357–363.

11 Hollett M.D., Jeffrey R.B., Nino-Murcia M. *et al.* (1995) Dual phase helical CT of the liver: value of arterial phase scans in the detection of small malignant hepatic neoplasms. *American Journal of Roentgenology* **164**, 879–884.

12 Baron R.L., Oliver J.H., III, Dodd J.D., III *et al.* (1996) Hepatocellular carcinoma: evaluation with biphasic, contrast enhanced helical CT. *Radiology* **199**, 505–511.

13 Oliver J.H., III, Baron R.L., Federle M.P. *et al.* (1996) Detecting hepatocellular carcinoma: value of unenhanced or arterial phase CT imaging or both used in conjunction with conventional portal venous phase contrast enhanced CT imaging. *American Journal of Roentgenology* **167**, 71–77.

14 Oi H., Murakami R., Kim T. *et al.* (1996) Dynamic MR imaging with early phase helical CT for detecting small intra-hepatic metastases of hepatocellular carcinoma. *American Journal of Roentgenology* **166**, 369–374.

15 Yamashita Y.Y., Mitsuzaki K.M., Yi T. *et al.* (1996) Small hepatocellular carcinoma in patients with chronic liver damage: prospective comparison of detection with dynamic MR imaging and helical CT of the whole liver. *Radiology* **200**, 79–84.

16 Dawson P., Adam A. & Banks L. (1993) Diagnostic iodised oil embolisation of liver tumours—the Hammersmith experience. *European Journal of Radiology* **16**, 201–206.

17 Saada J., Bhattacharya S., Dhillon A.P. *et al.* (1997) Detection of small hepatocellular carcinomas in cirrhotic livers using iodised oil computed tomography. *Gut* **41**, 404–407.

18 Robinson P.J.A. (1996) The characterisation of liver tumours by MRI. *Clinical Radiology* **51**, 749–761.

19 Bierman H.R., Steinbach H.L., White L.P. *et al.* (1952) Portal venopuncture percutaneous trans-hepatic approach. *Proceedings of the Society of Experimental Biology in Medicine* **79**, 550–552.

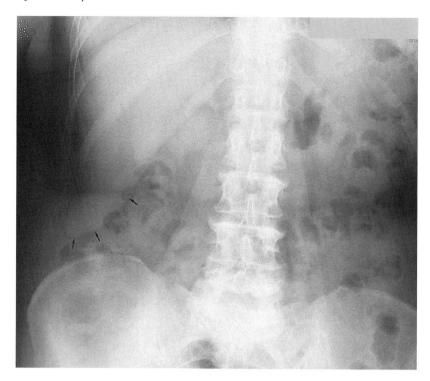

Fig. 7.1 **Normal liver.** The inferior margin of the normal liver (arrows) is visible on this control film for an intravenous pyelogram examination in a patient with no clinical evidence of liver disease. The inferior margin is a little lower than usual, but it emphasizes the difficulty in trying to assess liver size by plain radiography. This is much more accurately done by cross-sectional imaging.

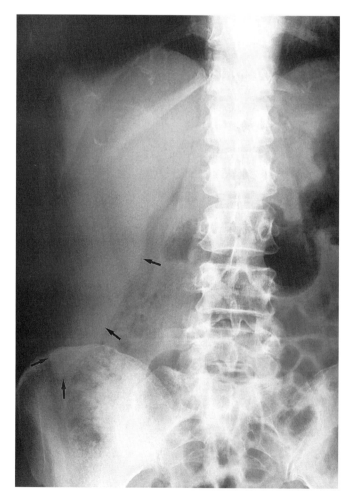

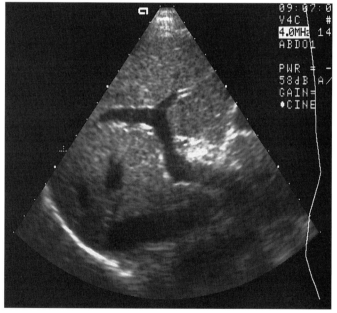

Fig. 7.3 **Normal liver.** A 4 MHz sagittal scan in the plane of the inferior vena cava shows the portal vein entering the liver and dividing into the left and right branches. Patency of the portal vein can be readily established by the use of colour Doppler or spectral Doppler.

Fig. 7.2 **Normal liver, Riedel's lobe.** The inferior border of the right lobe of liver is seen to extend downwards well into the right iliac fossa (arrows) in a patient with no clinical features of liver disease. This is a well-recognized normal variant.

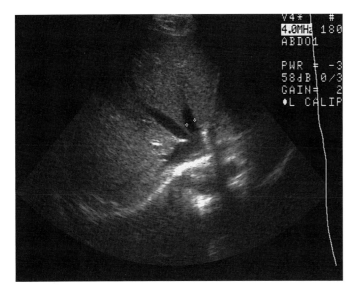

Fig. 7.4 Normal hepatic veins. A 4 MHz transverse scan through the liver of a 15-year-old boy, with no evidence of liver or heart disease, shows the normal convergence of the hepatic veins on the inferior vena cava. The left hepatic vein (with markers) measures less than 8 mm and the middle hepatic vein measures 9 mm in diameter.

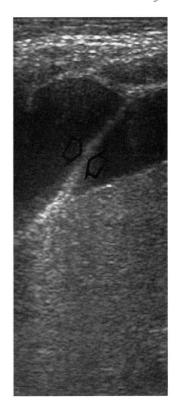

Fig. 7.5 Falciform ligament. This double layer of peritoneum is not normally visible on ultrasound (5 MHz transducer). However, if the liver is separated from the diaphragm by ascitic fluid, as in this case, the falciform ligament may be visualized (open arrowheads).

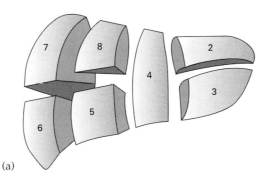

(a)

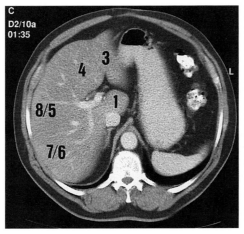

(c)

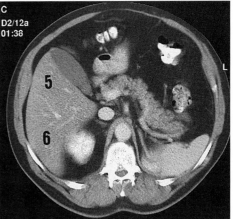

(d)

(b)

Fig. 7.6 (a) Diagram of exploded anterior view of the liver showing the numbered segments described by Couinaud [2]. Segment 1 (caudate lobe) is hidden by segment 4. (b) A spiral CECT through the liver in a plane superior to the portal vein bifurcation showing segments 1, 2, 4, 7 and 8. (c) A spiral CECT through the liver in the plane of the right portal vein showing segments 1 and 3–8. (d) A spiral CECT through the inferior aspect of the liver showing only segments 5 and 6.

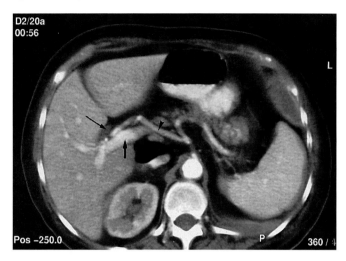

Fig. 7.7 Normal porta hepatis and structures in the lesser omentum. A spiral contrast-enhanced CT (CECT) (with 10 mm collimation) through the plane of the coeliac axis illustrates the course of the portal vein (thick arrow), the hepatic artery (arrowhead) and the common hepatic duct (thin arrow).

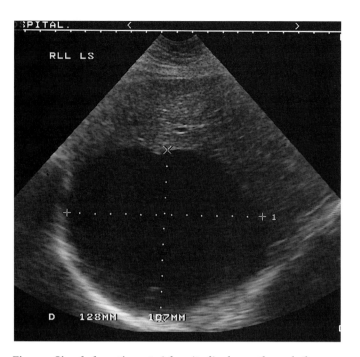

Fig. 7.9 Simple hepatic cyst. A longitudinal scan through the right lobe of liver shows a very well-circumscribed echo-free intrahepatic lesion, measuring almost 13 cm in maximum diameter, the appearance being characteristic of a simple cyst.

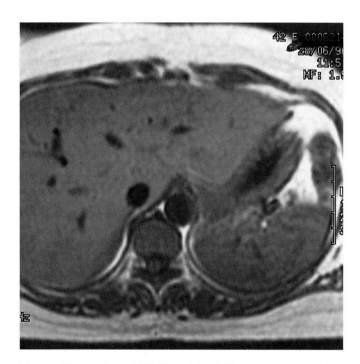

Fig. 7.8 Normal liver, MRI. T_1-weighted SE transverse scan. The vessels appear as a signal void as they course through the liver parenchyma.

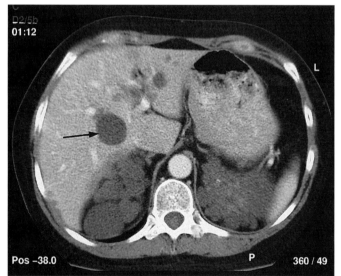

Fig. 7.10 Polycystic liver and renal disease. A spiral CECT scan through the upper abdomen in a 57 year-old male patient with chronic renal failure on haemodialysis because of polycystic renal disease. Both kidneys have been almost entirely replaced by numerous cysts, and several cysts are shown within the liver, which contrast with the normally enhancing liver parenchyma (arrow).

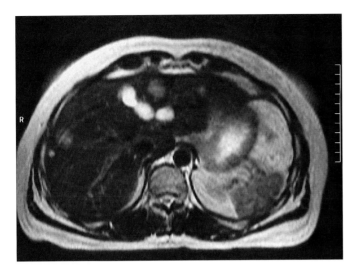

Fig. 7.11 Multiple liver cysts. A 54-year-old female patient with known breast carcinoma had equivocal appearance of cysts on ultrasound. An axial T$_2$ FSE MRI scan of the liver shows multiple, well-defined, high-signal masses of varying size in both lobes of the liver. A coronal T$_1$ GRE showed well-circumscribed, thin-walled cysts of low signal. (Courtesy of Dr Graeme Houston.)

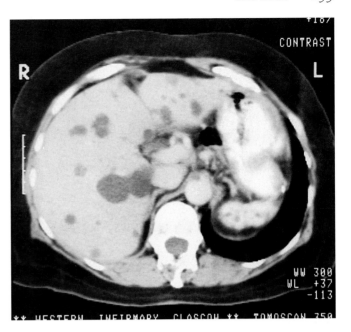

Fig. 7.12 Caroli's disease. This rare condition consists of communicating cavernous ectasia of intrahepatic bile ducts. This produces segmental intrahepatic ductal dilatation. The diagnosis had previously been established at laparotomy and cholecystectomy. Multiple, well-circumscribed, low-attenuation lesions of varying size are shown within the liver. Several renal cysts were visible on lower sections, there being an association between Caroli's disease and renal cysts.

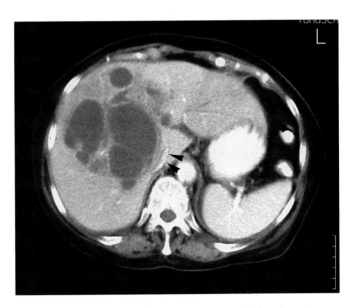

Fig. 7.13 Multiple liver abscesses. A 78-year-old female patient gave a history of nausea, vomiting and weight loss over several weeks. A spiral CECT shows multiple, interconnecting, low-attenuation lesions within the right lobe of liver, associated with considerable compression of the IVC (arrowheads). Pus was drained by percutaneous intervention.

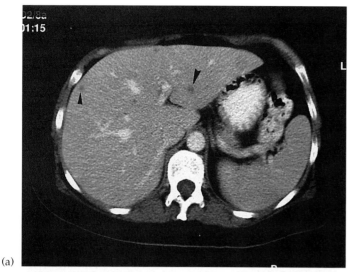

(a)

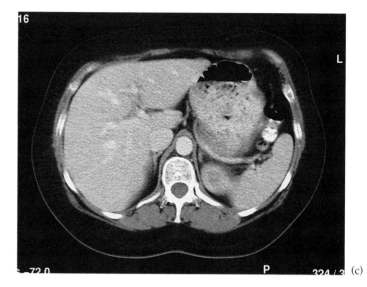

(c)

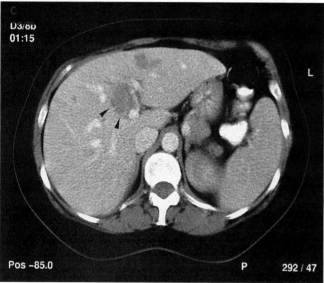

(b)

Fig. 7.14 Liver candidiasis. A 35-year-old female patient with acute myeloid leukaemia developed clinical features of fungal infection. (a) A spiral CECT shows multiple small focal lesions scattered throughout the liver (arrowheads). Similar lesions were also shown in other sections of the spleen. The appearance is typical of candidiasis. (b) A repeat scan 4 weeks later shows fewer lesions, but one lesion lying lateral to the left branch of the portal vein is seen to have enlarged (arrowheads) and a second lesion lying anteriorly in the left lobe has also increased in size. (c) A further repeat, 4 months after (a), shows complete resolution of the fungal infection.

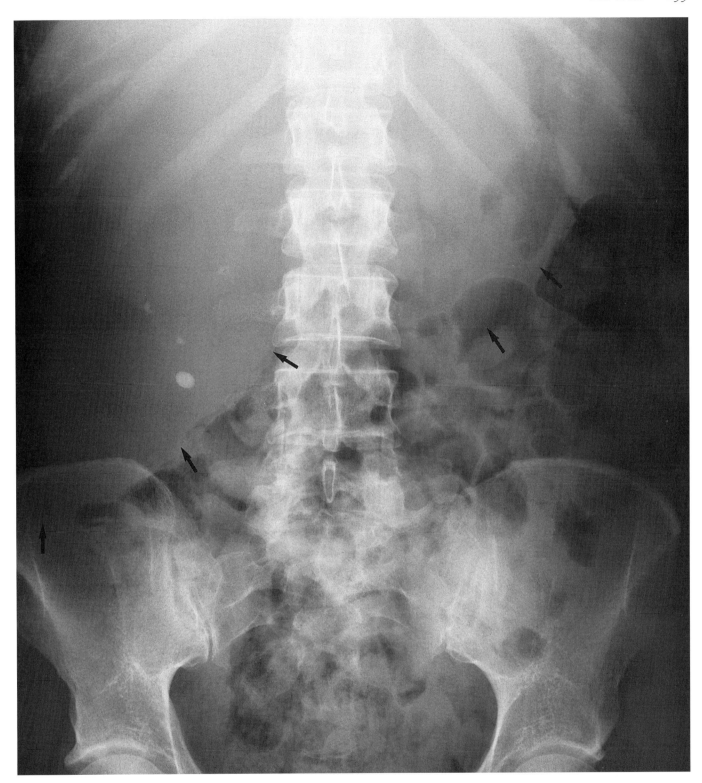

Fig. 7.15 Hepatomegaly due to metastatic liver disease. This 39-year-old female patient had a short history of weight loss, anorexia and an obvious mass in the right upper quadrant. The plain abdominal film suggests a substantial degree of hepatomegaly, the inferior margin being indicated by the arrows. A calcified gallstone is shown and, in addition, several smaller foci of calcification are visible. These were associated with very extensive metastatic liver disease. Biopsy revealed poorly differentiated adenocarcinoma. No primary tumour was identified.

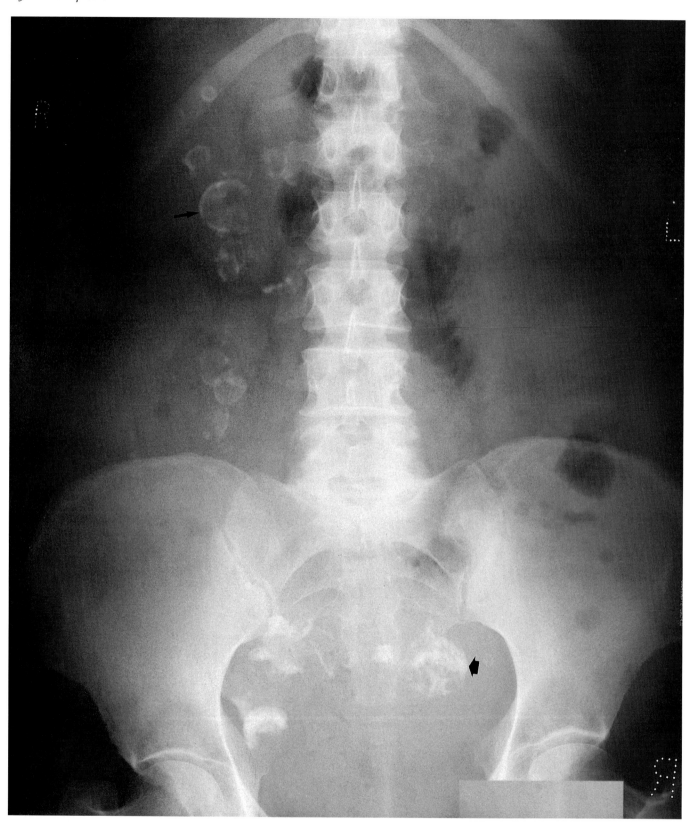

Fig. 7.16 Metastatic liver disease. A plain abdominal film in a patient with advanced ovarian carcinoma; calcification in the primary lesion is indicated by the arrowhead. The liver is enlarged and multiple calcified liver metastases are visible (arrow). Calcification is a feature in less than 5% cases of metastatic liver disease.

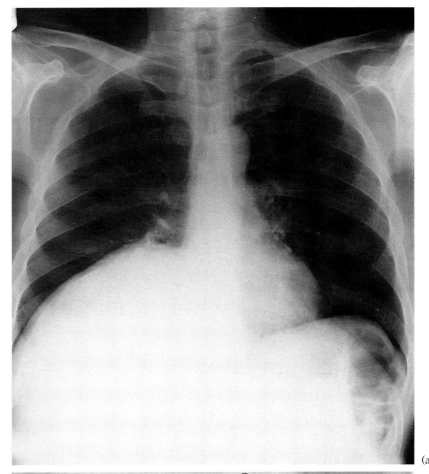

(a)

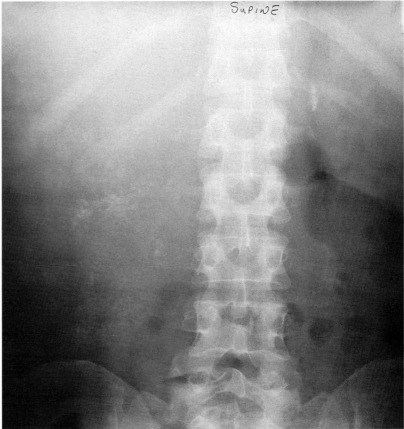

(b)

Fig. 7.17 Metastatic liver disease. (a) A chest X-ray of a 74-year-old male patient with a history of colonic carcinoma shows quite marked elevation of the right hemidiaphragm, in keeping with hepatomegaly, and widespread stippled calcification is just visible. (b) There is very extensive stippled and slightly confluent calcification in the right upper quadrant on this plain abdominal film. This was due to mucin-secreting metastatic adenocarcinoma.

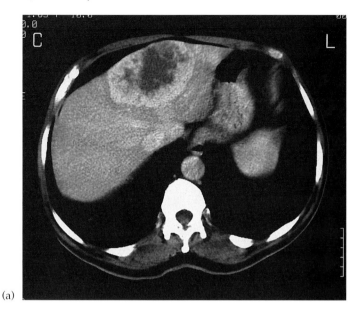

(a)

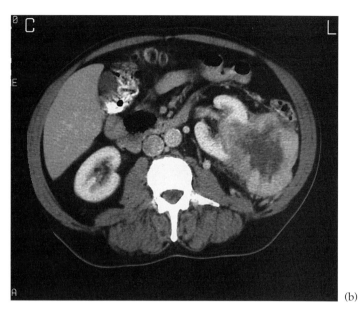

(b)

Fig. 7.18 Metastatic liver disease. (a) A 61-year-old male patient presented with left upper quadrant pain and a palpable mass. He was noted to have polycythaemia. A spiral CECT through the liver shows one of several enhancing mass lesions, with evidence of central necrosis. (b) The primary lesion was a carcinoma arising in the left kidney, the morphology of which is remarkably similar to the metastasis in (a). Multiple pulmonary metastases were also present.

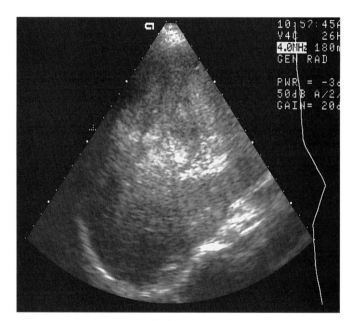

Fig. 7.19 Metastatic liver disease. Ultrasound scan in a male patient with a 23-year history of inflammatory bowel disease. Abnormal liver function tests raised a clinical suspicion of primary sclerosing cholangitis, but, on ultrasound, the liver was found to be enlarged and largely replaced by metastatic disease, some of which is calcified. The biopsy indicated mucin-secreting adenocarcinoma.

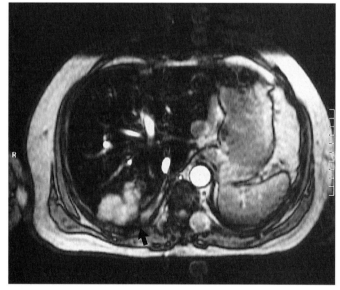

Fig. 7.20 Metastatic liver disease from primary gastric carcinoma with extracapsular spread. A 56-year-old male patient with resected gastric carcinoma had, at his 3 years' follow-up, an axial T_1 GRE MRI scan of the liver using superparamagnetic ferric oxide contrast (Endorem). There is a peripheral metastasis in the posterior inferior segment of the right lobe of the liver, which shows extracapsular spread (arrow). Surgical confirmation. (Courtesy of Dr Graeme Houston.)

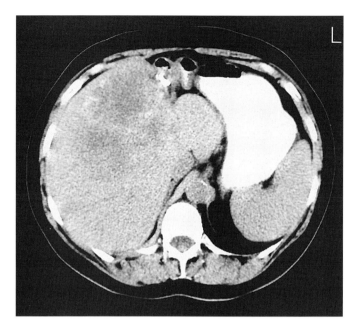

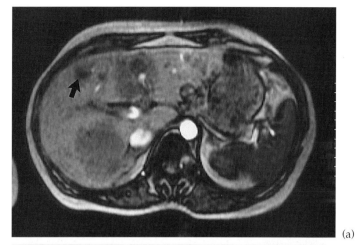

(a)

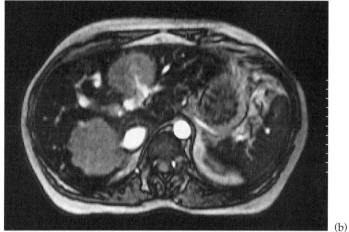

(b)

Fig. 7.21 Metastatic liver disease. This 62-year-old female patient had a past history of colonic resection for adenocarcinoma, together with partial left hepatic lobectomy for metastatic disease, as well as recent right upper quadrant pain and weight loss. The spiral CT (without contrast enhancement) shows partial resection of the left lobe. The right lobe is enlarged, with a very extensive area of reduced attenuation and with poor marginal definition and amorphous calcification, in keeping with mucin-secreting adenocarcinoma. The caudate lobe is hypertrophied.

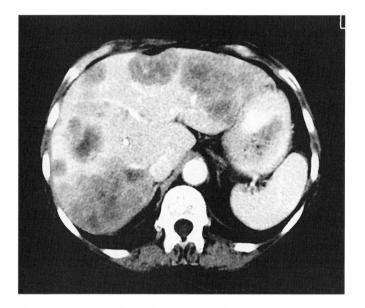

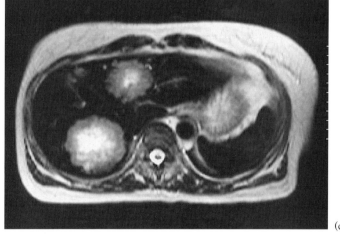

(c)

Fig. 7.23 Metastatic liver disease from colonic primary. A 68-year-old female with colonic carcinoma had focal lesions in the liver on ultrasound. (a) Axial T_1 GRE MRI scan of the liver, (b) axial T_1 GRE and (c) axial T_2 FSE after superparamagnetic ferric oxide contrast (Endorem). There are two large (5 cm, 4 cm) metastases in each lobe of the liver, with central high signal on the T_2-weighted sequence, in keeping with central liquefaction. A further smaller 1.5 cm metastasis is shown anteriorly in the right lobe (arrow). (Courtesy of Dr J. Graeme Houston.)

Fig. 7.22 Metastatic liver disease. A spiral CECT of a 70-year-old female patient with a history of mastectomy 5 years previously and clinical hepatomegaly. It shows multiple low-attenuation lesions throughout the liver, in keeping with metastatic deposits. The histology was positive.

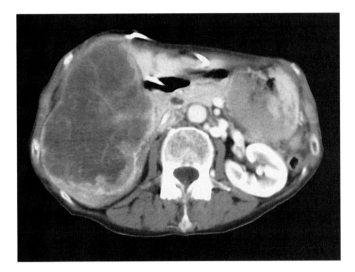

Fig. 7.24 Metastatic liver disease. A very large solitary metastasis is shown in this spiral CECT in a patient with known colon cancer. The margin of the lesion enhances with contrast, but most of it is liquefied as a result of necrosis.

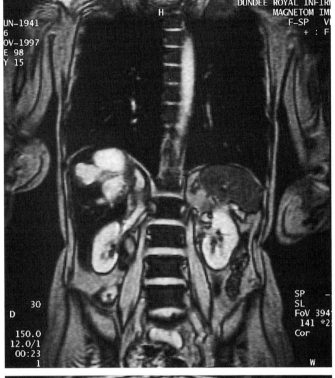

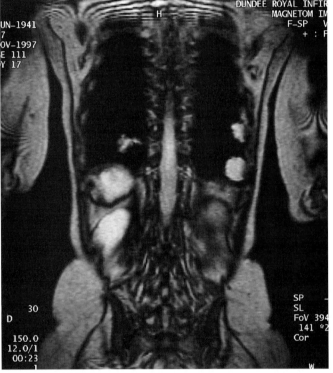

Fig. 7.25 Metastatic liver and lung disease from a colonic primary. A 48-year-old female patient with colonic carcinoma: (a and b) coronal T$_2$ GRE MRI scan of the liver using superparamagnetic ferric oxide contrast (Endorem). There are multiple lesions of varying size in the right lobe of the liver and two intrapulmonary lesions, consistent with metastases. (Courtesy of Dr Graeme Houston.)

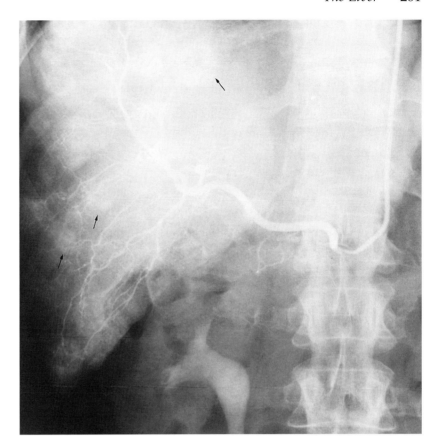

Fig. 7.26 Metastatic liver disease. Ovarian carcinoma treated by hysterectomy and bilateral salpingo-oophorectomy, with a relapse following chemotherapy. Selective hepatic arteriography shows multiple, faintly enhancing lesions throughout the liver, in keeping with metastatic deposits (arrows). Direct arteriography is no longer used as a primary diagnostic method in metastatic liver disease, but may be combined very successfully with CT scanning to produce the most sensitive currently available diagnostic test for metastatic liver disease.

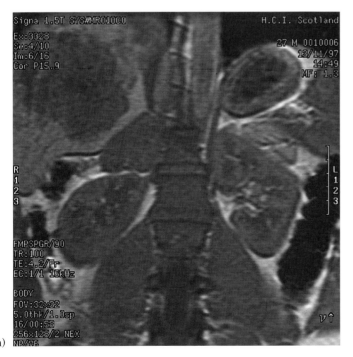

(a)

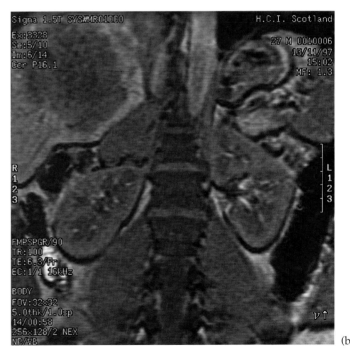

(b)

Fig. 7.27 Colorectal carcinoma with hepatic and adrenal metastases. A 30-year-old male patient with advanced rectosigmoid carcinoma had coronal T_1-weighted gradient echo images obtained with fat and water signal (a) 'in phase' and (b) 'out of phase'. The decrease in signal from the retroperitoneal fat and vertebral marrow on the out-of-phase imaging is apparent. The adrenal lesion has an unchanged signal, inferring that it contains little fat and is very likely to represent a metastatic deposit rather than a benign adrenal lesion. (Courtesy of Dr Alasdair Taylor.)

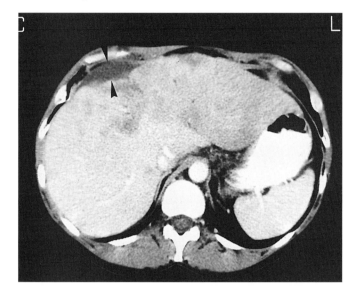

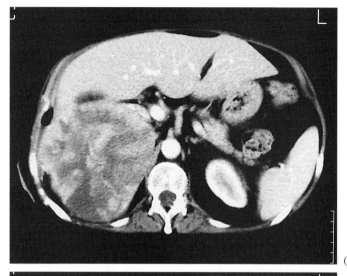

Fig. 7.28 Metastatic liver disease with subcapsular fluid collection. A spiral CECT of a 37-year-old female patient with ovarian carcinoma and metastatic liver disease shows extensive but rather poorly defined metastatic liver disease. A subcapsular fluid collection is shown anteriorly (arrowheads), apparently resulting from tumour necrosis.

(a)

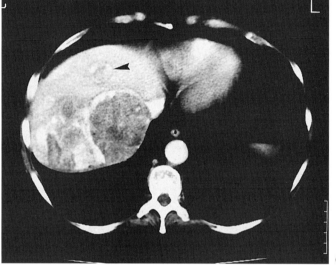

(b)

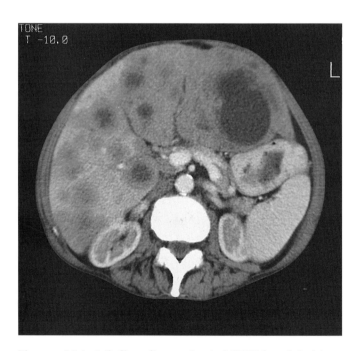

Fig. 7.30 Metastatic liver disease. (a) This spiral CECT shows a 9 cm mass lesion arising in the right adrenal gland with uneven attenuation. The biopsy showed this to be adrenal carcinoma. (b) As well as direct extension of the partly calcified primary lesion into the liver, separate metastatic deposits are shown, one of which is arrowed.

Fig. 7.29 Metastatic liver disease. A spiral CECT (70 s delay) in a 58-year-old male patient with advanced bladder carcinoma. Numerous metastatic deposits are shown in the liver of varying size and attenuation, which is particularly reduced centrally, in keeping with necrosis/liquefaction.

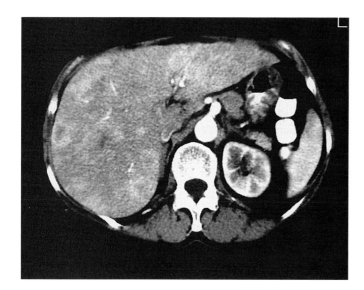

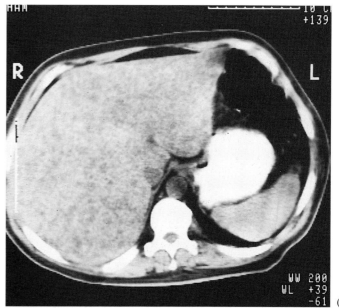

(a)

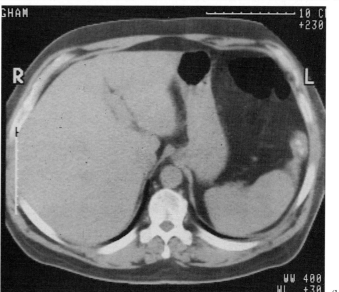

(b)

Fig. 7.31 Metastatic liver disease. A spiral CECT in a 67-year-old female patient with proved primary carcinoid tumour in the stomach shows widespread metastatic liver disease. This was subsequently treated by embolization with Ivalon and Lipiodol.

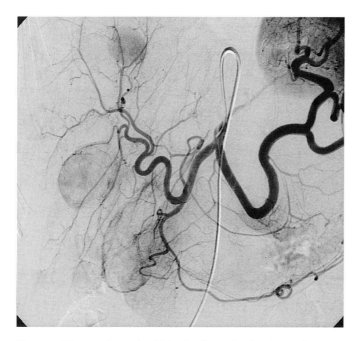

Fig. 7.32 Metastatic carcinoid in the liver. A selective coeliac arteriogram shows multiple hypervascular metastases. The patient presented with symptoms of carcinoid syndrome. (Courtesy of Dr Richard D. Edwards.)

Fig. 7.33 Hepatic lymphoma. (a) Incremental CT through the liver without contrast enhancement. Numerous areas of reduced attenuation are shown within the liver, but no splenomegaly or lymphadenopathy. (b) In response to chemotherapy, the liver disease has completely resolved 3 months later.

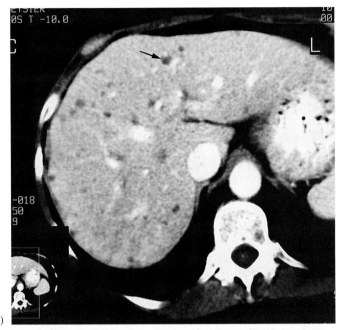

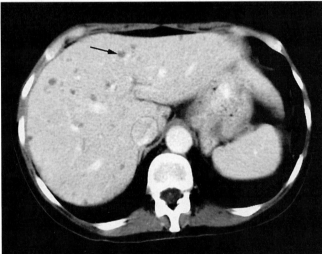

Fig. 7.34 Multiple biliary hamartoma. (a) Spiral CECT shows numerous low-attenuation lesions (arrow) throughout the liver, each measuring a few millimetres in diameter. The liver biopsy was negative, apart from biliary hamartoma. (b) The patient was fit and well 4 months later, and the CT appearance of the liver is unchanged. Ultrasound in this patient revealed no abnormality and, in particular, there was no evidence of hepatic cysts.

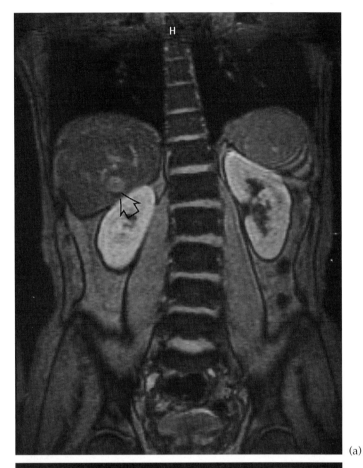

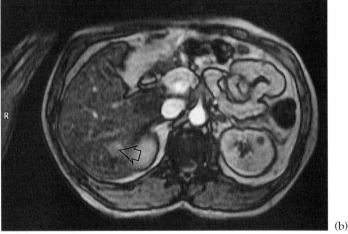

Fig. 7.35 Hepatocellular carcinoma and cirrhosis. This 64-year-old male patient was hepatitis C positive and had a raised α-fetoprotein. (a) This coronal T_1 GRE and (b) axial T_1 GRE of the liver, after superparamagnetic ferric oxide contrast (Endorem), show a focal 1.5 cm lesion in the posterior inferior segment of the right lobe of liver (arrows) and relatively poor liver parenchymal signal reduction. This is in keeping with cirrhosis (surgical confirmation). (Courtesy of Dr J. Graeme Houston.)

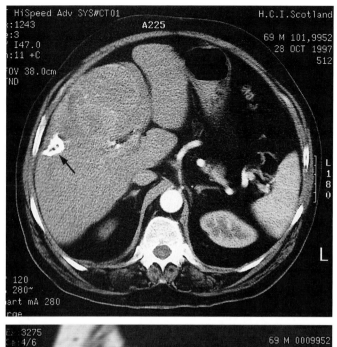

(a)

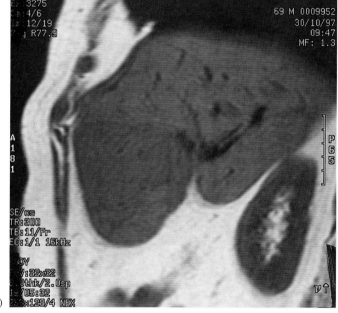

(b)

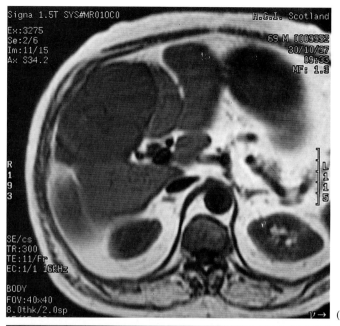

(c)

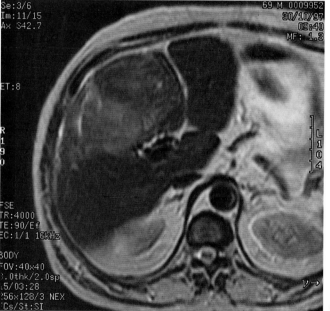

(d)

Fig. 7.36 Hepatocellular carcinoma. (a) The spiral CECT shows a large well-circumscribed solid mass lesion with relatively little enhancement lying anterior in the right lobe of the liver. Some focal calcification (arrow) lying adjacent to the lesion was the result of a previous liver injury. (b) The T_1-weighted sagittal MRI scan confirms the presence of a solid, well-circumscribed, mass lesion anteriorly in the liver. (c) The same lesion is visible in a transverse-section T_1-weighted image. (d) FSE T_2-weighted image. The lesion was successfully resected surgically and the diagnosis confirmed. There was no evidence of cirrhosis. (Courtesy of Dr Alasdair Taylor.)

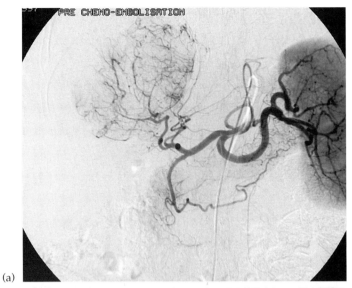

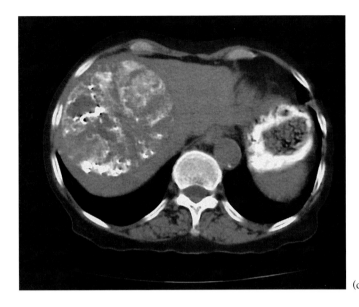

(a)

(c)

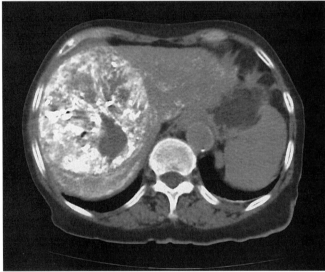

(b)

Fig. 7.37 Hepatocellular carcinoma. This 79-year-old female patient had histologically proved primary biliary cirrhosis and hepatoma. (a) Selective coeliac angiography using DSA shows a moderately vascular liver tumour, the histology of which was a very well-differentiated hepatoma. (b) A CT scan on the same day as hepatic artery embolization with Lipiodol, which was given with Adriamycin, shows marked retention of the Lipiodol by the hepatoma and minimal retention by the normal liver parenchyma. (c) A repeat CT scan 6 weeks later shows a moderate reduction in the size of the hepatoma, which still retains a substantial amount of the Lipiodol. The liver parenchyma is clear. (Courtesy of Dr Richard D. Edwards.)

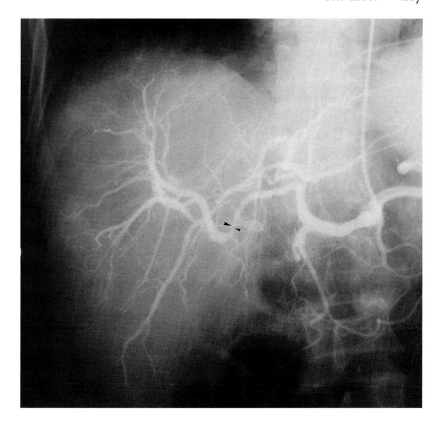

Fig. 7.38 Hepatocellular carcinoma. Coeliac angiography in histologically proved hepatoma shows substantial narrowing of the hepatic artery at the level of the liver hilum (arrowheads), in keeping with tumour encasement. The arterial tree has been accessed by a left brachial approach.

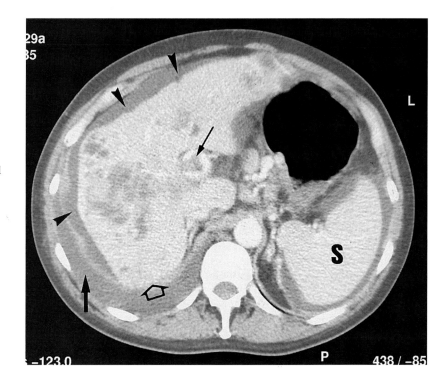

Fig. 7.39 Hepatitis C cirrhosis, hepatocellular carcinoma, portal hypertension and portal vein thrombosis. A 46-year-old male patient developed chronic hepatitis C with a past history of excess alcohol. A previous liver biopsy indicated cirrhosis. This spiral CECT shows an irregularly contracted liver containing multiple areas of reduced attenuation during the portal venous enhancement phase, in keeping with hepatocellular carcinoma (positive biopsy). An irregular filling defect is shown within the portal vein (thin arrow) and gastric varices are seen to enhance with contrast. The patient died of variceal bleeding. S, spleen; thick arrow, pleural effusion; closed arrowheads, ascites; open arrowhead, bare area of the liver.

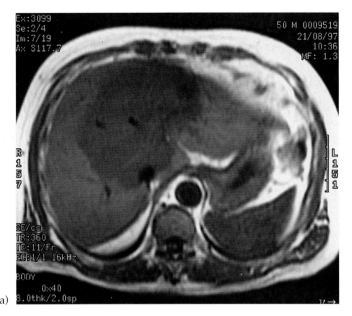

(a)

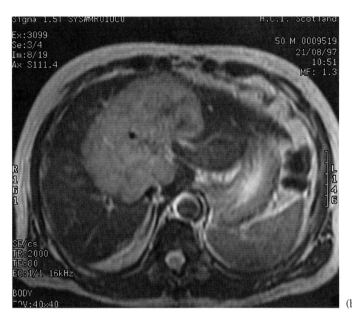

(b)

Fig. 7.40 Intrahepatic cholangiocarcinoma. A 50-year-old male had progressive right upper quadrant discomfort for 6 months. (a) T_1-weighted and (b) T_2-weighted spin echo MRI axial sections demonstrated a large, relatively well-circumscribed, central hepatic lesion, with a conspicuous lack of bile-duct dilatation. Histology of an ultrasound-guided biopsy demonstrated cholangiocarcinoma. (Courtesy of Dr Alasdair Taylor.)

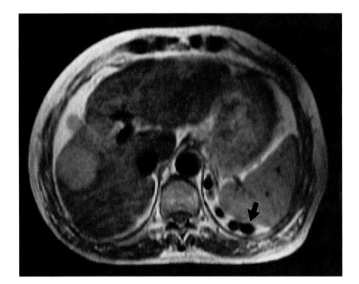

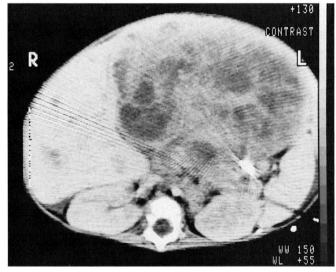

Fig. 7.41 Hepatocellular carcinoma and cirrhosis. A 54-year-old male patient presented with haematemesis and raised α-fetoprotein. The axial T_1 GRE MRI of liver with gadolinium (0.1 mmol/kg) enhancement shows a focal, 5 cm, enhancing mass in the right lobe of the liver, with irregularly enlarged liver and serpiginous vessels with a flow void posterior to the liver, in keeping with portal hypertension and collateral varices (arrow). Surgical confirmation. (Courtesy of Dr J. Graeme Houston.)

Fig. 7.42 Hepatoblastoma. This contrast-enhanced incremental CT scan in a 2-year-old child with progressive abdominal distension shows a huge mass lesion within the liver, predominantly in the left lobe, but with satellite lesions in the right lobe and with para-aortic lymphadenopathy, which on higher sections extended into the posterior mediastinum. The artefact is produced by the nasogastric tube. Histological confirmation.

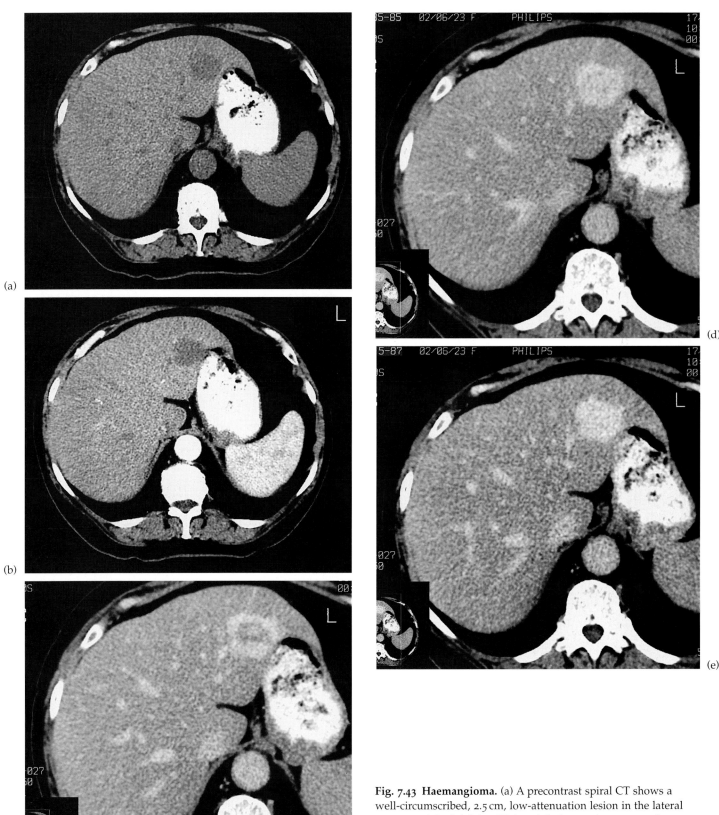

(a)

(b)

(c)

(d)

(e)

Fig. 7.43 Haemangioma. (a) A precontrast spiral CT shows a well-circumscribed, 2.5 cm, low-attenuation lesion in the lateral segment of the left lobe. (b) Arterial-phase enhancement shows very slight nodular peripheral enhancement. (c–e) The venous phase at 70 s delay and further sections through the same lesion over several minutes show gradual infilling of the lesion with contrast, which is characteristic of haemangioma.

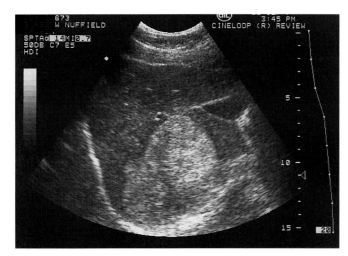

Fig. 7.44 Giant haemangioma. A 40-year-old female patient presented with vague right upper quadrant discomfort. A 9 cm, relatively well-defined, echogenic mass lesion is shown posteriorly in the liver on this sagittal section, consistent with a giant haemangioma. The internal echoes are the result of multiple septations. A CT scan in this patient showed typical changes of haemangioma, with characteristic centripetal contrast enhancement over several minutes. Surgical resection of this lesion confirmed the diagnosis.

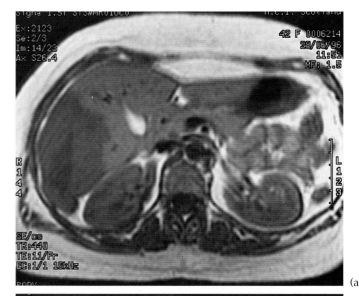

(a)

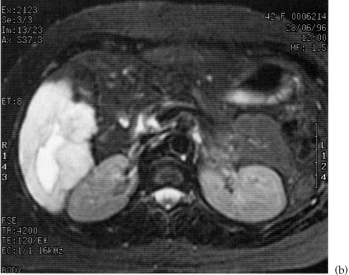

(b)

Fig. 7.45 Giant hepatic haemangioma. A 42-year-old female patient presented with a 1–2-year history of right upper quadrant pain. (a) A T$_1$-weighted axial MRI scan shows an irregular, but moderately well-defined, large area of reduced signal intensity in the right lobe of the liver. (b) A T$_2$-weighted FSE MRI scan shows a very high signal intensity, which is typical of haemangioma. The central zone of still higher signal intensity is atypical and was found to be fluid filled at histology of the resected specimen, possibly as a result of thrombosis or infarction during pregnancy. (Courtesy of Dr Alasdair Taylor.)

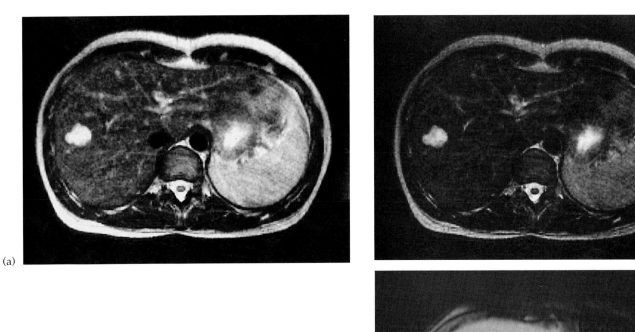

(a)

(b)

(c)

Fig. 7.46 Liver haemangioma. A 68-year-old female patient with colonic carcinoma: (a) first echo, in dual-echo FSE, shows high signal; (b) this is maintained on the second echo, dual-echo FSE MRI scans. (c) Five minutes post gladolinium enhancement (0.1 mmol/kg), the gradient echo T$_1$ shows enhancement. (Courtesy of Dr J. Graeme Houston.)

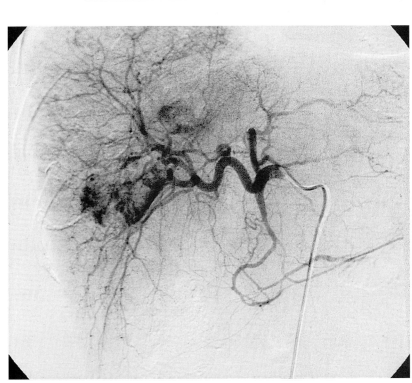

Fig. 7.47 Multiple liver haemangiomata. A 30-year-old female patient with no clinical evidence of malignancy had multiple echogenic hepatic lesions on ultrasound, consistent with haemangiomata. Selective hepatic arteriography using DSA shows multiple vascular lesions. Diagnostic angiogram prior to embolization. (Courtesy of Dr Richard D. Edwards.)

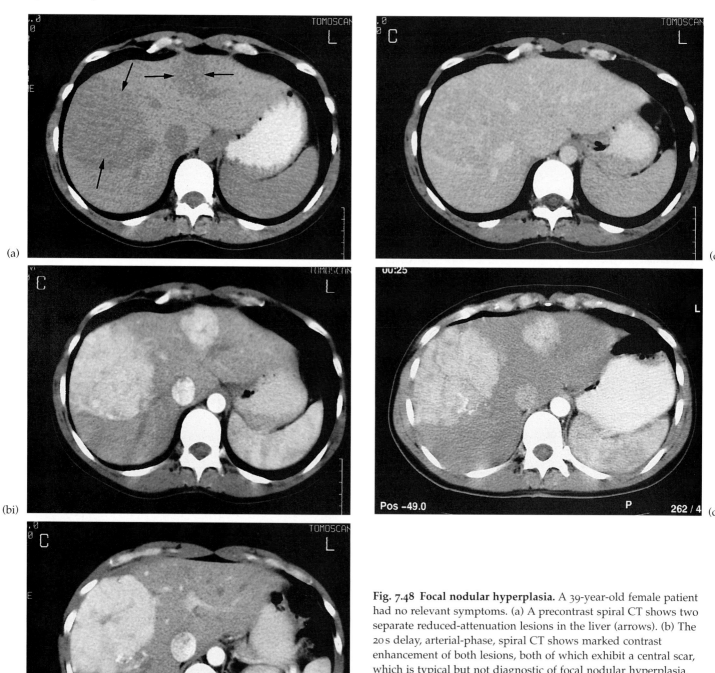

(a)

(bi)

(bii)

(c)

(d)

Fig. 7.48 Focal nodular hyperplasia. A 39-year-old female patient had no relevant symptoms. (a) A precontrast spiral CT shows two separate reduced-attenuation lesions in the liver (arrows). (b) The 20 s delay, arterial-phase, spiral CT shows marked contrast enhancement of both lesions, both of which exhibit a central scar, which is typical but not diagnostic of focal nodular hyperplasia. (bii) is 2 cm distal to (bi). (c) An equilibrium-phase scan at 2.5 min from the beginning of the injection shows that both lesions are virtually isodense with the normal liver parenchyma, such that they could easily have been overlooked had the scan been performed only at this stage. (d) A repeat examination (arterial phase) 5.5 months later shows no change in either lesion. Diagnosis was confirmed by laparoscopic biopsy.

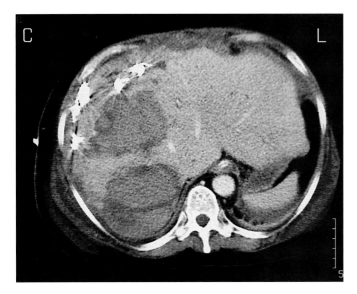

Fig. 7.49 Intrahepatic haemorrhage. A 49-year-old female patient on long-term warfarin therapy developed abdominal pain and anaemia. The patient became shocked and required emergency surgery, at which time an extensive subcapsular haematoma was evacuated. Spiral CECT in the postoperative period shows artefacts produced by the surgical packs. Two well-defined intrahepatic haematomata are shown in the right lobe.

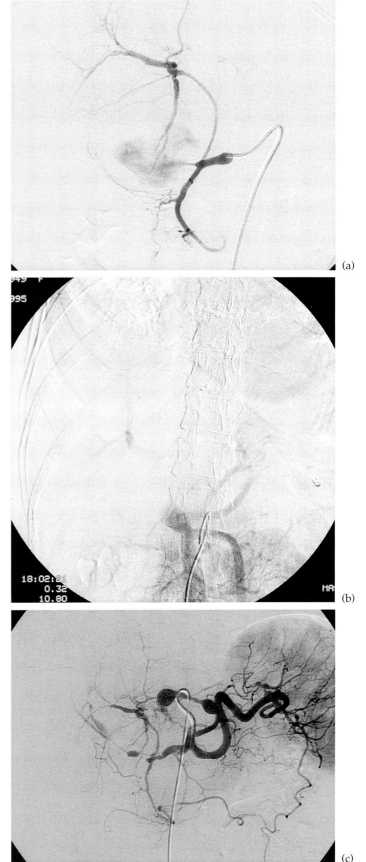

(a)

(b)

(c)

Fig. 7.50 Liver trauma resulting in pseudoaneurysms of the hepatic artery. (a) Selective hepatic arteriogram in a patient who sustained severe blunt liver trauma. There is avulsion of the right hepatic artery with a large pseudoaneurysm, which compresses the portal vein (b). (c) Postoperative angiogram demonstrates two intrahepatic pseudoaneurysms arising from the left hepatic artery. (Courtesy of Dr Richard D. Edwards.)

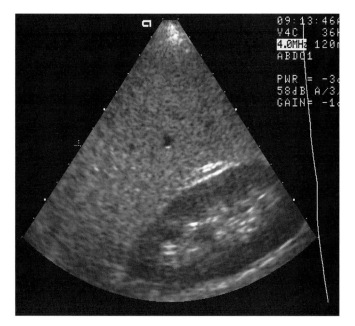

Fig. 7.51 Fatty liver. Longitudinal scan of the right lobe of the liver in the plane of the right kidney in a patient with a long history of excessive alcohol intake and clinical hepatomegaly. The echo density of the liver is increased relative to the renal parenchyma and there is reduced vascular detail, consistent with fatty change. Other causes of fatty infiltration include obesity, diabetes, steroid therapy, chemotherapy, hepatitis, parenteral nutrition and liver transplantation.

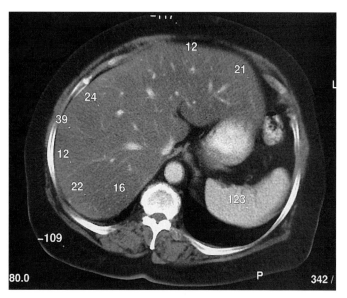

Fig. 7.53 Fatty liver associated with obesity. A spiral CECT scan shows markedly reduced attenuation values in the liver, despite the presence of IV contrast. The contrast between the liver parenchyma and the vessels is marked and the attenuation is much lower than in the contrast-enhanced spleen.

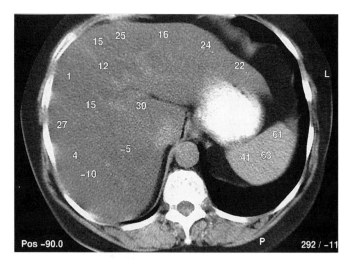

Fig. 7.52 Fatty liver. Spiral CT without contrast shows a diffuse reduction in attenuation indicated by multiple Hounsfield values, which vary between −10 and +30 (normal = 50–70). In contrast, the attenuation of the spleen is normal.

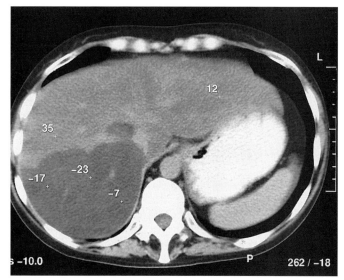

Fig. 7.54 Focal fatty infiltration of the liver. Sometimes fatty infiltration is distinctly focal, with a clear demarcation from normal or near-normal liver parenchyma. In this spiral CT without contrast enhancement, the right lobe posteriorly is very markedly reduced in attenuation, whereas the remainder of the liver shows less severe change. The 43-year-old female patient had a history of excessive alcohol intake and pancreatitis.

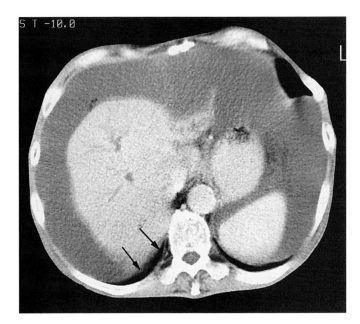

Fig. 7.55 Cryptogenic cirrhosis. Spiral CECT in an elderly male patient with progressive abdominal distension. The liver is small and a large volume of ascites is present. However, contact is maintained between the posterior surface of the liver and the diaphragm (arrows), the 'bare area' since this region is not peritonealized.

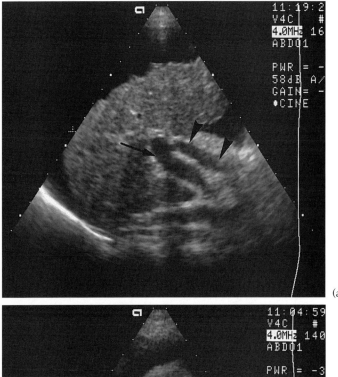

(a)

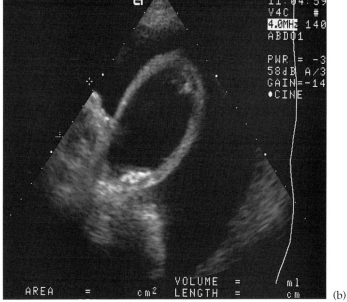

(b)

Fig. 7.56 Primary biliary cirrhosis. (a) A longitudinal scan of the right upper quadrant shows that the liver is grossly contracted, irregular in outline and uneven in texture. The portal vein (arrow) was shown to be patent by spectral Doppler and the direction of blood flow within it was normal. The bile duct (arrowheads) lies anterior to the portal vein in the hepatoduodenal ligament. (b) A longitudinal ultrasound scan through the gallbladder shows low-attenuation calculi within it and thickening of the wall, which could be due to chronic cholecystitis or cirrhosis or both. There was no clinical evidence of acute cholecystitis. In primary biliary cirrhosis, the male/female ratio is 1/9, the immunoglobulin M is increased in 95% and antimitochondrial antibodies are present in 85–100% of cases.

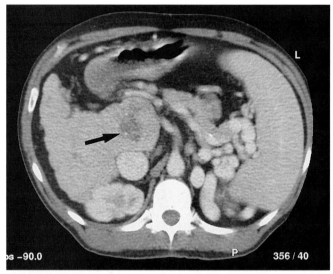

(a)

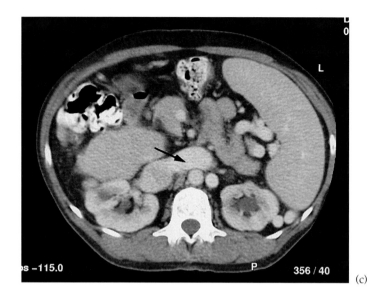

(c)

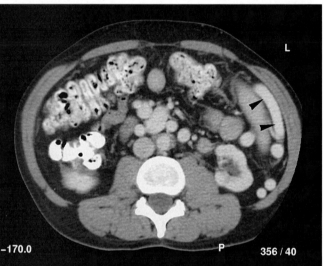

(b)

Fig. 7.57 Cirrhosis with portal hypertension. (a) A spiral CECT of a 45-year-old male patient with cirrhosis shows a contracted irregular liver, with a regenerative nodule in the caudate lobe (arrow). The spleen is seen to be enlarged and multiple contrast-enhanced perisplenic varices are shown. (b) A more distal section also shows numerous varices, one of which is interposed between the spleen and the abdominal wall (arrowheads). In an unenhanced scan, the central abdominal varices might be mistaken for enlarged lymph nodes. (c) The markedly enlarged left renal vein (arrow) and distended inferior vena cava indicate the distal extent of the portosystemic (lienorenal) shunt. This mechanism has a more favourable prognosis than oesophagogastric varices.

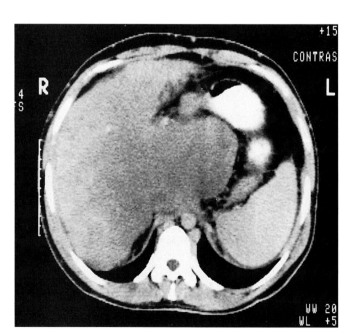

Fig. 7.58 Alcoholic cirrhosis and thrombosis of the IVC. A 40-year-old male patient had a long history of excess alcohol intake, abdominal swelling and gross bilateral lower-limb oedema. The liver is uneven in attenuation, there is contraction of the right and left lobes and massive regeneration of the caudate lobe, which is seen to extend well beyond the midline. The IVC was found to be occluded and the hemiazygos and, to a lesser extent, the azygos veins are seen to be distended.

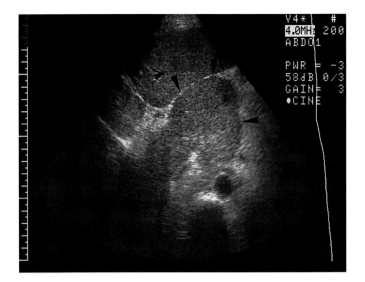

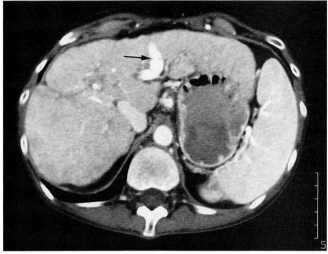

(a)

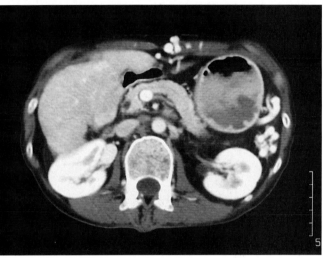

(b)

Fig. 7.59 Alcoholic liver disease. A transverse US scan through the liver shows marked hypertrophy of the caudate lobe (arrowheads) in another patient with alcoholic cirrhosis. The inferior vena cava was found to be compressed but patent. The caudate lobe should not be confused with lymphadenopathy.

Fig. 7.60 Cirrhosis with portal hypertension. (a) Spiral CECT shows recanalization of the umbilical vein (arrow). The liver is uneven in attenuation and irregular in outline, in keeping with cirrhosis. (b) The contrast-enhanced varicose recanalized umbilical vein is shown within the anterior abdominal wall. Gastrorenal collateral veins are also shown. The normal pancreas, pancreatic duct and common bile duct are clearly visible.

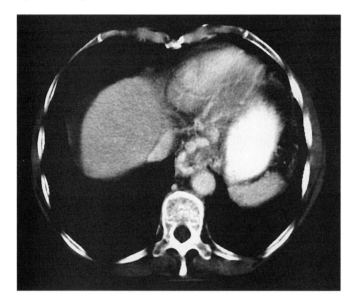

Fig. 7.61 Cirrhosis with portal hypertension. The spiral CECT of a 74-year-old female patient with cirrhosis complicating chronic hepatis C shows engorged oesophagogastric varices.

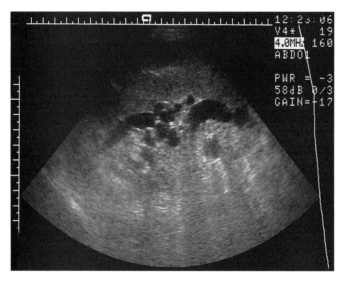

Fig. 7.62 Cryptogenic cirrhosis with portal hypertension. A longitudinal US scan of the left upper quadrant shows extensive varicosity in the region of the hilum of the spleen.

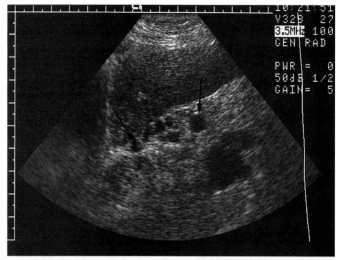

(a)

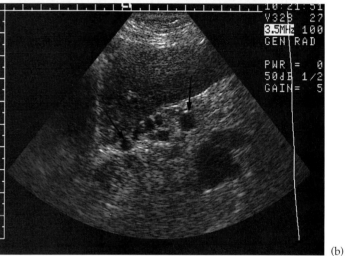

(b)

Fig. 7.63 Cirrhosis secondary to haemochromatosis. A female patient with Waldenström's macroglobulinaemia was treated by repeated blood transfusions, resulting in haemochromatosis and cirrhosis with portal hypertension. (a) A longitudinal US scan through the left lobe of the liver shows multiple varices involving the oesophagogastric junction and proximal stomach (arrows). These were confirmed endoscopically. (b) A transverse US scan shows a grossly distended splenic vein and junction of the superior mesenteric vein and splenic vein. This is a sign of portal hypertension. The patient's spleen measured 16 cm in diameter.

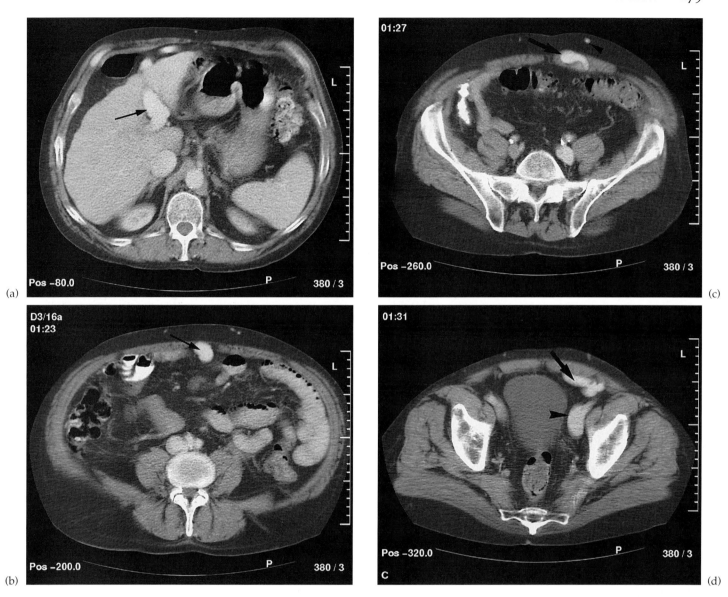

(a)

(b)

(c)

(d)

Fig. 7.64 Cirrhosis with recanalization of the umbilical vein.
This male patient with alcoholic cirrhosis was known to have
portal hypertension. (a) The umbilical vein has recanalized
(arrow). (b) The contrast-filled umbilical vein is shown within the
anterior abdominal wall (arrow) above the umbilicus. (c) The
contrast has drained into the distended inferior epigastric vein
(arrow) and also the subcutaneous superficial epigastric vein
(arrowhead). (d) In the pelvis, the inferior epigastric vein is again
shown (arrow) before draining into the external iliac vein
(arrowhead), completing the spontaneous portosystemic shunt.

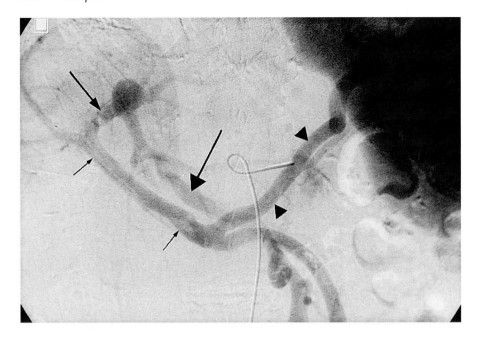

Fig. 7.65 Portal hypertension with recanalization of the umbilical vein. The venous phase of a DSA after splenic artery injection of contrast shows an opacified splenic vein (arrowheads), portal vein (small arrows), left portal vein (medium arrow) and recanalized umbilical vein (large arrow). (Courtesy of Dr Richard D. Edwards.)

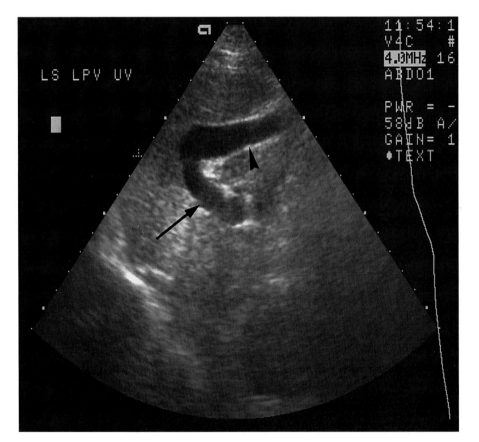

Fig. 7.66 Portal hypertension with recanalization of the umbilical vein. This 42-year-old female patient had alcoholic liver disease and hepatitis C but no history of gastrointestinal bleeding. A longitudinal US scan through the liver shows the left portal vein (arrow), which was shown on Doppler to drain blood into the recanalized umbilical vein (arrowhead). This vessel could be traced as far as the umbilicus, where it anastomosed with systemic collaterals. Clinically, there was no visible caput medusae.

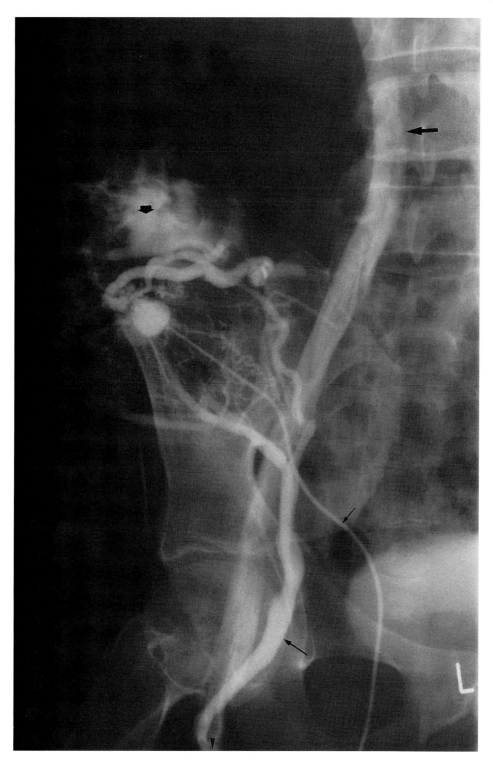

Fig. 7.67 Portal hypertension with ileostomy varices. The patient had had a long history of non-specific ulcerative colitis, treated by panproctocolectomy. Eight years later, he became jaundiced and primary sclerosing cholangitis was diagnosed. This progressed to cirrhosis with portal hypertension, resulting in recurrent bleeding from varices related to his ileostomy. A direct-injection venogram into a varix shows extensive varicosity around the ileostomy in the right iliac fossa. These are seen to drain into a large circumflex iliac vein (long thin arrow), which is a tributary of the long saphenous vein, the junction being indicated by the small arrowhead. There is extensive opacification of the common femoral, external and common iliac veins and IVC (large black arrow). The smallest arrow indicates the injection catheter (on skin surface), and some extravasation of contrast is shown (large arrowhead).

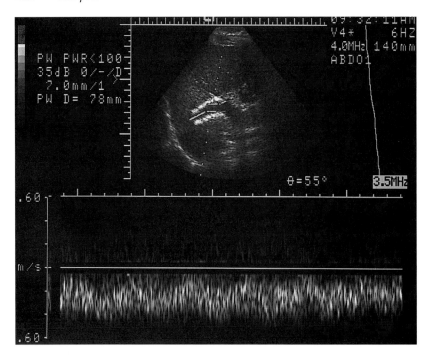

Fig. 7.68 Follow-up of a transjugular intrahepatic portosystemic shunt. Longitudinal US scan of the liver with a spectral Doppler sample volume within the metal stent, the walls of which are markedly echogenic, indicates blood flow in the stent, with a velocity of 0.5 m/s (18 months postprocedure).

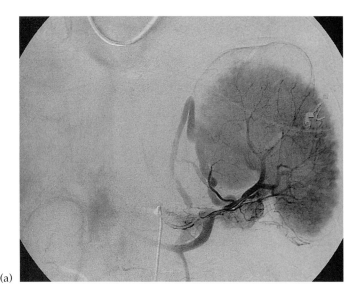

(a)

(b)

Fig. 7.69 Segmental portal hypertension, distal splenic vein thrombosis. A portosystemic shunt via the left renal vein is present. (a) A selective contrast injection into the splenic artery has opacified the spleen which is drained by a large collateral. This fills the proximal portion of the splenic vein, the distal segment being occluded. (b) A separate injection of contrast into the left renal vein shows a large connection with the splenic vein tributary from which the contrast fills the portal vein. (Courtesy of Dr Richard D. Edwards.)

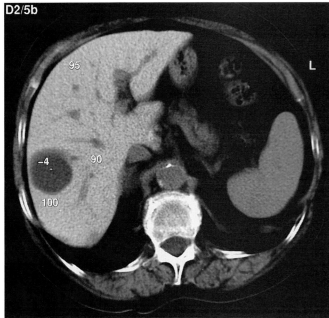

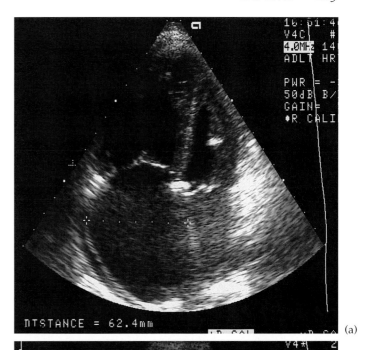

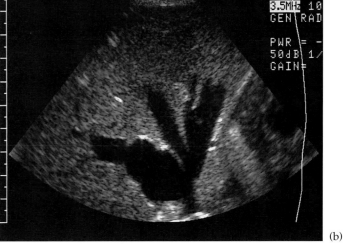

(a)

(b)

Fig. 7.70 Haemochromatosis. An unenhanced spiral CT of the liver in a 66-year-old female patient with a serum ferritin greater than 4000 µg/l (normal = 12–200 µg/l). A liver biopsy showed grade 4 iron deposition. The liver is markedly increased in attenuation, varying between 90 and 100 HU (normal = 50–70 HU). A simple cyst is also present within the liver with HU −4. The differential diagnosis of increased liver attenuation on CT includes Wilson's disease, amiodarone therapy and glycogen-storage disease.

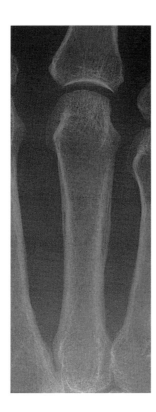

Fig. 7.71 Hypertrophic osteoarthropathy complicating primary biliary cirrhosis. A female patient with proved primary biliary cirrhosis had a history of pain in her hands and wrists. Plain films of her hands show a periosteal reaction affecting the metacarpals and phalanges, particularly the left middle metacarpal. The radius and ulna on both sides were also affected.

Fig. 7.72 Hepatic venous engorgement complicating right-sided heart failure. This lifelong smoker had severe chronic obstructive airway disease and hepatomegaly. (a) In four-chamber view cardiac ultrasound the right side of the heart is seen to be markedly dilated, the right atrium measuring 62 mm transversely. This is associated with tricuspid regurgitation on Doppler sampling. (b) In a transverse ultrasound section of the upper abdomen, the hepatic veins are seen to be markedly engorged.

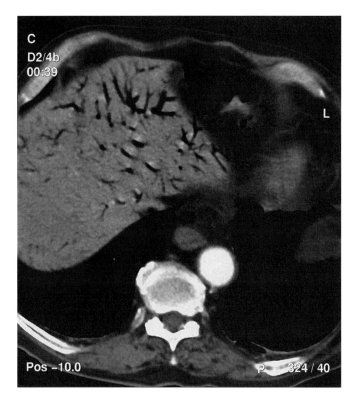

Fig. 7.73 Gas (air) in the portal vein. An 83-year-old male patient was referred for CT pneumocolon immediately after an incomplete colonoscopy, at which a necrotic tumour was found at the splenic flexure. A spiral CECT through the liver shows extensive filling of the portal vein branches with air, which is seen to extend almost to the surface of the liver. The patient was not acutely ill and, in particular, had no clinical features of sepsis. There was spontaneous resolution. Gas in the portal vein complicating bowel infarction has a much more serious prognosis.

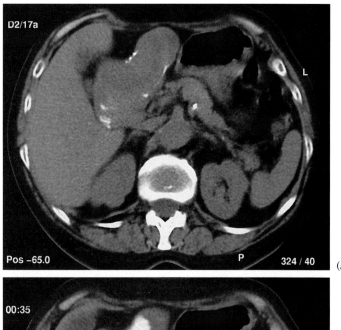 (a)

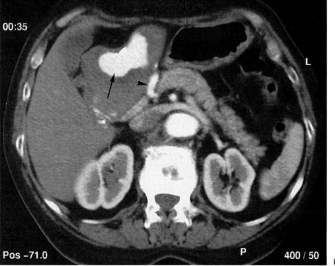 (b)

Fig. 7.75 Hepatic artery aneurysm. A 66-year-old female patient with several months history of right upper quadrant discomfort was examined. The diagnosis was readily made by ultrasound, including colour Doppler and spectral Doppler. However, in order to plan definitive treatment, a spiral CT was performed (a). A large well-circumscribed lobulated mass lesion is shown extending from the porta hepatis to the anterior abdominal wall. Mural calcification is an important sign. (b) An arterial-phase scan shows marked contrast enhancement of the false lumen of the aneurysm (arrow), which is almost completely surrounded by very extensive mural thrombus. The hepatic artery is indicated by the arrowhead. This lesion should not be confused with a porcelain gallbladder.

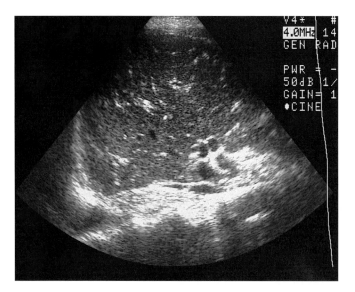

Fig. 7.74 Multifocal liver calcification in chronic renal failure and haemodialysis. The longitudinal ultrasound section of the liver shows a widespread echogenic linear branching pattern, in keeping with vascular calcification. Similar and more marked changes were also present in the spleen.

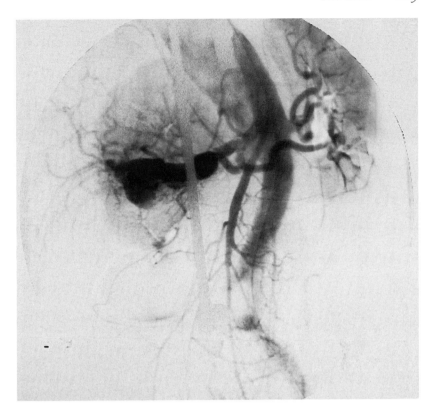

Fig. 7.76 Hepatic artery aneurysm in Marfan's syndrome. A large aneurysm of the common hepatic artery can be seen; a Harrington rod is also present. (Courtesy of Dr Richard D. Edwards.)

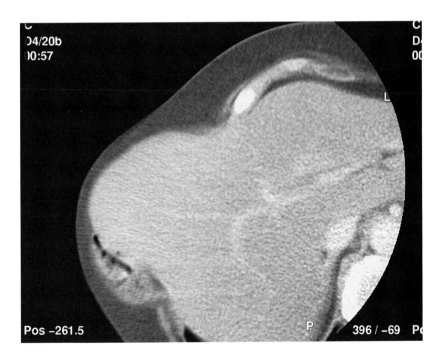

Fig. 7.77 Post-surgical intercostal hernia of the liver and hepatic flexure of the colon. This elderly patient was found to have a firm non-tender swelling in the right upper quadrant of the abdomen. A spiral CECT shows extensive intercostal herniation of the right lobe of the liver, together with hepatic flexure of the colon which was more obvious on lower sections.

8: The Gallbladder and Biliary Tract

Anatomy

The pear-shaped reservoir of bile known as the gallbladder is approximately 8 cm in length, with a capacity of 25–50 ml. It lies in a fossa on the inferior surface of the right lobe of the liver and is covered on its inferior surface with peritoneum, which binds it closely to the liver. Its fundus may project beyond the lower margin of the liver, in which case it has complete peritoneal investment. Occasionally, the peritoneal attachments may be much looser, affording a considerable degree of mobility, with an attendant risk of herniation or torsion. The term 'floating gallbladder' is sometimes applied. The gallbladder is divided into the fundus, the body and the neck, which is continuous with its cystic duct. The neck may include a localized dilatation, Hartmann's pouch. The fundus and body are related on their medial and inferior aspects to the first part and the beginning of the second part of the duodenum and, on the lateral side, the gallbladder is related to the hepatic flexure of the colon and the beginning of the transverse colon. The wall of the gallbladder has an inner layer of mucosa, which is thrown into a series of relatively tall folds, which form a honeycomb pattern. These are gradually effaced as the gallbladder distends. The surface epithelium of the mucous membrane is supported by an areolar lamina propria containing a rich capillary plexus.

Absence or agenesis of the gallbladder is rare—0.03–0.07% of the population [1, 2]. Between 1/3000 and 1/12 000 of the population exhibit duplication of the gall-bladder [1, 2]. Minor, more common anomalies and variations include folding, kinking and septation, and much less commonly the gallbladder may have an ectopic location—for example, under the left lobe of the liver, which is commoner than an intrahepatic site, which is commoner than a retrohepatic position [2]. Very rarely, the gallbladder may be located within the falciform ligament, within the interlobar fissure and sometimes a diverticulum of the gallbladder may be present.

Anatomical variations in the biliary tree are numerous [3] and intrahepatic anomalies are more frequent than the extrahepatic biliary tree. The biliary tree has no anastomotic connections, as there are in the portal venous system, so that there is no intrinsic means of bypassing an obstruction. In 40% of people, the right hepatic duct is absent and the right-sided tributaries may be connected with the left duct or the common hepatic duct (CHD) [4]. In 3%, all the segmental ducts converge at the origin of the CHD. The CHD and common bile duct (CBD) together measure 4–6 cm in length, the length of each being very variable, depending on the point of insertion of the cystic duct. In the wall of the duodenum, there is a special aperture in the muscular layer through which the common duct passes to join the pancreatic duct of Wirsung, at the end of which a small dilatation occurs (the ampulla of Vater). The sphincter of Oddi consists of smooth-muscle fibres situated around the termination of both the distal common duct and pancreatic duct as well as the ampulla. Its histology differs from the muscular layer of the wall of the duodenum. The CBD, unlike the gallbladder, has only a glandular mucosa and a wall of connective tissue, with very few muscle fibres. The helical arrangement of the mucosa within the cystic duct is referred to as the spiral valve of Heister. The dual functions of relaxation of the sphincter of Oddi and of contraction of the gallbladder are dependent on a dual autonomic nerve supply, provided by the sympathetic and parasympathetic fibres. Sympathetic fibres are transmitted by the right splanchnic nerve, and the parasympathetic supply is derived from branches of the vagus nerves beyond the stomach. The CBD and pancreatic duct are usually conjoined distally and drain via a single papilla into the duodenum in 98% of cases [5]. Close but separate bile-duct and pancreatic-duct orifices may be seen opening through the same papilla in 0.5% and widely separate orifices in 1.5% [5]. Other workers, however, report close but separate bile-duct and pancreatic-duct orifices in as many as 30–40% of patients and widely separate orifices in 3.4% [1].

Plain film radiography

Plain abdominal X-rays are of limited value in biliary-tract disease, but 20–30% of gallstones are opaque on plain films. Occasionally, gas-containing fissures are shown within gallstones [6]. This feature may also be apparent on CT scanning [7]. Calcification of the gallbladder wall—'porcelain gallbladder'—when present is an indication of chronic cholecystitis. 'Limey bile', so called because of the high calcium content in biliary sludge, is also a sign of chronic cholecystitis. Plain X-rays are also useful in showing gas in the biliary tree. Intramural gas is a feature of emphysematous cholecystitis. The combination of gas in the biliary tree and signs of small-bowel obstruction should suggest gallstone ileus. Plain films may also reveal pancreatic calcification in chronic pancreatitis, but this method is less sensitive than CT scanning.

Oral cholecystography

The gallbladder may be opacified with orally administered contrast medium, for example sodium ipodate (Biloptin) and calcium ipodate (Solubiloptin). The test depends on the lipid-soluble contrast medium being readily absorbed into the bloodstream and transported to the liver bound to albumin; from there it is excreted in the bile. Opacification of the gallbladder depends on the cystic duct being patent.

Oral cholecystography (OCG) used to be the primary method of investigating the gallbladder, but is now seldom employed, having been very largely replaced by ultrasound. Nevertheless, the accuracy of OCG in a functioning gallbladder is about 85–90% [1, 8, 9]. However, non-visualization cannot be assumed to be an indirect sign of gallstones [10]. In patients in whom US has been technically unsatisfactory on more than one occasion or if there is a mismatch between negative US findings and the patient's signs and symptoms, OCG may be of use. In addition, knowledge that the gallbladder is functioning is a necessary precursor to certain forms of gallstone therapy—for example, extracorporeal shock-wave lithotripsy [11] and the dissolution of gallstones using chenodeoxycholic acid and ursodiol [12].

Ultrasound

Gallstones are normally demonstrated with remarkable ease within the gallbladder with US, which is rapid, safe, repeatable and inexpensive. Nevertheless, there are significant pitfalls, and false-positive results can be obtained, particularly by the inexperienced operator. Gallstones typically cast strong acoustic shadows. Changes in the patient's posture usually result in a change in the position of the stones, but they are occasionally found to be adherent to the mucosa, which may cause confusion with cholesterol polyps. The accuracy of US in gallstone diagnosis is very high in expert hands—for example, 98% [1] and 96% [13]. Care must be taken not to confuse the echoes produced by the spiral valve of Heister in the cystic duct with small cystic-duct stones. Ultrasound is also valuable in the diagnosis of acute and chronic cholecystitis [14]. Colour Doppler and power

Doppler may demonstrate an increased vascularity in the gallbladder wall in acute cholecystitis [14].

In the jaundiced patient, US should be the first-line imaging method in virtually every case, since it is the easiest means of confirming or excluding intrahepatic and extrahepatic bile-duct dilatation. Dewbury [15] found the normal common duct to measure 2–5 mm. However, in another normal series, 11% of normal subjects had a duct diameter of greater than 6 mm and 4% were greater than 7 mm [16]. It is widely accepted that the normal duct increases in size with increasing age and, in our experience, a duct diameter of 8 mm in elderly patients may be a normal finding. In expert hands, the level of obstruction in the biliary tree may be predicted by US with a high degree of accuracy; for example, in one prospective study of 65 patients, Gibson *et al.* [17] showed that the level of obstruction was correctly indicated in 95% of cases and the cause in 88%.

ENDOLUMINAL ULTRASOUND

Endoluminal US is analogous to intravascular US. Both techniques depend on the availability of miniaturized technology, with a US transducer delivered via a catheter. The transducers in use are either of a rotating mechanical type or electronically switched phased array. Using a very high frequency of 12.5–20 MHz, the biliary tract is accessed percutaneously via a transhepatic 7 or 8 F sheath [18].

Cholangiography

INTRAVENOUS CHOLANGIOGRAPHY

Opacification of the extrahepatic biliary tree may be achieved by the slow IV infusion over 20–30 min of either ioglycamide (Biligram) or iotroxime (Biloscopin). Even under favourable conditions, including conventional tomography, the contrast density by this method is relatively poor. The technique has very largely been superseded by more accurate, more rapid and safer techniques, including US. In jaundiced patients, IV cholangiography is of very little value. In one series [19], when the bilirubin level was higher than 0.18 mg/l, no ducts could be visualized by this method. The contrast medium is also moderately toxic, with a mortality of 1/5000 patients [20]. Intravenous cholangiography has, however, been combined with considerable success with CT scanning [21].

PERCUTANEOUS TRANSHEPATIC CHOLANGIOGRAPHY

Percutaneous transhepatic cholangiography (PTC) involves the direct percutaneous puncture, under fluoroscopic control, of the biliary tree, using a fine-bore needle. The safety of the method has been greatly enhanced by the introduction of the Chiba needle [22]. With a high level of expertise, 98% of dilated ducts and 80% of normal ducts may be punctured [1]. This method, of course, enables the biliary tree to be opacified regardless of the presence of jaundice. The coagulation status of the patient needs to be satisfactory, corrected if necessary by vitamin K given over several days prior to the procedure or, on the day of the test, a transfusion of fresh frozen plasma and platelets.

ENDOSCOPIC RETROGRADE CHOLANGIOGRAPHY

The widespread use of the excellent technique of endoscopic retrograde cholangiography, which very frequently also includes examination of the pancreatic duct, has represented a very major advance in the investigation and management of biliary-tract disease. This was facilitated by the development of fibreoptic duodenoscopes in the 1970s. This somewhat invasive method provides relatively easy access to the biliary tree and pancreatic duct and, at the same time, pathology may be detected in the stomach or duodenum. It also provides an opportunity to obtain a biopsy or cytological evidence of malignancy. In most patients with obstructive jaundice, endoscopic retrograde cholangiopancreatography (ERCP) should be the investigation of choice after US, and it will establish the cause in the vast majority of cases. While PTC is more invasive, it has the advantage of showing the intrahepatic biliary tree more clearly. The mortality from ERCP is about 0.2% [23], related principally to septicaemia following cholangitis or pancreatitis. In patients having ERCP, there is a significant risk of acute pancreatitis. A transient increase in serum amylase occurs in between 40% and 75% of cases immediately following ERCP, but clinical pancreatitis occurs in less than 7% [1].

Computerized tomography scanning

The clinical application of CT to biliary-tract diagnosis has advantages and disadvantages. The disadvantages, compared with US, are its reduced availability, much greater cost and very substantial radiation dose. It is fairly clear that CT is inferior to US in detecting uncalcified gallstones [24]. However, it is of particular value in ultrasonically difficult patients—for example, the obese or those where access is restricted by bowel gas. It therefore has a complementary role to that of US. For detecting and staging malignant biliary-tract tumours, CT is the method of choice, and it has a useful role in the differential diagnosis of biliary-tract lesions. The usefulness of CT has been enhanced by the advent of spiral (helical) scanning, in which, during a single breath-hold, a substantial volume of tissue can be imaged. Impressive vascular and soft-tissue contrast enhancement is possible because of the shorter scanning time, and potentially subtle radiological signs—for example, vascular encasement by tumour—may be much more clearly shown. It is also possible to produce high-quality multiplanar reconstructions. The combination of IV cholangiography with spiral CT has also been used with good effect to produce

3-D images of the biliary tract [25]. Using the same technology, spiral CT angiography is being used increasingly to determine the resectability of cholangiocarcinoma and pancreatic cancer, with consecutive arterial- and portal-venous-phase contrast-enhanced studies during a single examination, using fourth-generation scanners.

Magnetic resonance imaging

In current practice, MRI plays no role in the diagnosis of gallstones, almost all of which may be demonstrated by US. An exciting role for MRI in the biliary tree, however, is emerging. The advent of MR cholangiography provides a 3-D reconstruction of the biliary tract without the need for contrast medium [26]. It is not yet clear whether MR cholangiography will routinely replace diagnostic ERCP. A vital positive feature of ERCP is that it provides ready access to interventional techniques, such as stone extraction and stent insertion, at the time of the diagnostic procedure. At the present time, outcome analysis and the cost-effectiveness of MRI need to be further evaluated [27].

Angiography

The surgical resectability of neoplasms involving the biliary tract depends to a large extent on the presence or absence of vascular encasement by the tumour. Selective digital-subtraction angiography has a role in assessing these patients, so that those with unresectable disease are not subjected to unnecessary surgery. In addition, involvement of the portal vein may be confirmed or excluded by portal venography, which is usually part of a combined procedure beginning with arteriography.

Angiography may also be of value in the investigation of patients with bleeding into the biliary tree (haemobilia)—for example, secondary to interventional techniques, including liver biopsy.

References

1 Adam A., Roddie M.E. & Bowley N.B. (1997) The biliary tract. In: Grainger R.G. & Allison D.J. (eds) *Diagnostic Radiology*, 3rd edn. New York: Churchill Livingstone, 1201–1234.
2 Dahnert W. (1996) *Radiology Review Manual*, 3rd edn. Baltimore: Williams & Wilkins, 497.
3 Hayes M.A., Goldenberg I.S. & Bishop C.C. (1958) The developmental basis for bile duct anomalies. *Surgery, Gynaecology and Obstetrics* 107, 447–456.
4 Rabischong P. & Pissas A. (1997) Anatomy. In: Rossi P. & Bezzi M. (eds) *Biliary Tract Radiology*. Berlin: Springer, 3–11.
5 Bartram C.I. & Kumar P. (1981) *Clinical Radiology in Gastroenterology*. Oxford: Blackwell Scientific Publications, 30.
6 Meyers M.A. & O'Donohue N. (1973) The Mercedes Benz sign: insight into the dynamics of formation and disappearance of gallstones. *American Journal of Roentgenology* 119, 63–70.
7 Dunne M.G. & Johnston M.L. (1980) Gas within gallstones on CT. *Americal Journal of Roentgenology* 134, 1064–1066.

8 Karani J. (1998) The biliary tract. In: Sutton D. (ed.) *A Textbook of Radiology and Imaging*, 6th edn. New York: Churchill Livingstone, 955–980.

9 Bazzocchi M., Quaia E, Zuiani C. *et al.* (1997) Oral cholecystography. In: Rossi P. & Bezzi M. (eds) *Biliary Tract Radiology*. Berlin: Springer, 33–37.

10 Mujahed Z. (1976) Factors interfering with the opacification of a normal gallbladder. *Gastro-intestinal Radiology* **1**, 183–185.

11 Nealon W.H., Urrutia F., Fleming D. *et al.* (1991) The economic burden of gallstone lithotripsy, will cost determine its fate? *Annals of Surgery* **213**, 645–649.

12 Fromm H. (1989) Gallstone disolution therapy with ursodiol. Patient selection. *Digestive Disease Science* **34** (Suppl. 12), 365–385.

13 Cooperberg P.L. & Gibney R.G. (1987) Imaging of the gallbladder. *Radiology* **163**, 605–613.

14 Bazzochi M., Zhiani C., Rigamonti A. *et al.* (1997) Ultrasonography of the gallbladder. In: Rossi P. & Bezzi M. (eds) *Biliary Tract Radiology*. Berlin: Springer, 39–51.

15 Dewbury K.C. (1980) Visualisation of normal biliary ducts with ultrasound. *British Journal of Radiology* **53**, 774–780.

16 Parulekar S.G. (1979) Ultrasound evaluation of common bile duct size. *Radiology* **133**, 703–707.

17 Gibson R.N., Yeung E., Thompson J.N. *et al.* (1986) Bile duct obstruction: radiologic evaluation of level, cause and tumour resectability. *Radiology* **160**, 43–47.

18 Brambs H.-J. (1997) Endoluminal ultrasonography of the biliary tree. In: Rossi P. & Bezzi M. (eds) *Biliary Tract Radiology*. Berlin: Springer, 121–127.

19 Eubanks B., Martinez C.R., Mehigan D. *et al.* (1982) Current role of intravenous cholangiography. *Americal Journal of Surgery* **143**, 731–733.

20 Ansell G. (1970) Adverse reactions to contrast agents: scope of problem. *Investigative Radiology* **5**, 374–391.

21 Paivansalo M., Merikanto J., Lahde S. *et al.* (1988) Radiographic diagnosis of bile duct cysts, retrospective analysis of 13 cases. *Acta Radiologica* **29**, 657–660.

22 Okuda K., Tanikawa K., Emura T. *et al.* (1974) Non-surgical percutaneous transhepatic cholangiography—diagnostic significance in medical problems of the liver. *American Journal of Digestive Diseases* **19**, 21–36.

23 Bilbao M.K., Dotter C.T., Lee T.G. *et al.* (1976) Complications of ERCP: a study of one thousand cases. *Gastro-enterology* **70**, 314–320.

24 van Hoe L., van Beckevoort D. & Baert A.L. (1997) CT of the gallbladder. In: Rossi P. & Bezzi M. (eds) *Biliary Tract Radiology*. Berlin: Springer, 53–57.

25 Stockberger S.M., Was J.L., Scherman S. *et al.* (1994) Intravenous cholangiography with helical CT, comparison with endoscopic retrograde cholangiography. *Radiology* **192**, 675–680.

26 Bret P.M. & Reinhold C. (1997) MRI of the gallbladder. In: Rossi P. & Bezzi M. (eds) *Biliary Tract Radiology*. Berlin: Springer, 59–69.

27 Reinhold C. & Bret P.M. (1997) MRI of the bile ducts. In: Rossi P. & Bezzi M. (eds) *Biliary Tract Radiology*. Berlin: Springer, 101–120.

28 McLean A. & Fairclough P. (1996) Endoscopic ultrasound—current applications. *Clinical Radiology* **51**, 83–98.

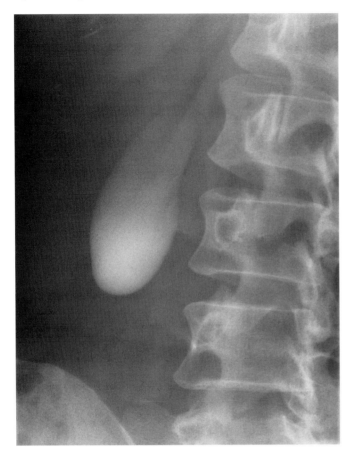

Fig. 8.1 Normal oral cholecystogram. Erect oblique view of a normally opacified gallbladder.

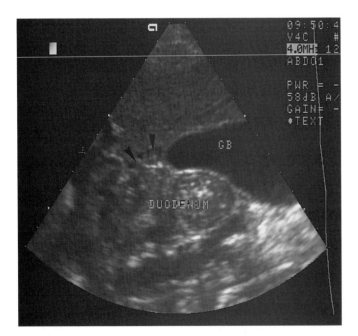

Fig. 8.2 Normal gallbladder, ultrasound. A longitudinal US scan (4 MHz) shows the normal echo-free lumen of the gallbladder (GB). The spiral valve is just visible (arrowheads).

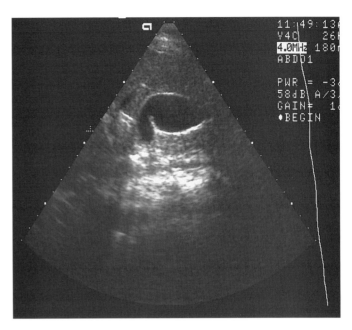

Fig. 8.3 Normal postural folding of the gallbladder. The US scan shows a postural kink in the posterior wall of the gall-bladder. This was seen to alter with changes in posture and only in this way can it be distinguished from a septum.

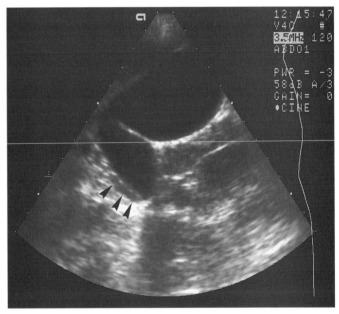

Fig. 8.4 Congenital gallbladder septum. A clearly defined linear partition is shown within the gallbladder, partly dividing the lumen. This showed no change with posture. The cystic duct is shown (arrowheads).

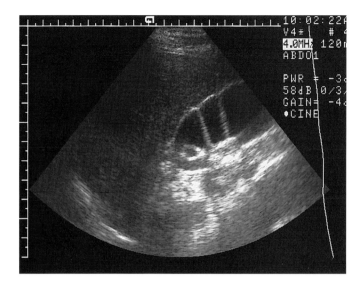

Fig. 8.5 Multiple gallbladder septa. The longitudinal US scan shows two well-defined transverse partitions dividing the gallbladder.

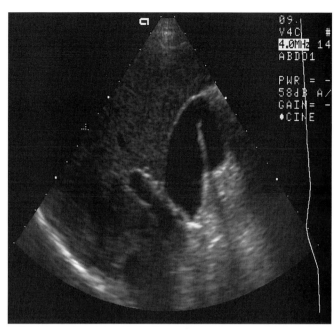

Fig. 8.6 Phrygian cap gallbladder septum. This is a normal variant, consisting of a septum involving the fundus.

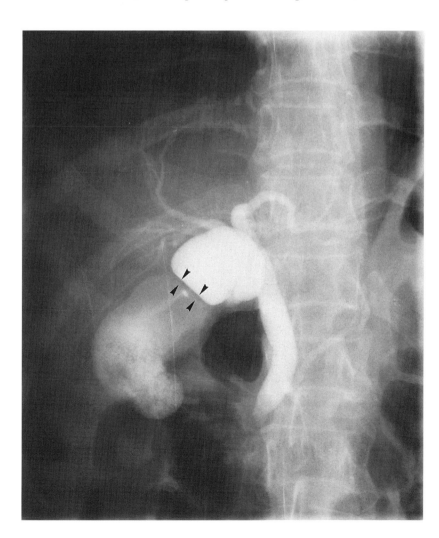

Fig. 8.7 Gallbladder septum, ERCP. A late film following the removal of the endoscope shows contrast in the biliary tree and in the gallbladder, there being a marked difference in contrast density on the two sides of the congenital septum (arrowheads), resulting from slow retrograde filling beyond the septum. (Courtesy of Dr Richard D. Edwards.)

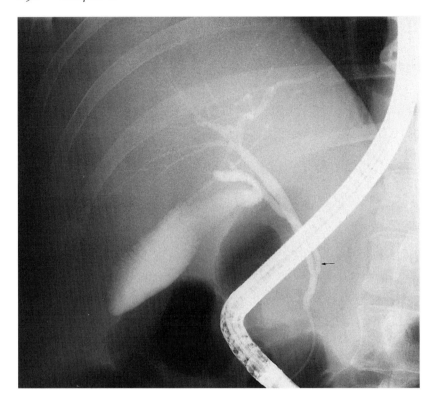

Fig. 8.8 Normal gallbladder and biliary tree, ERCP. The bile duct has been cannulated and the biliary tree has been outlined with contrast, with obvious patency of the cystic duct and normal gallbladder filling. The so-called 'spiral cystic duct' is seen to cross the bile duct and has an unusually low insertion into the medial side of the common duct 2.5 cm above the ampulla. This is normal variant.

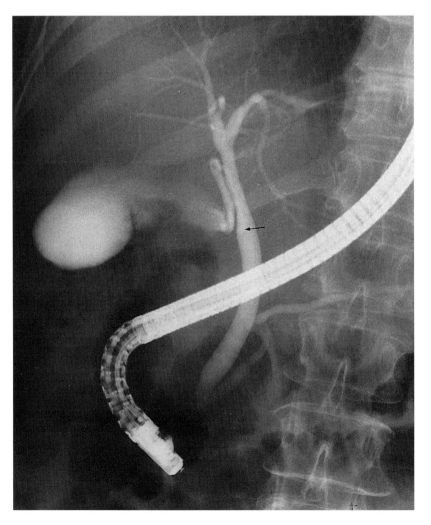

Fig. 8.9 Normal gallbladder, ERCP. The biliary tree and pancreatic duct have been opacified with contrast. The cystic duct has an unusually tortuous course, travelling upwards adjacent to the CHD before turning downwards to be inserted into the bile duct at the same level as its origin (arrow). Gallstone-related inflammation of the cystic duct may cause extrinsic obstruction of the CHD (Mirizzi's syndrome). In addition, the potential for injury to the CHD during cholecystectomy is obvious in this situation.

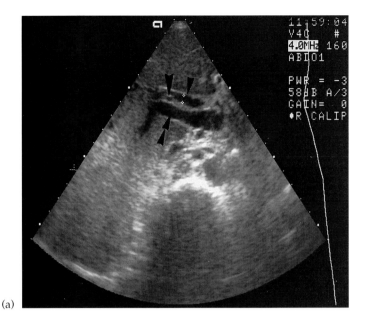

(a)

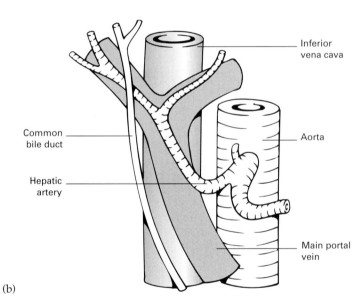

(b)

Common bile duct

Hepatic artery

Inferior vena cava

Aorta

Main portal vein

Fig. 8.10 Normal bile duct, ultrasound. (a) The relationship of the normal bile duct to the hepatic artery and portal vein in the hepatoduodenal ligament is shown. Small arrowhead, common duct; large arrowhead, hepatic artery in cross-section; double arrowhead, portal vein. (b) The anatomical relationship between the hepatic artery, bile duct, portal vein and inferior vena cava (IVC) is shown.

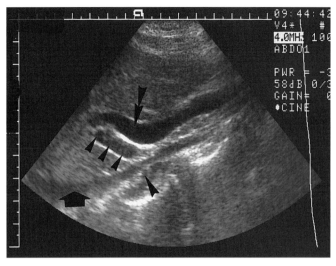

Fig. 8.11 Moderate bile-duct dilatation without obstruction, post-cholecystectomy. Longitudinal US scan in the plane of the IVC (broad arrow) with the right renal artery shown in transverse section posterior to it (large arrowhead). Anterior to the IVC, the portal vein is shown (small arrowheads). The moderately dilated CBD is visible anterior to the portal vein (double arrowhead).

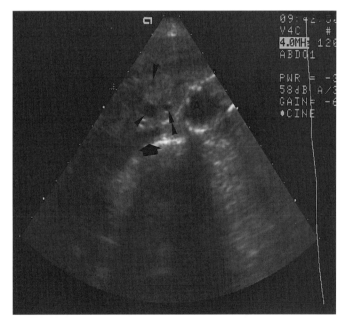

Fig. 8.12 Normal distal bile duct. Transverse US scan through the head of the pancreas shows the IVC posteriorly (broad arrowhead), the CBD in transverse section (small arrowhead), the pancreatic duct in transverse section (double arrowhead) and the gastroduodenal artery in cross-section (large arrowhead). A, aorta.

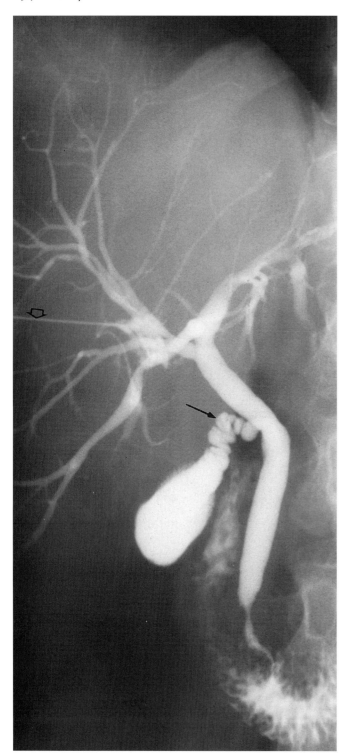

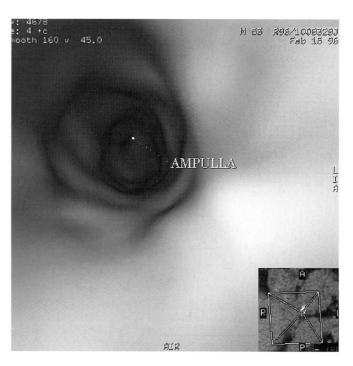

Fig. 8.14 Normal CT cholangiography. Virtual cholangioscopy has been created by 3-D reconstruction of a CT cholangiogram. The ampulla is indicated. This elegant technique has much potential, but is too time-consuming for routine use at the present time. (Courtesy of Dr Marie Callaghan.)

Fig. 8.13 Normal biliary tree, PTC. A bile-duct tributary has been punctured with a Chiba needle (open arrowhead) and contrast injected percutaneously. The normal intramural course of the distal end of the bile duct is shown. The normal spiral valve of Heister is also visible (arrow). Contrast is seen in the normally contracted duodenum.

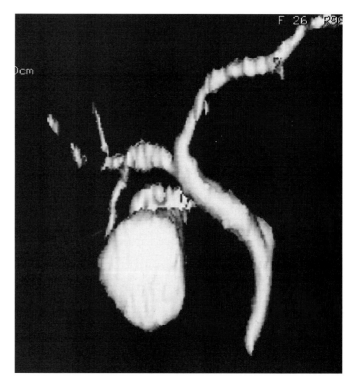

Fig. 8.15 Normal CT cholangiogram. A shaded surface 3-D reconstruction has been employed to display the biliary tree, including a posterior spiral cystic duct entering the bile duct on its medial side. (Courtesy of Dr Marie Callaghan.)

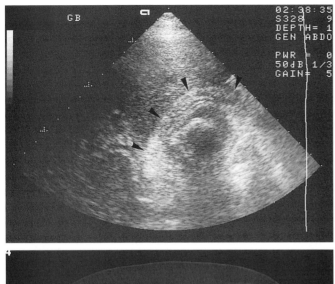

(a)

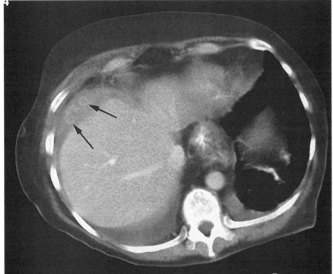

(bi)

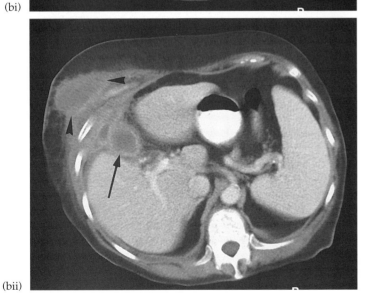

(bii)

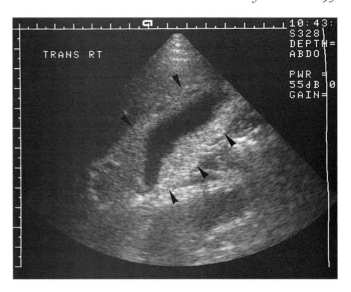

Fig. 8.17 Acalculous cholecystitis. This US scan of the right upper quadrant in a patient with acute pain there shows gross thickening and reduction in the marginal definition of the gallbladder wall (arrowheads), in the absence of any evidence of calculi. In cases of acute cholecystitis, 10% have no evidence of gallstones. (Courtesy of Dr Wilma Kincaid.)

Fig. 8.18 Emphysematous cholecystitis. This plain abdominal X-ray of the right upper quadrant shows gas within the lumen of the gallbladder, together with extensive intramural gas. There is no evidence of opaque gallstones.

Fig. 8.16 Acute cholecystitis. (a) This patient had a sudden onset of severe right upper quadrant pain, nausea, pyrexia and raised white-cell count. The US scan of the right upper quadrant shows marked swelling of the gallbladder wall, the perimeter of which is indicated by the arrowheads. At least one calculus is shown within the lumen of the gallbladder. (Courtesy of Dr Wilma Kincaid.) (b) Acute cholecystitis leading to spontaneous gallbladder rupture: (i) gallstones are visible within the right anterior subphrenic space (arrows); (ii) the gallbladder wall is thickened (arrow) and an inflammatory mass is seen to extend through an intercostal space into a subcutaneous abscess (arrowheads).

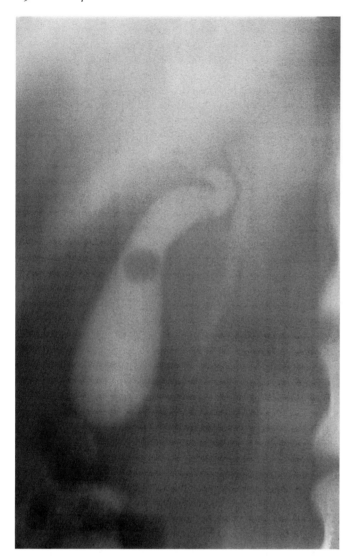

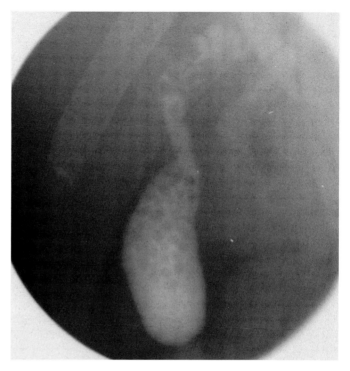

Fig. 8.20 Gallstones causing biliary colic. This oral cholecystogram during an attack of biliary colic shows contrast within the gallbladder and cystic duct, with numerous small radiolucent calculi within the gallbladder and also within the cystic duct. The attack of biliary colic was precipitated by giving a fatty meal.

Fig. 8.19 Gallbladder calculus. Oral cholecystography with conventional tomography shows normal opacification of the gallbladder, indicating patency of the cystic duct. A clearly defined 1 cm calculus is shown within the gallbladder. The bile duct is faintly opacified and is of normal calibre.

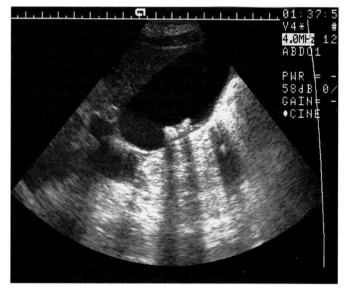

Fig. 8.21 Gallbladder calculi, ultrasound. This longitudinal US scan shows several echogenic calculi with prominent acoustic shadowing. In this case, there is no evidence of gallbladder wall thickening to suggest either acute or chronic cholecystitis.

The Gallbladder and Biliary Tract

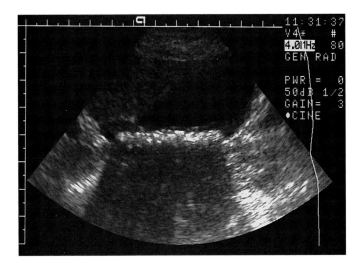

Fig. 8.22 Numerous small gallbladder calculi. This US scan shows numerous tiny calculi forming a layer on the posterior wall of the gallbladder and associated with a broad apron of acoustic shadowing.

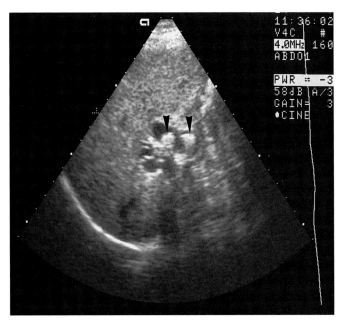

Fig. 8.24 Cystic-duct calculi, ultrasound. An oblique scan through the porta hepatis shows two calculi (arrowheads) within the cystic duct. The gallbladder, which also contained calculi, and the bile duct were clearly shown on separate sections.

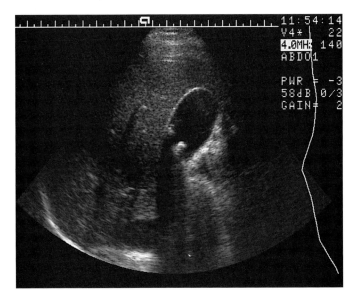

Fig. 8.23 Gallstones associated with hereditary spherocystosis. This US scan of a 24-year-old female patient who had a splenectomy at the age of 10 years and recent dyspepsia shows gallbladder calculi. The patient also had a 6 cm mass in her left upper quadrant, which was apparently the result of hyperplasia of an accessory spleen following her previous splenectomy.

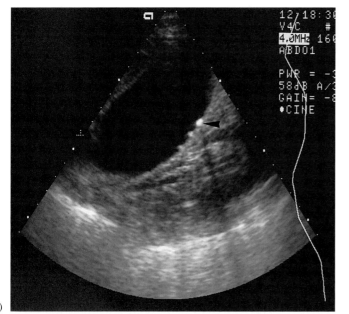

(a)

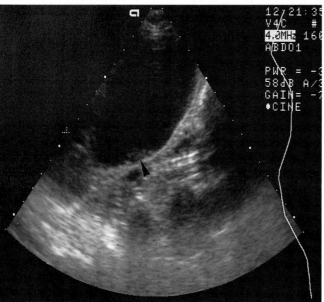

(b)

Fig. 8.25 Fixed intramural calculi and mobile gallstones.
(a) Several tiny fixed calculi are seen to be adherent to the wall of the gallbladder. One shows acoustic shadowing (arrowhead). These were unaffected by changes in position. (b) In the same patient, multiple tiny calculi of low reflectivity and without acoustic shadowing were seen to be highly mobile (arrowhead).

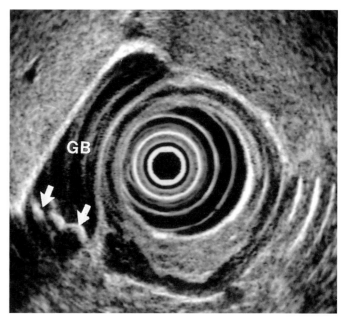

Fig. 8.26 Gallbladder calculi, endoscopic ultrasound. In patients in whom transabdominal US is difficult (due to obesity), gallbladder (GB) calculi (arrows) can be easily seen on endoscopic US. In patients with recurrent acute pancreatitis, gallbladder microlithiasis is more easily diagnosed on endoscopic US than with transcutaneous scanning. (Courtesy of Dr Alison McLean.)

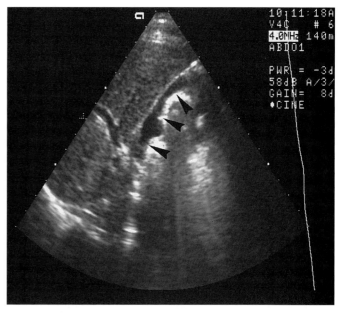

Fig. 8.27 Gallbladder artefact, ultrasound. A longitudinal scan through the gallbladder shows echogenic material (arrowheads) with poorly developed acoustic shadowing, raising the possibility of gallbladder calculi. On real time, however, there is obvious peristalsis in this area, indicating that these changes are the result of an extrinsic impression on the gallbladder wall from the adjacent duodenum.

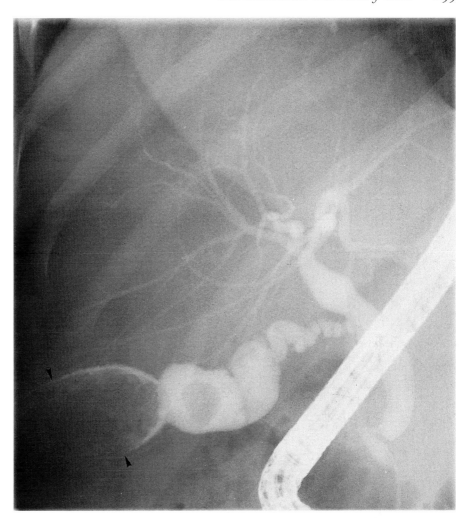

Fig. 8.28 Large fundal gallstone, ERCP.
Normal filling of the fundus of the
gallbladder by contrast is largely
prevented by a large irregular stone
(arrowheads). A smaller calculus is shown
in the body of the gallbladder.

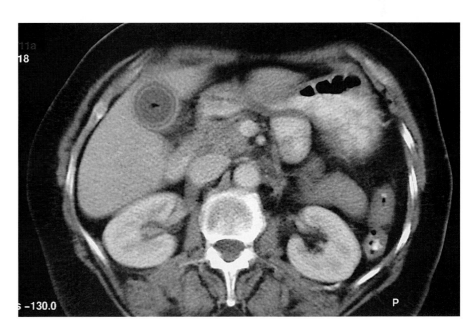

Fig. 8.29 Gallstone containing gas.
A spiral contrast-enhanced CT (CECT)
shows a small central collection of gas
within a gallstone, which is seen to fill the
lumen of the gallbladder.

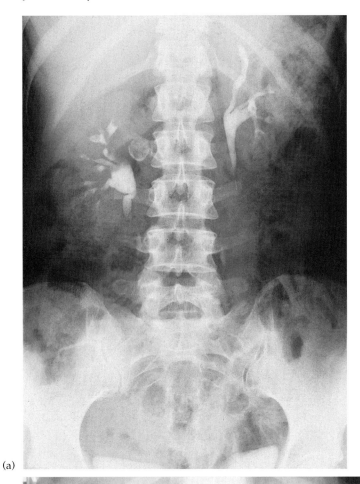

(a)

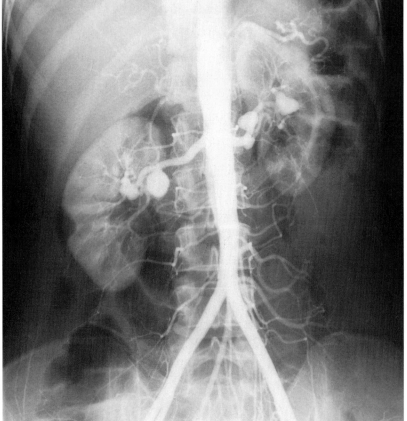

(b)

Fig. 8.30 Calcified opacity mimicking a gallstone. (a) An IV urogram shows a normal pyelogram on each side. There is curvilinear calcification projected over the transverse process of L2 on the right side. The gallbladder was found to be normal. (b) Renal arteriography shows multiple renal artery aneurysms, one of which corresponds with the calcified opacity in a patient with pseudoxanthoma elasticum.

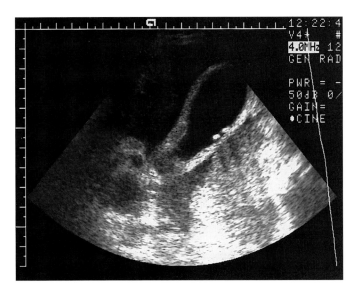

Fig. 8.31 Gallbladder wall thickening in primary biliary cirrhosis. This female patient with proved primary biliary cirrhosis, portal hypertension and ascites was found to have a thick-walled gallbladder on US. She also has two small gallstones with acoustic shadowing. The gallbladder wall thickening could be due to cirrhosis or chronic cholecystitis or both.

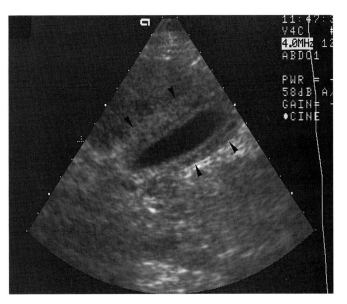

Fig. 8.32 Gallbladder wall thickening in primary biliary cirrhosis. The US of this gallbladder shows gross thickening of the wall in a patient with proved primary biliary cirrhosis (arrowheads). There was no evidence of gallstones and the patient had no clinical features of cholecystitis.

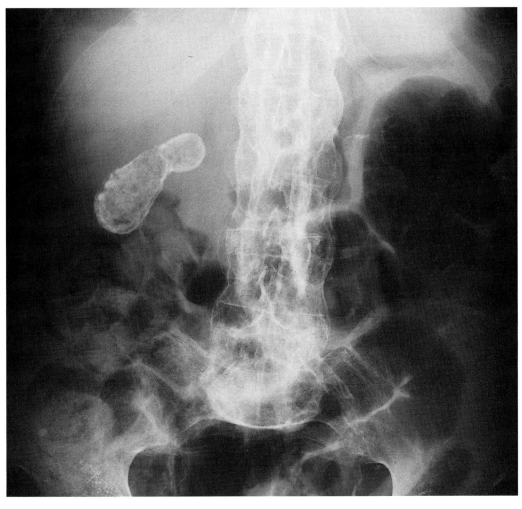

Fig. 8.33 Gallbladder wall calcification in chronic cholecystitis (porcelain gallbladder). An 82-year-old male patient with a long history of gallbladder dyspepsia had a plain film which shows extensive, slightly uneven, gallbladder wall calcification. This condition predisposes to gallbladder cancer. This patient also has far advanced ankylosing spondylitis.

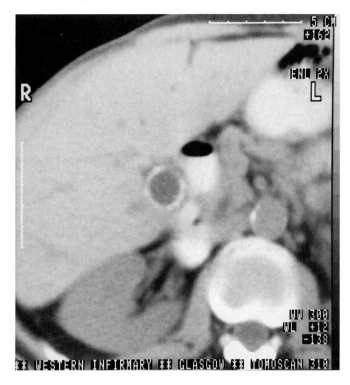

Fig. 8.34 Chronic cholecystitis (porcelain gallbladder). A CT scan without IV contrast enhancement in another patient shows moderate calcification of the gallbladder wall.

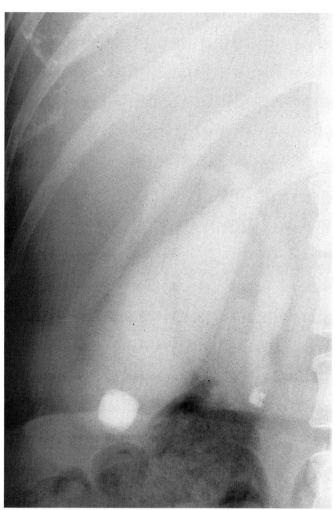

Fig. 8.36 Milk of calcium bile (limey bile). This plain film of the right upper quadrant, without any kind of contrast medium administration, shows diffuse opacification of the gallbladder and bile duct, resulting from opaque bile. A calculus is shown in the gallbladder and also in the bile-duct.

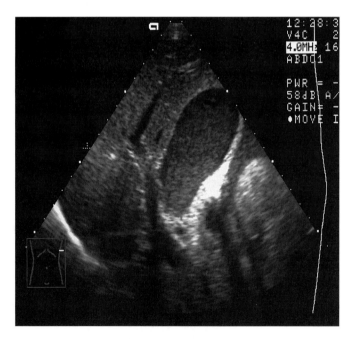

Fig. 8.35 Viscous bile. An ultrasound of a 42-year-old male patient, 12 days postoperation for small-bowel perforation and peritonitis. The wall of the gallbladder is normal on US, but there is a diffuse increase in echogenicity of the bile within it. This is due to calcium bilirubinate and cholesterol crystals associated with biliary stasis. It occurs in prolonged fasting, hyperalimentation, cystic-duct obstruction, haemolysis and cholecystitis.

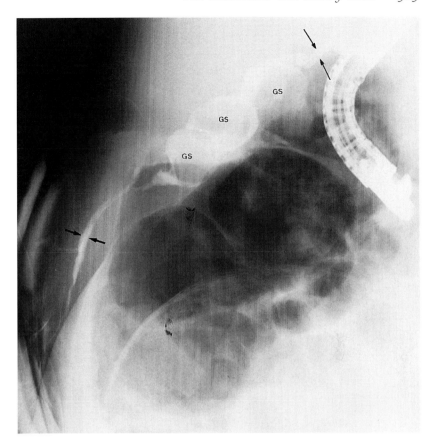

Fig. 8.37 Chronic cholecystitis complicated by cutaneous biliary fistula. The ERCP shows contrast filling of the gallbladder via the cystic duct (thin arrows). At least three large calculi are shown in the gallbladder (GS). Contrast is seen to escape from the fundus of the gallbladder and reaches the skin surface via a fistula (broad arrows). The patient had previously discharged small gallstones via this fistula. (Courtesy of Dr Peter Mills.)

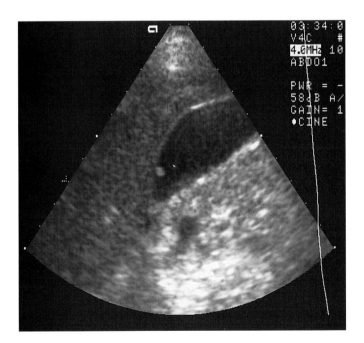

Fig. 8.38 Cholesterol polyp in the gallbladder. A tiny structure is seen to be attached to the wall of the gallbladder, with no evidence of acoustic shadowing and with no change in posture. Cholesterol polyps are relatively common and frequently multiple.

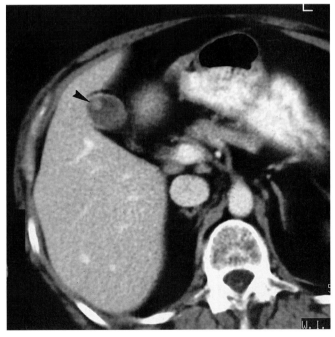

Fig. 8.39 Cholesterol polyp in the gallbladder. Spiral CECT scan of another patient shows a fixed polyp (arrowhead) attached to the roof of the gallbladder wall.

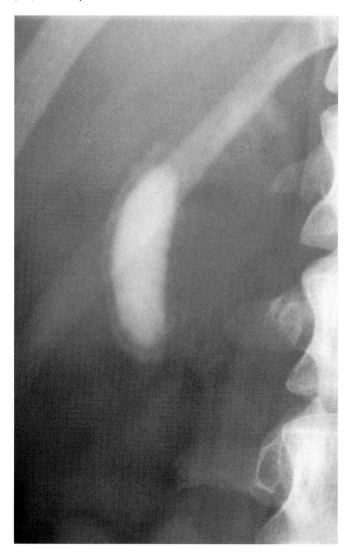

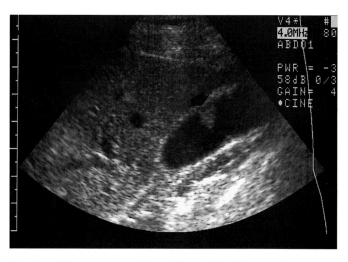

Fig. 8.42 **Adenomatous polyp of the gallbladder.** An ultrasound of the right upper quadrant shows an 8 mm diameter, soft-tissue, mass lesion (arrowhead) arising from the roof of the gallbladder. The lesion was found to be solitary.

Fig. 8.40 **Adenomyomatosis of the gallbladder.** Oral cholecystography shows contrast in the lumen of the gallbladder, together with filling of the tiny Rokitanksi–Aschoff sinuses within the thickened wall.

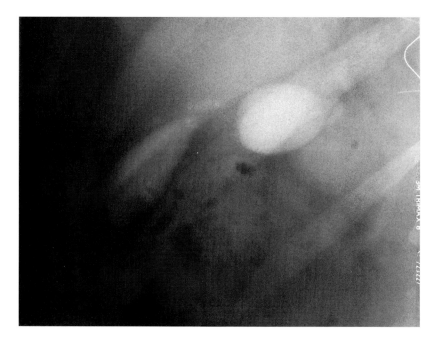

Fig. 8.41 **Adenomyomatosis of the gallbladder associated with duplication of the gallbladder.** One of a pair of gallbladders is seen to opacify normally. The second is also seen to opacify, but multiple Rokitanski–Aschoff sinuses are seen to fill, in keeping with adenomyomatosis. (Courtesy of Dr Richard D. Edwards.)

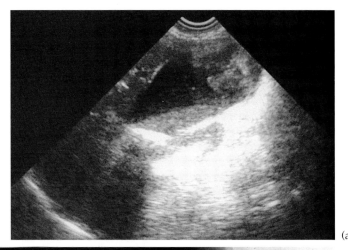

(a)

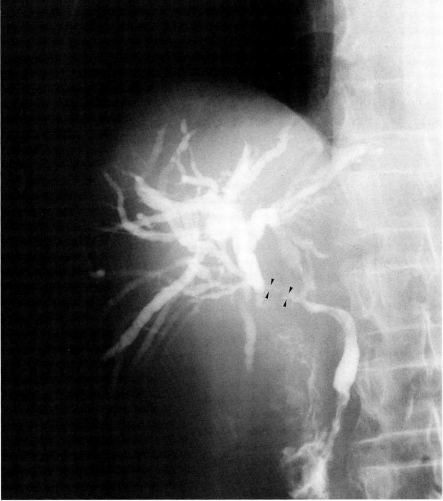

Fig. 8.43 Carcinoma of the gallbladder.
A 65-year-old male patient presented
with right upper quadrant pain. (a) On
ultrasound, gallstones and a constant
filling defect in the gallbladder were
shown. The patient declined definitive
treatment and 6 months later became
jaundiced. (b) The PTC at this stage
shows an irregular stricture of the
biliary tree in the hilum of the liver
(arrowheads). The differential diagnosis
includes primary cholangiocarcinoma,
inflammatory stricture and extrinsic
compression from lymphadenopathy.

(b)

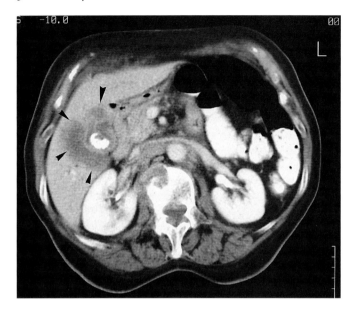

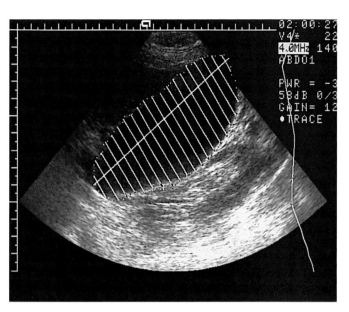

Fig. 8.44 Carcinoma of the gallbladder. An ultrasound in a 74-year-old female patient with anorexia, weight loss and a dull pain in her right upper quadrant showed a solid mass lesion involving the gallbladder. She subsequently became jaundiced. A spiral CECT shows a mass lesion replacing the gallbladder wall (arrowheads) with a central calcified gallbladder calculus. Separate sections showed coeliac nodal disease, as well as retroperitoneal lymphadenopathy.

Fig. 8.46 Distension of the gallbladder. This US scan shows a markedly distended gallbladder, which is otherwise normal. The patient has no evidence of biliary-tract obstruction. The estimated volume of the gallbladder, using a modified Simpsons' formula for left-ventricular volume estimation during cardiac US, indicates a volume of almost 200 ml (normal volume = 20–50 ml).

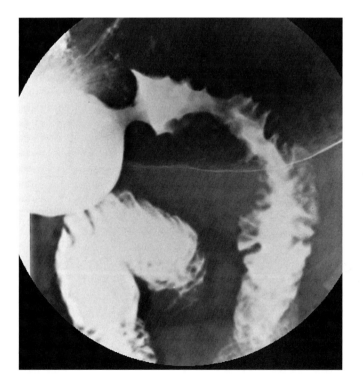

Fig. 8.45 Recurrence of gallbladder cancer invading the duodenum. This female patient had elective cholecystectomy for what was thought to be chronic cholecystitis. The histology of the gallbladder specimen indicated carcinoma. Following chemotherapy, the patient was symptom-free for 12 months, but developed nausea and copious vomiting. Endoscopy indicated deformity of the first and second parts of the duodenum. A double-contrast barium meal with IV glucagon shows loss of distensibility of the first and proximal second parts of duodenum, with gross deformity of the duodenal mucosa, in keeping with tumour infiltration. This was managed by palliative gastrojejunostomy.

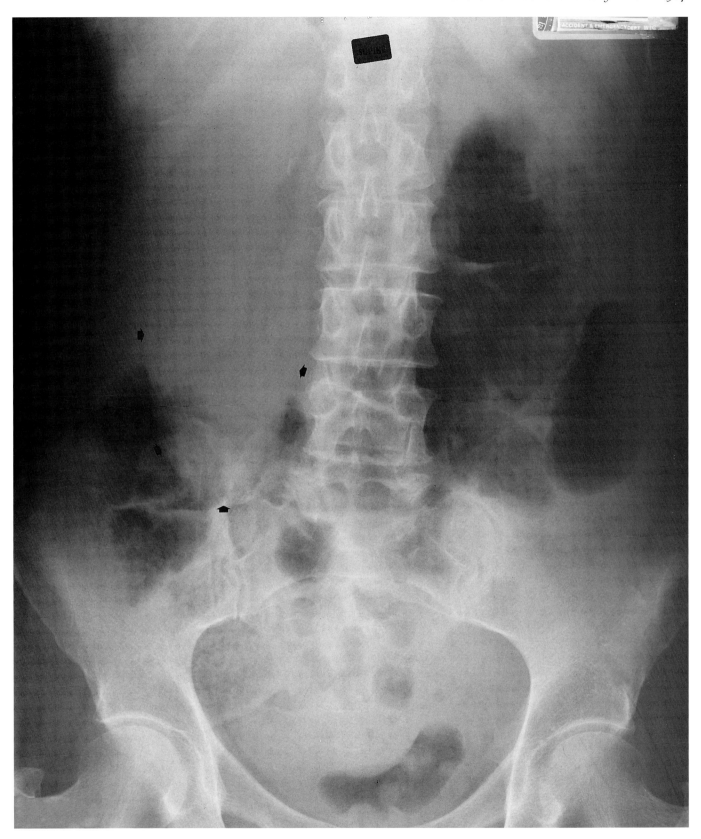

Fig. 8.47 Gallbladder distension secondary to biliary-tract obstruction. A plain abdominal X-ray shows a diffuse, soft-tissue swelling in the right side of the abdomen (arrowheads), associated with downward displacement of the hepatic flexure of the colon. The plain-film appearance is non-specific. The gallbladder distension in this case was due to gross biliary-tract obstruction secondary to recurrent carcinoma of the stomach.

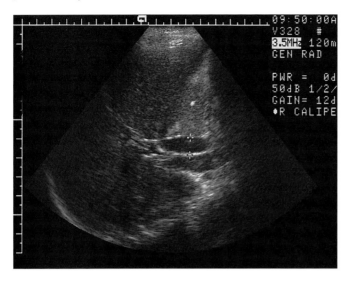

Fig. 8.48 Dilatation of the common bile duct, ultrasound. A US scan through the hepatoduodenal ligament shows mild dilatation of the CBD (9 mm between crosses) anterior to the portal vein.

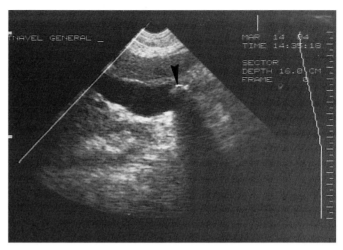

Fig. 8.50 Biliary-tract obstruction by a gallstone. An 87-year-old female patient had a 4-week history of obstructive jaundice. The US scan shows a grossly distended CBD (2.7 cm), at the distal end of which there is a large calculus (arrowhead) with acoustic shadowing.

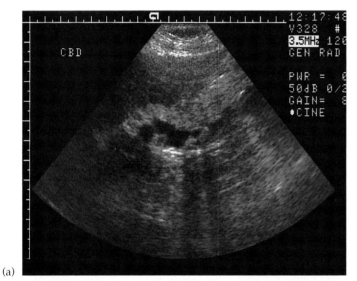

(a)

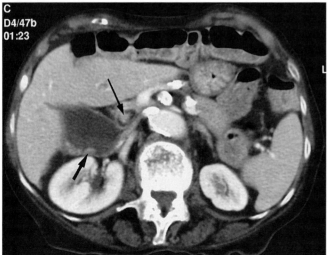

(b)

Fig. 8.49 Gallstones in the dilated bile duct. (a) A US scan shows several echogenic calculi with acoustic shadowing within a moderately dilated CBD. (b) In another patient, a previous US scan detected biliary tract dilatation without a visible cause in a clinical context of haemolytic anaemia and jaundice. This spiral CECT shows one of several stones (thin arrow) in a dilated bile duct as well as multiple calculi (thick arrow) within a distended gallbladder, an exception to Courvoisier's law.

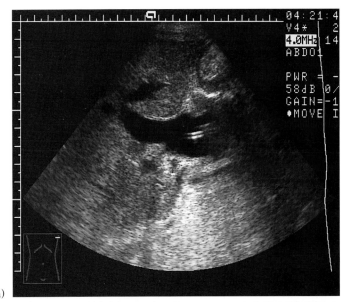

(a)

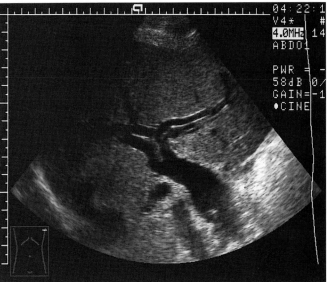

(b)

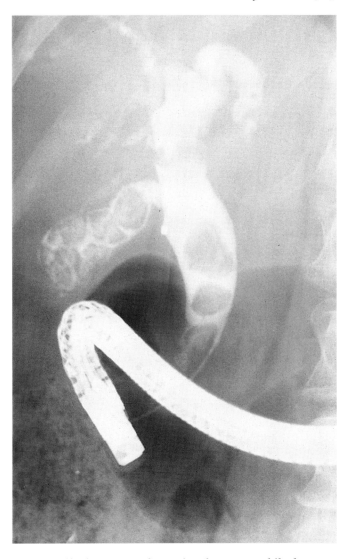

Fig. 8.52 Bile-duct stones obstructing the common bile duct, ERCP. The bile duct has been cannulated and contrast injected. Multiple, large, radiolucent calculi are shown within the CBD and at least one calculus is shown in the common hepatic duct. Stones within the gallbladder are also outlined by contrast.

Fig. 8.51 Biliary-tract obstruction due to calculi, bile-duct stent *in situ*. An ERCP of an elderly male patient with biliary-tract obstruction demonstrated a large impacted bile-duct calculus, which could not be removed. A plastic stent was inserted, but the serum bilirubin has remained elevated. (a) The bile duct is seen to be markedly dilated and the upper end of the stent is visible. (b) The bile duct is seen to be much wider than the portal vein, and intrahepatic biliary dilatation is shown. These changes imply that the stent is blocked.

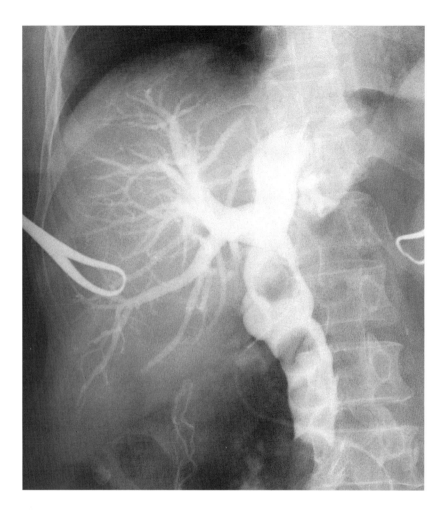

Fig. 8.53 Biliary-tract obstruction with bile-duct calculi, operative cholangiography. Direct puncture of the common duct and injection of contrast at operation shows massive dilatation of the biliary tree, with multiple, very large, bile-duct calculi. Only a trace of contrast is seen to have reached the duodenum.

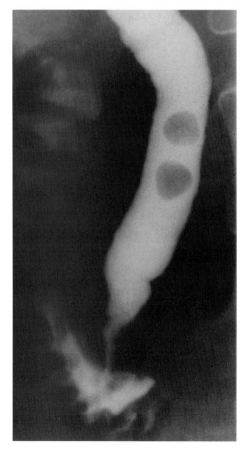

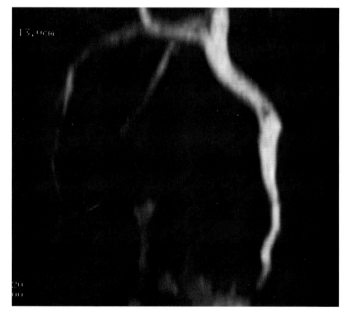

Fig. 8.55 Computerized tomography cholangiography, 3-D reconstruction with maximum-intensity projection. The biliary tree is densely opacified with IV contrast. A small radiolucent calculus is visible. (Courtesy of Dr Marie Callaghan.)

Fig. 8.54 Retained bile-duct stones following cholecystectomy, T-tube cholangiography. Two radiolucent calculi are visible in the densely opacified CBD. The sphincter of Oddi is patent and contrast is seen in the duodenum.

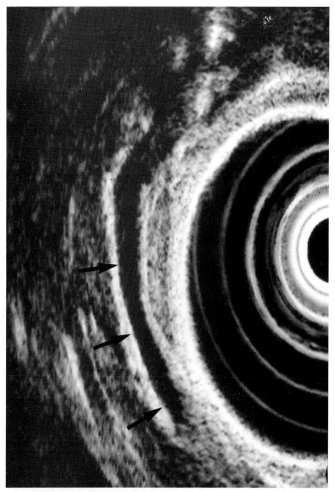

(a)

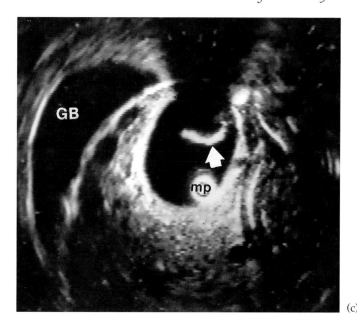

(c)

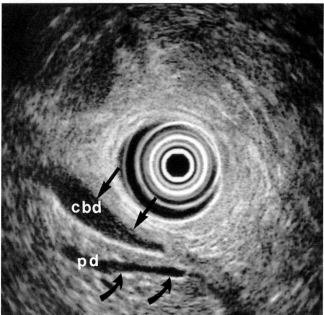

(b)

Fig. 8.56 Bile-duct imaging, endoscopic ultrasound. (a) The normal common bile duct (cbd; straight arrows) can usually be visualized on endoscopic US, and (b) can be traced down to its junction with the pancreatic duct (pd; curved arrows) at the level of the ampulla. Endoscopic US represents a non-invasive method of investigation of the cause of obstructive jaundice, without the risk of the postprocedure complications that accompany ERCP. Miniprobes may be passed directly into the common bile duct, with better definition of intraduct pathology (stone or tumour). (c) An intraduct stone (arrow) is seen via a miniprobe (mp), with a clearly defined acoustic shadow. GB, gallbladder. (Reprinted from [28] with permission; courtesy of Dr Alison McLean.)

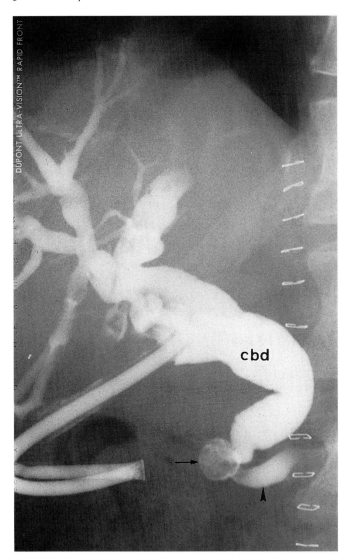

Fig. 8.57 Gallstone impacted in the ampulla of Vater, T-tube cholangiogram. Following cholecystectomy and bile-duct exploration with T-tube drainage, a postoperative cholangiogram shows dilatation of the biliary tree and also of the pancreatic duct (arrowhead), caused by a 1 cm calculus impacted in the ampulla (arrow). cbd, common bile duct.

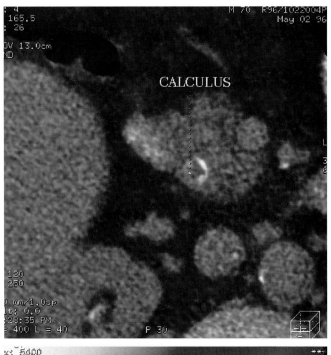

(a)

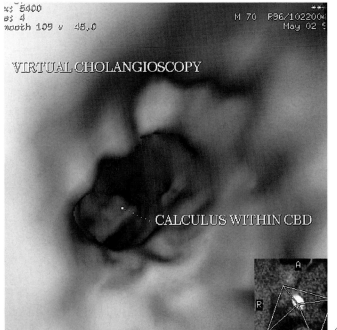

(b)

Fig. 8.58 Bile-duct stones, CT cholangiography. (a) A spiral CT (IV Biloscopin 100 ml) through the head of the pancreas shows a stellate filling defect (calculus) surrounded by contrast in the intrapancreatic portion of the bile duct. (b) The same calculus is demonstrated within the bile duct, using a 3-D reconstruction technique—virtual cholangioscopy. (Courtesy of Dr Marie Callaghan.)

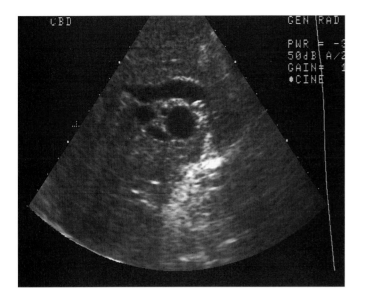

Fig. 8.59 Bile-duct calculus following liver transplantation. A female patient, who, 1 year previously had had a liver transplant for primary biliary cirrhosis, recently developed right upper quadrant pain. The oblique US scan through the liver shows moderate dilatation of the bile duct to 11 mm. At least one low-density stone is visible within the bile duct.

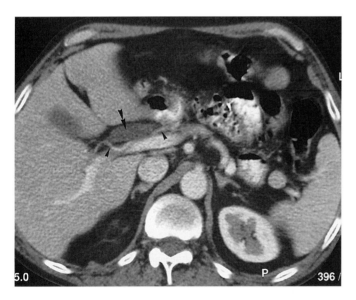

Fig. 8.60 Biliary obstruction associated with chronic pancreatitis. A spiral CECT in a patient with known chronic pancreatitis at the level of the hilum of the liver shows considerable dilatation of the bile duct to 14 mm (double arrowhead). The course of the hepatic artery is indicated by the small arrowheads anterior to the contrast-filled portal vein. Pancreatic calcification was visible on the lower sections.

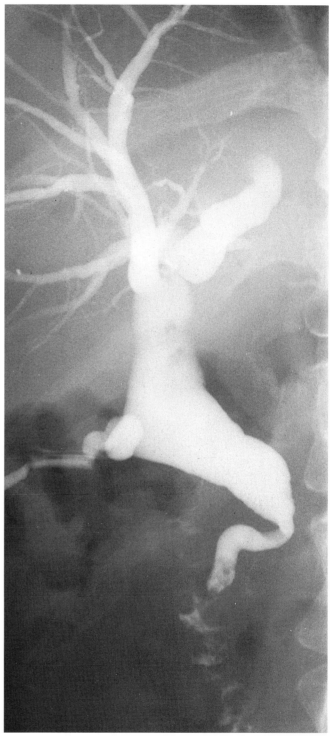

Fig. 8.61 Biliary obstruction associated with recurrent pancreatitis. A T-tube cholangiogram, with the tube partly extruded, shows considerable dilatation of the biliary tree and deformity and constriction of the distal CBD. Several small radiolucent calculi are shown within the distal end of the bile duct, but some contrast drainage into the duodenum is apparent.

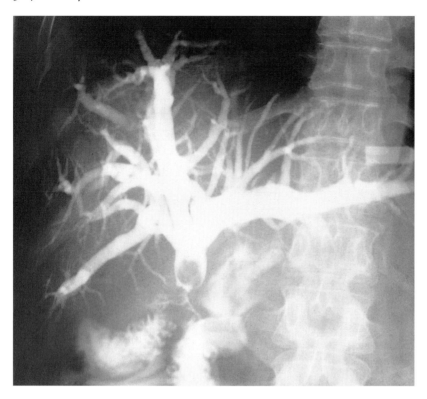

Fig. 8.62 Bile-duct calculus associated with choledochojejunostomy for a benign stricture. A PTC shows fairly marked dilatation of the biliary tree. The anastomosis between the common hepatic duct and a loop of jejunum is seen to be tightly stenosed and, immediately proximal to the anastomosis, a 1.5 cm radiolucent calculus has formed.

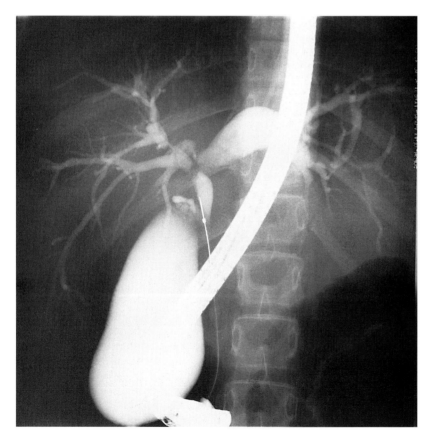

Fig. 8.63 Primary sclerosing cholangitis. The patient has a history of ulcerative colitis and abnormal liver-function tests. The ERCP shows a rather complex stricture at the upper end of the common hepatic duct, with quite marked dilatation of the left hepatic duct and, to a lesser extent, the right hepatic duct above this level. The appearance is indistinguishable from cholangiocarcinoma, but, in this case, an ERCP performed 12 months previously had an identical appearance. (Courtesy of Dr Peter Mills.)

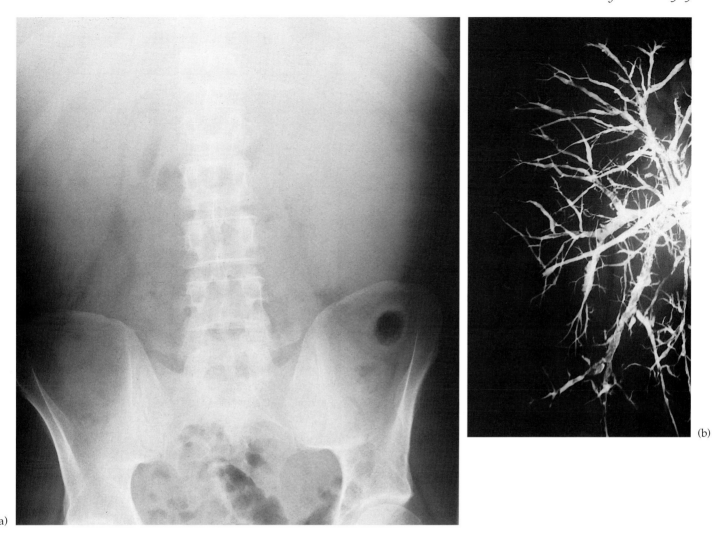

(a)

(b)

Fig. 8.64 Primary sclerosing cholangitis and micronodular cirrhosis. A 5-year history of progressive liver failure and portal hypertension in a 34-year-old male patient was followed by massive bleeding from the oesophageal varices. (a) A supine abdominal X-ray shows a marked soft-tissue swelling in the left side of the abdomen, in keeping with gross splenomegaly. The liver is also seen to be enlarged. (b) A post-mortem cholangiogram, in which numerous bile-duct tributaries show tapering strictures and segments of sacculation, consistent with sclerosing cholangitis. The histology demonstrated micronodular cirrhosis.

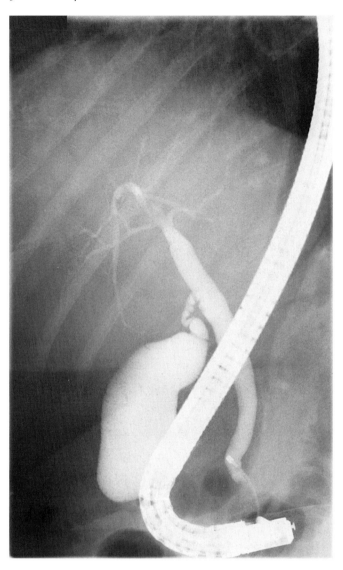

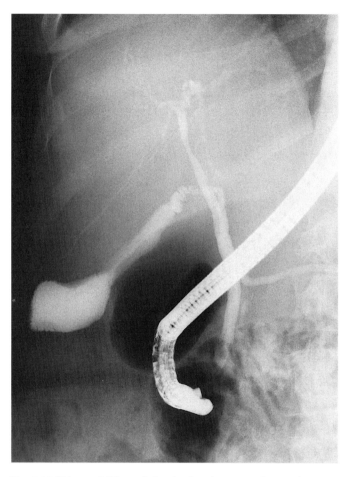

Fig. 8.66 Primary biliary cirrhosis. Another case of proved primary biliary cirrhosis in a patient with even more marked pruning of the intrahepatic bile ducts. The extrahepatic biliary tree has a normal appearance. (Courtesy of Dr Peter Mills.)

Fig. 8.65 Primary biliary cirrhosis. An ERCP was performed in a female patient with progressive deterioration in liver function, who had antimitochondria antibodies. The extrahepatic biliary tree is normal, but the bile-duct tributaries are sparse and attenuated, producing a 'pruned-tree' appearance. Histological confirmation. (Courtesy of Dr Peter Mills.)

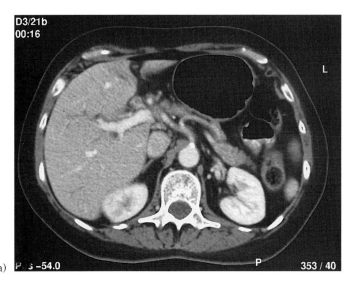

(a)

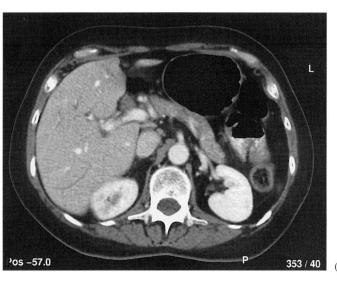

(b)

Fig. 8.67 Cholangiocarcinoma. A recent PTC in a 66-year-old female patient with obstructive jaundice demonstrated a hilar stricture. At the same time, biopsy confirmation of cholangiocarcinoma was obtained. (a) The spiral CECT shows biliary-tract dilatation within the liver. (b) A relatively discrete mass lesion is shown more distally in the hilum of the liver, anterior to the portal vein.

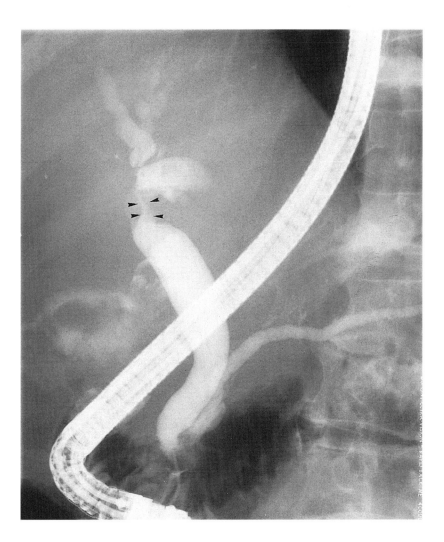

Fig. 8.68 Cholangiocarcinoma. A tight irregular stricture near the upper end of the common hepatic duct (arrowheads). The appearance is typical of a Klatskin tumour. (Courtesy of Mr Grant Fullarton.)

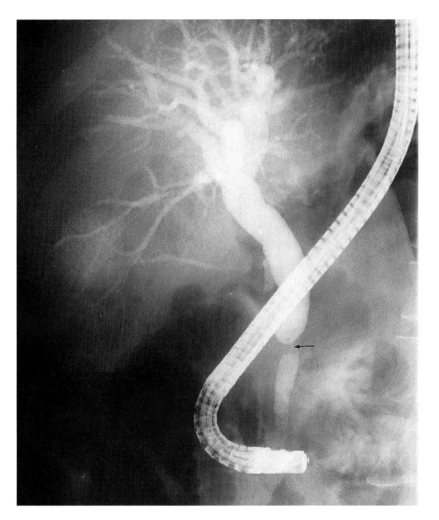

Fig. 8.69 Cholangiocarcinoma. An ERCP in a male patient with obstructive jaundice shows a short, very tight stricture of the CBD (arrow) 4 cm above the ampulla. There is marked dilatation of the biliary tree above this level. A Whipple's pancreaticoduodenectomy was performed and the diagnosis confirmed histologically. (Courtesy of Mr Grant Fullarton.)

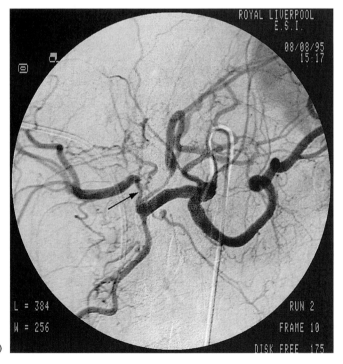

(a)

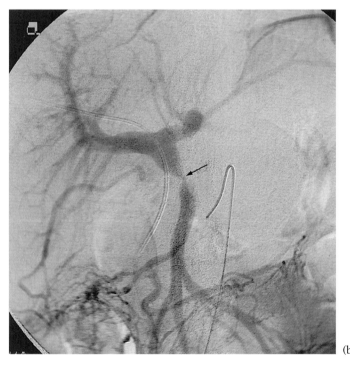

(b)

Fig. 8.70 Cholangiocarcinoma with vascular encasement.
(a) This coeliac arteriogram demonstrates irregular areas of arterial encasement of the right and left hepatic arteries and proximal gastroduodenal artery. Arrow, right hepatic artery.

(b) The portal venous phase of a superior mesenteric arteriogram shows focal stenosis of the portal vein (arrow) due to cholangiocarcinoma. An internal/external biliary drain is present. (Courtesy of Dr Richard D. Edwards.)

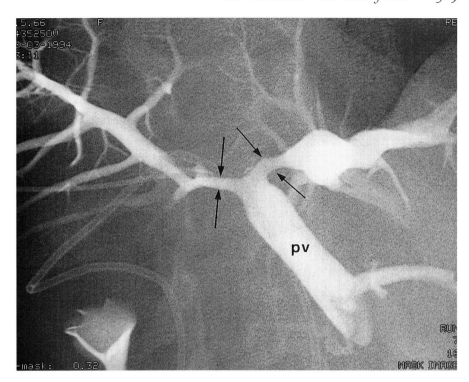

Fig. 8.71 Cholangiocarcinoma with portal vein encasement. Direct portal venography demonstrates tumour encasement of the portal venous bifurcation. The left gastric vein is dilated (arrows). An internal/external biliary drain is also seen. pv, portal vein. (Courtesy of Dr Richard D. Edwards.)

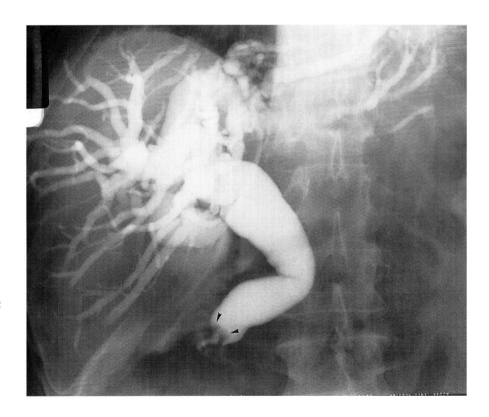

Fig. 8.72 Ampullary carcinoma. Transhepatic cholangiography in a patient with gross biliary-tract obstruction shows a small filling defect involving the ampulla (arrowheads). A trace of contrast is seen to enter the duodenum. This diagnosis may be mimicked by an impacted stone.

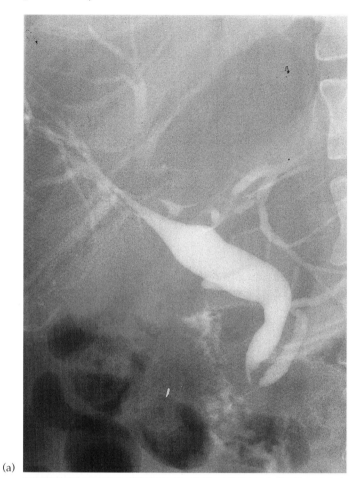

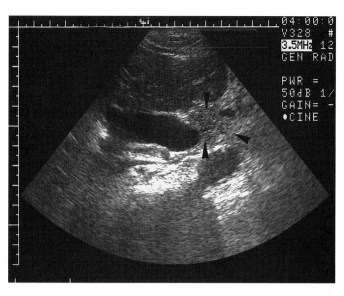

Fig. 8.74 Metastatic biliary-tract obstruction. This patient previously had a Hartmann's procedure for unresectable carcinoma of the rectum. The patient then developed partial small-bowel obstruction, right hydronephrosis and marked biliary-tract obstruction. The US scan of the right upper quadrant shows dilatation of the CBD, which is seen to be obstructed by a solid mass lesion at its distal end (arrowheads). The patient died after a short interval of generalized carcinomatosis.

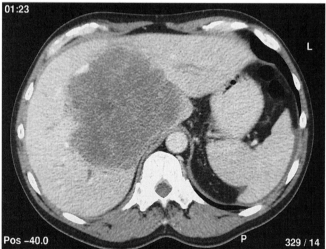

Fig. 8.73 Extrinsic biliary compression by malignant liver tumour. (a) The ERCP shows smooth extrinsic compression of the biliary tree within the liver, with a normal extrahepatic biliary tree. (b) The spiral CECT in the same patient shows an irregular, well-defined solid mass lesion within the liver. A US guided biopsy of this lesion indicated a rare yolk sac embryonic tumour, but metastatic carcinoma, hepatocellular carcinoma or intrahepatic cholangiocarcinoma could produce a similar appearance.

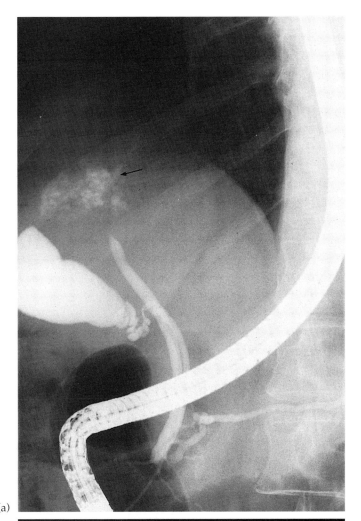

(a)

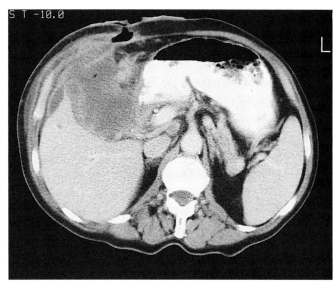

Fig. 8.76 Metastatic carcinoma involving the gallbladder. A 74-year-old male patient developed a massive recurrence of right renal carcinoma 9 years post nephrectomy. A spiral CECT through the upper abdomen shows extensive tumour infiltration involving the gallbladder and extending into the anterior abdominal wall. The histology of this mass was identical to that of the renal primary.

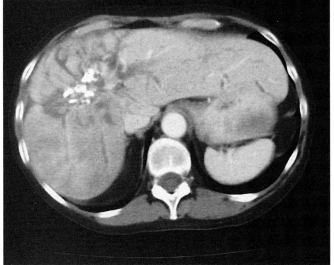

(b)

Fig. 8.75 Biliary obstruction associated with metastatic liver disease. A 61-year-old female patient had a history of mastectomy and recent jaundice. (a) The ERCP shows a normal extrahepatic biliary tree, but there is an irregular calcified mass within the liver (arrow), which is seen to prevent retrograde filling of the biliary tree within the liver. (b) A spiral CECT confirms the presence of calcification within the liver, associated with quite marked dilatation of the intrahepatic biliary tree. This was caused by metastatic breast carcinoma.

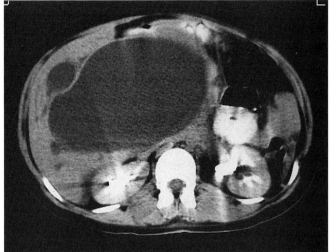

(ai)

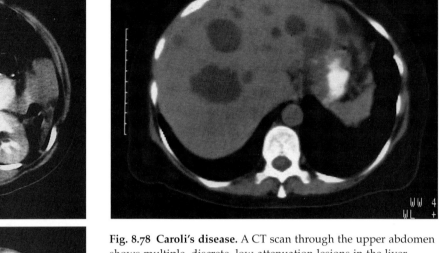

Fig. 8.78 Caroli's disease. A CT scan through the upper abdomen shows multiple, discrete, low-attenuation lesions in the liver. These are due to segmental biliary-tract dilatation. The diagnosis was established many years previously at laparotomy and cholecystectomy.

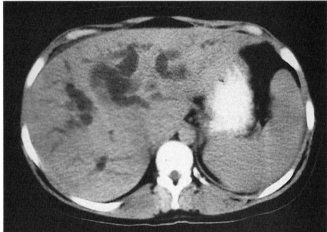

(aii)

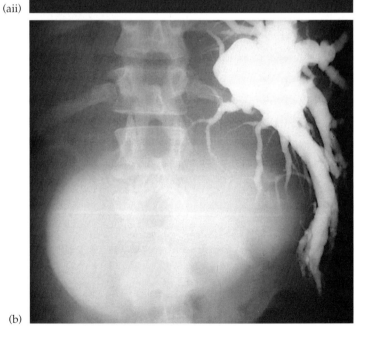

(b)

Fig. 8.77 Choledochal cyst. An enhanced CT scan shows (a) a large choledochal cyst with (b) secondary dilatation of the intrahepatic bile ducts, demonstrated by transhepatic cholangiography. (aii) is 6 cm superior to (ai). (Courtesy of Dr Richard D. Edwards.)

9: The Pancreas

Anatomy

From the foregut, ventral and dorsal pancreatic buds develop independently. They subsequently fuse, resulting in a single organ, in which there is usually union of the duct systems of the two buds. Eventually, the ventral bud contributes about 10% of the whole pancreas [1]. The pancreas in early fetal life consists of a series of branching ductules. From these, both acinar tissue and islet cells develop. In this remarkable feat of structural engineering, the whole pancreas—exocrine and endocrine—develops from foregut endoderm. The duct of the dorsal pancreas fuses with the ventral duct to form the main pancreatic duct (of Wirsung), which opens into the duodenum with the common bile duct (CBD) at the ampulla of Vater. The proximal section of the dorsal duct may atrophy or it may persist as the accessory pancreatic duct (Santorini), which opens into the duodenum at a higher level than the ampulla of Vater.

Various congenital anomalies of the pancreas are recognized. The head or tail are occasionally absent. Pancreatic tissue may be found in an ectopic location, such as the wall of the stomach or small bowel, gallbladder or spleen. An annular pancreas produces a smooth constriction of the second part of the duodenum. This may be either asymptomatic or, when there is a tight duodenal constriction, proximal obstruction presents in infancy [2]. Annular pancreas is probably due to a persistence of the left lobe of the ventral pancreas. Pancreas divisum occurs in 1–5% of individuals, and it refers to a failure of fusion of the dorsal and ventral buds. Endoscopic retrograde cholangiopancreatography (ERCP) readily demonstrates this anomaly. Characteristically, injection of contrast into the ampulla of Vater produces filling of only the ventral portion of the gland. Only when the accessory duct is injected with contrast does the dorsal duct system draining the body and tail become apparent.

The normal pancreas, which is about 15 cm in length, crosses the posterior abdominal wall obliquely from the concavity of the duodenal loop to the hilum of the spleen. Most of the pancreas is retroperitoneal, the tail lying within the layers of the lienorenal ligament. The head is covered anteriorly by the transverse colon and posteriorly it lies on the inferior vena cava and right renal vessels and is grooved by the CBD, which is often encircled by pancreatic tissue. The neck lies posterior to the pylorus and is covered anteriorly by the peritoneum of the lesser sac. Behind the neck, but in front of the uncinate process, the superior mesenteric vein (SMV) and the splenic vein unite to form the portal vein. The body of the pancreas extends to the left, upwards and posteriorly. It has a triangular cross-section and is related anteriorly to the lesser sac. The tail lies within the two layers of the lienorenal ligament at or close to the hilum of the spleen. The pancreas has a rich arterial blood supply. The anterior and posterior superior pancreaticoduodenal arteries, derived from the gastroduodenal artery, anastomose with the anterior and posterior inferior pancreaticoduodenal vessels, which usually arise by a common stem from the superior mesenteric artery (SMA). These vessels lie between the duodenum and pancreas and give off numerous branches to the pancreatic head. The posterior (dorsal) pancreatic artery arises either directly or indirectly from the coeliac artery or from the SMA. It passes downwards behind the neck and divides into right and left branches. The pancreas is also supplied by branches of the splenic artery.

The position, shape and size of the pancreas are remarkably variable, so that precise normal limits are very difficult to define. In addition, pancreatic size has been shown to decrease with advancing age [3]. According to Kreel and Sandin [4], the normal pancreas, based on CT criteria, measures: head 23 mm ± 3 mm, neck 19 mm ± 2.5 mm, body 20 mm ± 3 mm, tail 15 mm ± 2.5 mm. In another normal series, Muranaka et al. [5] said that the normal head measures 19.8–29.5 mm and the tail 12.1–21.4 mm.

Plain film radiography

Plain X-rays play a minor role in the diagnosis of pancreatic disease. In acute pancreatitis, many different radiological signs have been described, which in the individual case are of very little value [6]. On rare occasions, the presence of gas within the pancreas, usually in the form of multiple small bubbles producing a mottled appearance, is diagnostic of pancreatic abscess [7]. A localized paralytic ileus may be depicted by gas-filled loops of small bowel.

In chronic pancreatitis, focal calcification is due to the precipitation of calcium carbonate around the protein plugs in the duct system [8]. Calcification is likely to develop eventually over a number of years in most cases with chronic pancreatitis. Other causes of pancreatic calcification include hyperparathyroidism, cystic fibrosis, trauma and hereditary juvenile pancreatitis. In chronic pancreatitis, the presence of calcification implies major damage to the duct system.

Barium studies

Indirect evidence of pancreatic pathology, either inflammatory or neoplastic, may be manifested in changes in the stomach, duodenum, small bowel, large bowel and even the oesophagus. Widening of the duodenal loop is difficult to assess because it is subject to considerable normal variation, especially in obese patients, with a transverse gastric distribution and a rather long descending portion of duodenum. True widening may be caused by neoplasm or pancreatitis, including acute fluid collections and pseudocysts [9]. Lymphadenopathy can also widen the loop [10]. Aneurysms of the abdominal aorta and other retroperitoneal tumours may cause duodenal displacement, so that it should not be assumed that pancreatic disease is responsible. The 'reversed 3' sign of Frostberg [11] is a non-specific sign of pancreatic disease, originally described in malignancy, but more commonly a feature of pancreatitis.

Ultrasound

Ultrasound has become a valuable tool in pancreatic disease, particularly as a first-line investigation. The main limiting factor in transabdominal pancreatic ultrasound is the presence of intervening visceral gas and obesity or both. Under favourable conditions, however, much valuable information can be obtained using modern, grey-scale, real-time ultrasound with colour Doppler and spectral Doppler functions. Ultrasound measurements of the normal pancreas have been defined as 25 mm for the head and 15 mm for the body (maximum AP diameter) [12, 13]. The wide variation in the size of the normal pancreas is in part age-related. The calibre of the pancreatic duct increases with increasing age, but, in middle-aged or younger subjects, this should not exceed 2 mm [14]. With modern equipment, at least part of the pancreatic duct may be visualized in almost 90% of patients [2]. A fluid-filled stomach should not be confused with a pancreatic pseudocyst. Acute fluid collections, pseudocysts, cysts, abscesses and pseudoaneurysms should be searched for. The principal intra-abdominal vessels, including those related to the pancreas, can be scrutinized by Doppler-time velocity (spectral) wave-form signals and these can be affected by pancreatic disease. Spectral Doppler is complemented by colour Doppler and this provides anatomical information on the position of flowing blood and the relationship of vessels to mass lesions [2]. Pseudoaneurysms complicating pancreatitis or pancreatic surgery may be detected by this non-invasive technique.

The sensitivity of pancreatic ultrasound can be further enhanced by delivering the transducer very close to the surface of the pancreas—for example, endoscopically or intraoperatively, both of which facilitate much better resolution by virtue of the much higher ultrasound frequency—for example, 7–10 MHz.

Computerized tomography scanning

This method has become the principal investigation in cases with suspected or known inflammatory or neoplastic pancreatic pathology [15–17]. Spiral scanning has become particularly useful, arterial and portal venous enhancement phases being possible with a single bolus of contrast.

The pancreatic contour on CT is smooth in four out of five people and lobulated in one in five [18]. Diffuse or focal fatty replacement of the pancreas is common, particularly with advancing years. The normal pancreas has an attenuation of 30–50 Hounsfield units (HU).

In acute pancreatitis, contrast enhancement enables vital pancreatic tissue to be differentiated from non-enhancing necrotic tissue. Intrapancreatic and peripancreatic acute fluid collections are also readily demonstrated. Pancreatic cancer is usually visualized on contrast-enhanced scans as an area of reduced attenuation relative to normal pancreatic tissue. The high contrast levels afforded by spiral CT produce clear visualization of arterial and venous involvement by pancreatic disease. Three-dimensional rendering, using maximum-intensity projection or shaded-surface display techniques, may be useful in confirming vascular encasement or invasion [19]. Focal masses within the pancreas present a diagnostic and management dilemma. There may or may not be CT evidence of chronic pancreatitis, and biliary-tract obstruction may be present. Distinction from malignancy may be impossible [20].

Endoscopic retrograde pancreatography

While ultrasound, CT and MRI may be able to demonstrate pathology in the pancreatic duct, the detailed study of the duct system is best done with ERCP, not least because this valuable technique has the additional benefit of endoscopic intervention, where appropriate. The normal pancreatic duct is smooth and gradually tapers from the head to the tail. The maximum normal calibre [21] is 3–5 mm in the head, 2–3 mm in the body and 1–2 mm in the tail. Evenly distributed along the course of the main duct are the small lateral tributaries. In addition, larger tributaries draining the head and uncinate process are often visible. An accessory duct is found to be patent via the minor papilla in 30–60% of cases [21].

The diagnosis of chronic pancreatitis is confirmed by the deranged ductal morphology, as seen on endoscopic retrograde pancreatography. Strictures and occlusions are also found in pancreatic malignancy, and the clear distinction between inflammatory masses and neoplasm may be difficult or impossible on purely morphological grounds. About 60% of pancreatic pseudocysts complicating pancreatitis communicate with the duct system [8]. In this situation, injection of contrast via the duct system may introduce infection into a pseudocyst and carry a risk of septicaemia. Abnormalities in the filling pattern of the main duct may be due to lumbar spinal osteophytes or aneurysm, as well as tumours, cysts and chronic pancreatitis.

Magnetic resonance imaging

According to Haaga [22], the best two MRI sequences for pancreatic imaging are firstly, the standard spin-echo, T_1-weighted images, which give good anatomical information with a reasonably high signal intensity, and, secondly, a variety of breath-holding 'flash' images, which minimize motion artefact. In pancreatic malignancy, tumour masses are depicted as areas of decreased signal intensity within the gadolinium-enhanced pancreas. It may be possible to identify the pancreatic duct, duct dilatation and a level of obstruction if MR cholangiography sequences are included [20]. The introduction of breath-holding sequences allows imaging of the entire pancreas during one breath-hold with enhancement at the capillary stage, using gadolinium. In acute pancreatitis, the purpose of imaging methods is not to make the diagnosis, but to distinguish and, if possible, quantify the amount of viable pancreatic tissue from necrotic tissue. In addition, the task is to detect, observe and, if appropriate, plan the drainage of acute fluid collections. In acute pancreatitis, MRI can provide information comparable with CT [23]. Although MRI is capable of high-quality imaging in pancreatic disease, most workers at the present time prefer to rely on a combination of ultrasound, ERCP and CT, which are the mainstay of pancreatic imaging [22].

Angiography

Cross-sectional imaging and ERCP have reduced the need for angiography in pancreatic disease, but, in patients with inconclusive CT or ERCP results, angiography can make a vital contribution. Angiography may also be crucial in the diagnosis and management of pancreatic bleeding—for example, resulting from pancreatitis—and it also has a role in displaying the arterial and venous anatomy prior to pancreatic surgery. In particular, arteriography has a role in assessing the resectability of pancreatic tumours by confirming or excluding major arterial and venous encasement. The best technical results are achieved by experienced angiographers using selective and superselective catheter techniques with digital-subtraction angiography.

References

1 Foulis A.K. (1993) The pancreas. In: MacSween R.N.M. & Whaley K. (eds) *Muir's Textbook of Pathology*, 13th edn. London: Arnold, 791–803.
2 Garber S. & Lees W.R. (1993) The normal pancreas. In: Cosgrove D.O., Meire H. & Dewbury K.C. (eds) *Abdominal and General Ultrasound*. Edinburgh: Churchill Livingstone, 135–141.
3 Worthen N.G. & Beaubeau D. (1982) Normal pancreatic echogenicity: relation to age and body fat. *American Journal of Roentgenology* **139**, 1095–1098.
4 Kreel L. & Sandin B. (1973) Changes in pancreatic morphology associated with ageing. *Gut* **14**, 962–970.
5 Muranaka T., Teshima K., Honda H., Nanjo T., Hanada K. & Oshiumi Y. (1989) Computed tomography and histological appearance of pancreatic metastases from distant sources. *Acta Radiologica* **30**, 615–619.
6 Dans S., Parbhoo S.P. & Gibson M.J. (1980) The plain abdominal radiograph in acute pancreatitis. *Clinical Radiology* **31**, 87–93.
7 Field S. (1997) The plain abdominal radiograph—the acute abdomen. In: Grainger R.G. & Allison D.J. (eds) *Diagnostic Radiology*, 3rd edn. New York: Churchill Livingstone, 885–907.
8 Bartram C.I. & Kumar P. (1981) *Clinical Radiology in Gastroenterology*. Oxford: Blackwell Scientific Publications, 159.
9 Eisenberg R.L. (1994) Miscellaneous abnormalities in the stomach and duodenum. In: Gore R.M., Levine M.S. & Laufer I. (eds) *Textbook of Gastro-intestinal Radiology*. Philadelphia: W.B. Saunders, 717–741.
10 Zeman R.K., Schiebler M., Clark L.R. *et al.* (1985) The clinical and imaging spectrum of pancreatico-duodenal lymph node enlargement. *American Journal of Roentgenology* **144**, 1223–1227.
11 Frostberg N. (1938) Characteristic duodenal deformity in cases of different kinds of perivaterial enlargement of the pancreas. *Acta Radiologica* **19**, 164–173.
12 Niederau C., Sonnenberg A., Muller J. *et al.* (1983) Sonographic measurements of the normal liver, spleen, pancreas and portal vein. *Radiology* **149**, 537–540.
13 De Graff C., Taylor K.J.W., Simmonds B. *et al.* (1978) Grey scale echography of the pancreas: re-evaluation of normal size. *Radiology* **129**, 157–161.
14 Bryan P.J. (1982) Appearance of normal pancreatic duct. *Journal of Clinical Ultrasound* **10**, 63–66.
15 Freeny P.C., Traverso L.W. & Ryan J.A. (1993) Diagnosis and staging of pancreatic adenocarcinoma with dynamic computed tomography. *American Journal of Surgery* **165**, 600–606.
16 Freeny P.C. (1993) Incremental dynamic bolus computed tomography of acute pancreatitis: state of the art. *International Journal of Pancreatology* **13**, 147–154.
17 Freeny P.C. (1988) Radiology of the pancreas: two decades of progress in imaging and intervention. *American Journal of Roentgenology* **150**, 975–981.
18 Burgener F.A. & Kormano M. (1996) *Differential Diagnosis in Computed Tomography*. Stuttgart: Thieme Medical Publishers, 280–287.
19 Brink J.A., MacFarland E.G. & Heiken J.P. (1997) Helical/spiral computed body tomography. *Clinical Radiology* **52**, 480–503.
20 Megibow A.J. (1997) CT/MRI in pancreatic neoplasms. In: *Proceedings of the London CT/MRI Course*. Gleneagles, Scotland, 29–34.

21 Freeny P.C. (1994) Radiology of the pancreas. In: Freeny P.C. & Stevenson G.W. (eds) *Margulis and Burhenne's Alimentary Tract Radiology*, 5th edn. St Louis: Mosby, 1017–1026.

22 Haaga J.R. (1994) The pancreas. In: Hagga J.R., Lanzieri C.F., Sartoris D.J. *et al.* (eds) *Computed Tomography and Magnetic Resonance Imaging of the Whole Body*, 3rd edn. St Louis: Mosby, 1037–1130.

23 Ward J., Chalmers A.G., Guthrie A.J. *et al.* (1997) T_2 weighted and dynamic enhanced MRI in acute pancreatitis: comparison with contrast enhanced CT. *Clinical Radiology* **52**, 109–114.

24 McLean A. & Fairclough P. (1996) Endoscopic ultrasound—current applications. *Clinical Radiology* **51**, 83–98.

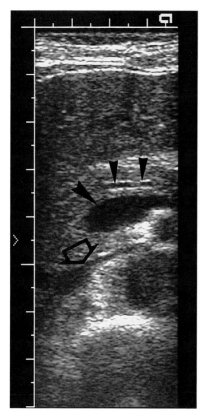

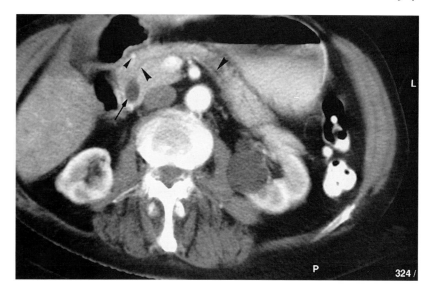

Fig. 9.3 Normal pancreatic duct, spiral CT. The course of the pancreatic duct in the body, neck and head of the pancreas is shown (large arrowheads). The intrapancreatic portion of the CBD is also shown (arrow). Any measurements of the CBD should be transverse and not anteroposterior because of its oblique course. Small arrowhead, gastroduodenal artery.

Fig. 9.1 Normal pancreas, ultrasound. A transverse US scan with a 5 MHz transducer through the head and the neck of the pancreas shows the pancreatic duct (small arrowheads), the confluence of the SMV and splenic vein (larger black arrowhead) and the junction of the left renal vein and inferior vena cava (open arrowhead) posterior to the head of pancreas.

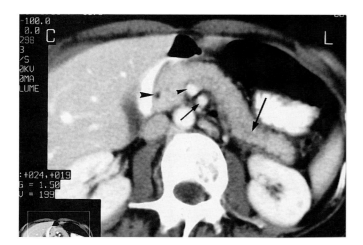

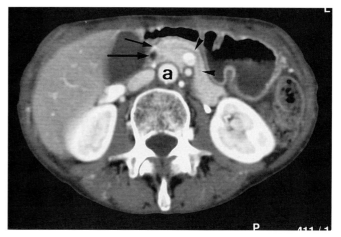

Fig. 9.2 Normal pancreas, CECT. On this 5 mm collimation spiral scan, the whole length of the normal pancreas is clearly visible. Only a short length of normal pancreatic duct is shown on this tomogram (large arrow). Large arrowhead, normal CBD; small arrowhead, SMV; smaller arrow, SMA.

Fig. 9.4 Congenitally short pancreas, spiral CECT. A 3 mm collimation, pitch one. The pancreas was found to be truncated, with no evidence on any of multiple sections of a tail. Uniform contrast enhancement of the pancreas is shown. a, aorta; large arrow, normal CBD; small arrow, gastroduodenal artery; arrowheads, pancreatic duct.

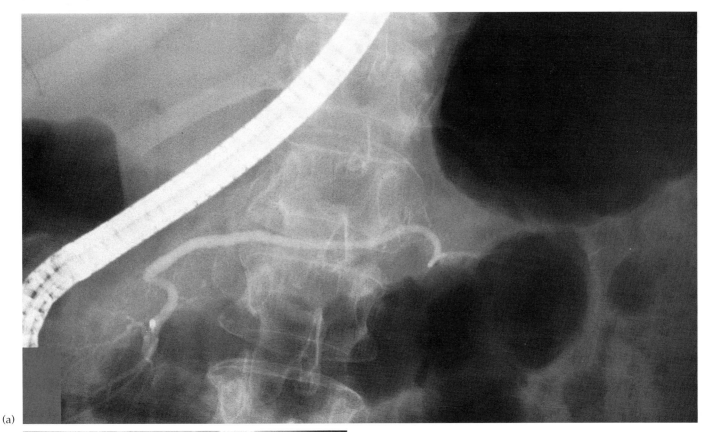

(a)

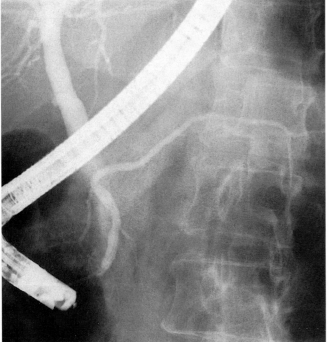

(b)

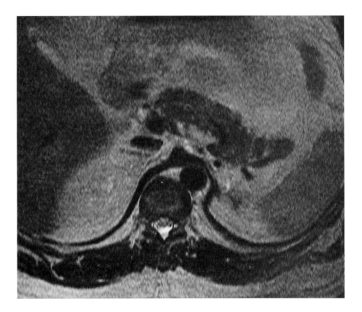

Fig. 9.6 Normal pancreas, MRI. Transverse FSE T$_2$ MRI scan of the pancreas demonstrating a high contrast between intermediate signal pancreas and fat. (Courtesy of Dr J. Graeme Houston.)

Fig. 9.5 Normal pancreatic duct, ERCP. (a) The pancreatic duct has been cannulated via a side-viewing endoscope and dilute contrast medium injected. The normal tapering structure of the main pancreatic duct is shown. Several tributaries from the head are clearly shown, but the smaller tributaries from the body and tail are scarcely visible. (b) In another normal study in a different patient, the main pancreatic duct is of smaller calibre, but the tributaries throughout the length of the pancreas are just visible.

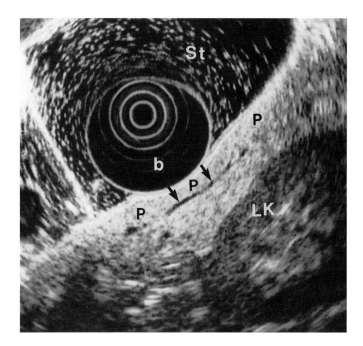

Fig. 9.7 Normal pancreas, endoscopic ultrasound. Visualization of the normal pancreas requires placement of the echo-endoscope in the second part of the duodenum to visualize the uncinate process and pancreatic head, with gradual withdrawal into the proximal duodenum to visualize the bile duct. The body and tail of the pancreas are visualized through the gastric wall. B, balloon surrounding scope; LK, left kidney; P, pancreas; St, water-filled stomach; black arrows, pancreatic duct. (Reprinted from [24] with permission; courtesy of Dr Alison McLean.)

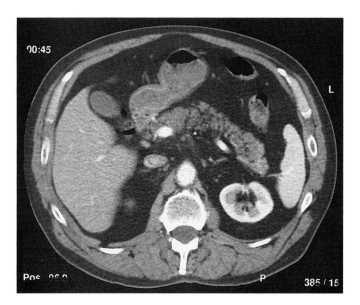

Fig. 9.8 Fatty infiltration of the pancreas. A spiral contrast-enhanced CT (CECT) scan shows mild multifocal fatty replacement of the pancreatic tissue. This is commonly observed with advancing age, but it is also related to diabetes, obesity, pancreatitis and cystic fibrosis.

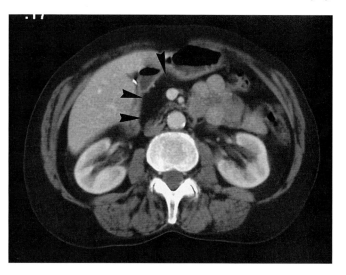

Fig. 9.9 Severe fatty replacement of the pancreas. A spiral CECT scan in a 60-year-old female patient shows very marked replacement of the head and neck of the pancreas by fat (arrowheads). The body and tail of pancreas were similarly affected.

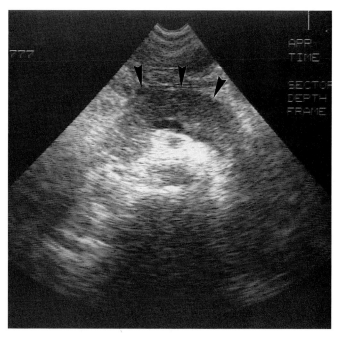

Fig. 9.10 Acute pancreatitis. Transverse upper abdominal US scan in a patient with sudden onset of severe abdominal pain and with a history of excessive alcohol intake. There is a high serum amylase. There is diffuse swelling of the pancreas (arrowheads), which shows a moderate reduction in echo density, in keeping with oedema. The AP diameter of the body of the pancreas measured 25 mm. The upper normal limit is 15 mm [12, 13].

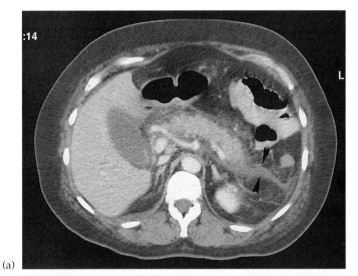

(a)

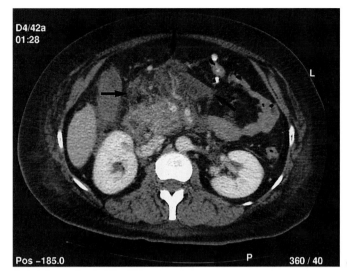

(c)

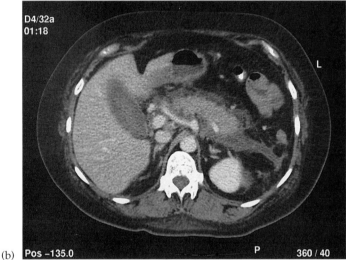

(b)

Fig. 9.11 Acute pancreatitis. (a) The spiral CECT shows satisfactory enhancement of pancreatic tissue, but there is some loss of marginal definition, in keeping with oedema, and there is moderate swelling of Gerota's fascia (between arrowheads). (b) A repeat scan 5 days later in the same patient shows more marked peripancreatic oedema and further thickening of the Gerota's fascia. (c) A more distal scan at the level of the uncinate process, which is swollen. There is evidence of extension of the inflammatory process into the fat of the mesentery (arrows).

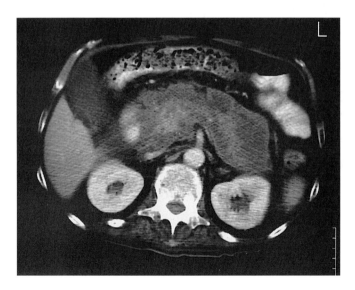

Fig. 9.12 Acute necrotizing pancreatitis. The spiral CECT shows poor uneven enhancement of pancreatic tissue with massive diffuse swelling, in keeping with oedema.

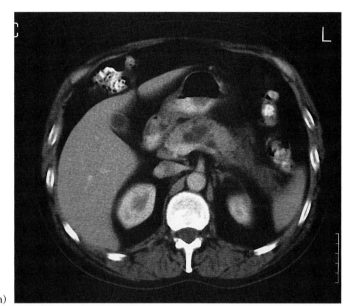

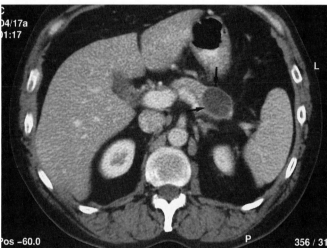

(a)

(b)

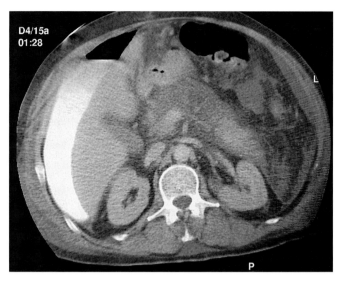

Fig. 9.14 Concurrent acute necrotizing pancreatitis and duodenal ulcer perforation. This spiral CECT was taken of a 65-year-old male patient with acute abdominal pain and collapse. Only the inferior part of the head and the tail of pancreas are seen to enhance, there being evidence of widespread necrosis of the remainder. In addition, there is orally administered contrast medium, together with air, in the right subphrenic space, which were due to a duodenal ulcer perforation, confirmed surgically.

Fig. 9.13 Acute necrotizing pancreatitis. There is a prominent history of alcohol abuse in this 47-year-old male patient. (a) The spiral CECT shows enhancement of the head and body, but a small loculated acute fluid collection is shown in the neck of the pancreas and there is a lack of enhancement of the tail, indicating necrosis. (b) The necrotic tail is seen, 15 months later, to have been replaced by a small well-circumscribed pseudocyst (arrows) immediately anterior to the left adrenal gland.

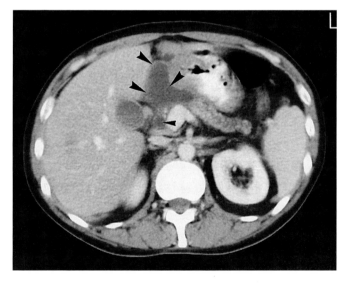

Fig. 9.15 Acute pancreatitis with acute fluid collection. Several days after the onset of acute pancreatitis, this spiral CECT shows a relatively well-defined acute fluid collection within the head of the pancreas (larger arrowheads). The bile duct is seen to be mildly dilated (small arrowhead); serum amylase 2000 units. The fluid collection increased in size over a 4-week period on subsequent ultrasound scans.

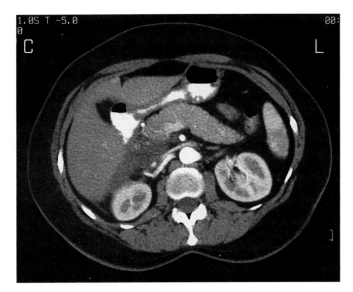

Fig. 9.16 Acute pancreatitis following ERCP. A spiral CECT showing that most of the head and the body and tail of the pancreas have a normal appearance. There is evidence of an acute fluid collection surrounding the head posteriorly and compressing the inferior vena cava.

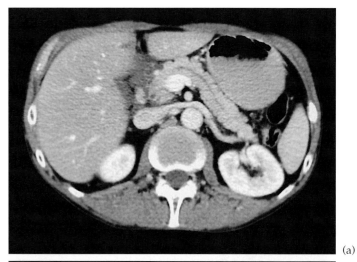

(a)

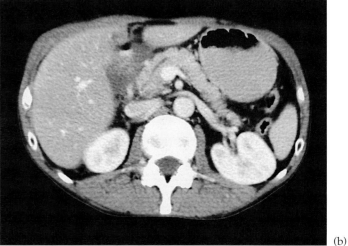

(b)

Fig. 9.18 Recurrent pancreatitis. (a) The pancreas is morphologically normal and, in particular, the pancreatic duct has a normal appearance. (b) Oedema of the adjacent soft tissues, including the duodenum, is more apparent here.

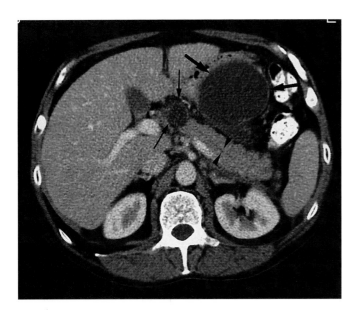

Fig. 9.17 Acute pancreatitis resulting in pseudocyst. Spiral CECT in a patient several weeks after the onset of acute pancreatitis. A small intrapancreatic pseudocyst is shown within the neck (thin arrows), without any evidence of pancreatic-duct obstruction. A larger, lesser-sac pseudocyst is also shown (large arrows). Arrowheads, pancreatic duct.

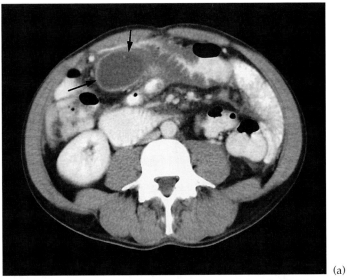

(a)

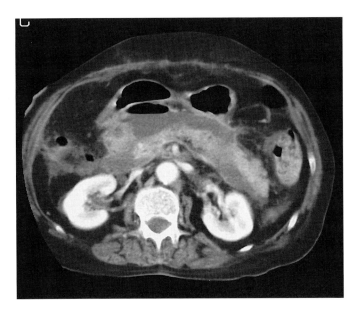

Fig. 9.19 Necrotizing pancreatitis with lesser-sac abscess. A spiral CECT shows partial necrosis with apparent separation of the body and tail. Gas and fluid are visible in the lesser sac anterior to the pancreas and posterior to the stomach.

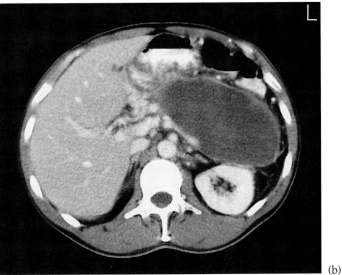

(b)

Fig. 9.21 Acute pancreatitis complicated by loculated pseudocyst. (a) Part of a complex pseudocyst is shown (arrows). Adjacent to it, a loop of small bowel is seen to be markedly oedematous. In addition, there is oedema surrounding the mesenteric vessels and the third part of the duodenum is compressed as it passes between the mesenteric vessels and the aorta. (b) A much larger left-sided pseudocyst is apparent at a higher level than (a).

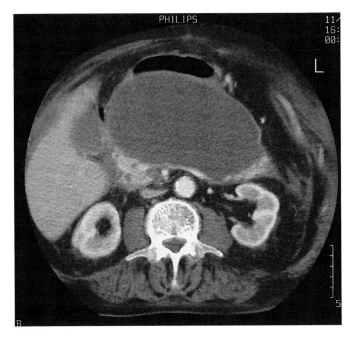

Fig. 9.20 Acute pancreatitis complicated by pseudocyst formation. On this spiral CECT, a large, well-circumscribed, unilocular, fluid collection is seen to have accumulated in the lesser sac, with part of the body and tail of the pancreas visible posteriorly. There is marked anterior displacement of the stomach (containing gas) and attenuation of the duodenal loop.

(a)
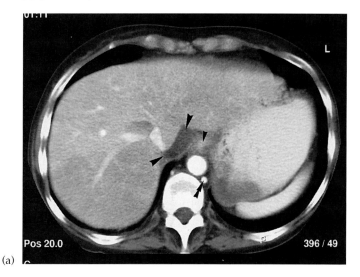

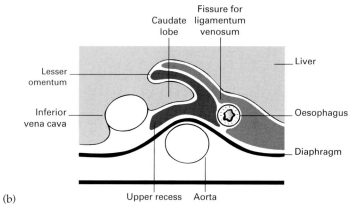
(b)

Fig. 9.22 Recurrent pancreatitis complicated by pseudocyst extending high into the superior recess of the lesser sac.
(a) There is loss of definition of the oesophagus, probably due to oedema (small arrowhead). The hemiazygos vein is shown (double arrowhead). The patient also has focal fatty change affecting the liver. Large arrowheads, lesser sac. (b) Diagram of the superior recess of the lesser sac.

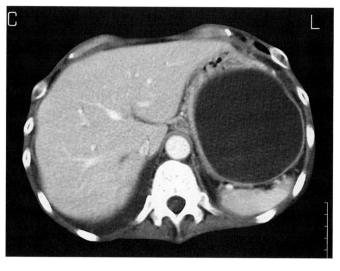

Fig. 9.23 Large unilocular pancreatic pseudocyst. This spiral CECT shows a well-circumscribed pseudocyst compressing the spleen backwards and the stomach forwards.

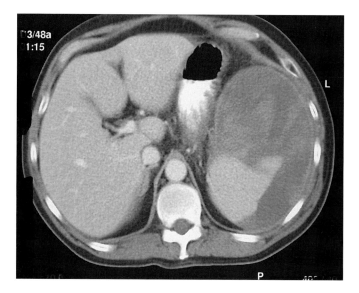

Fig. 9.24 Haemorrhagic perisplenic pseudocyst complicating pancreatitis. The patient had upper abdominal pain, pyrexia and a white-cell count of 17 000. A relatively well-circumscribed pseudocyst of uneven attenuation is shown surrounding the spleen and displacing the stomach medially. Bloodstained pseudocyst fluid was drained surgically.

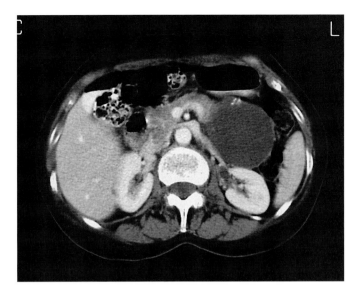

Fig. 9.25 Recurrent pancreatitis with pseudocyst. A well-circumscribed pseudocyst known to have been present for 6 months is associated with destruction of the distal part of the body and tail of the pancreas.

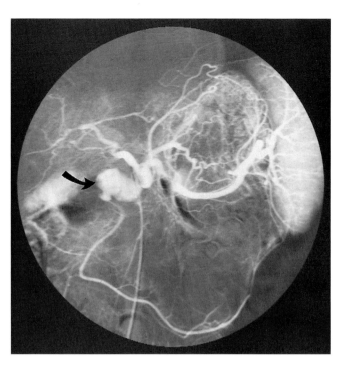

Fig. 9.27 Gastroduodenal artery pseudoaneurysm. Selective coeliac arteriogram showing gastroduodenal artery pseudoaneurysm (curved arrow). This occurred as a complication of acute pancreatitis. (Courtesy of Dr Richard D. Edwards.)

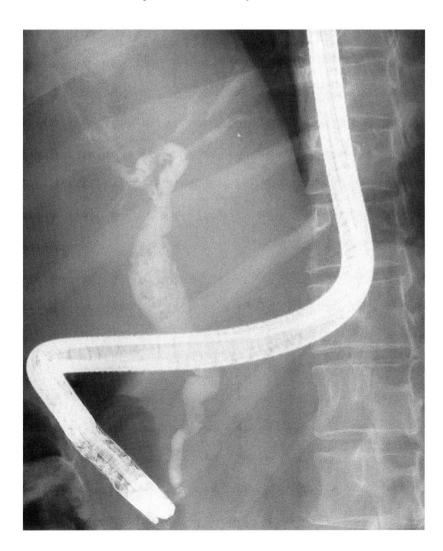

Fig. 9.26 Recurrent pancreatitis with biliary-tract stones and obstruction. An ERCP in a patient with recurrent pancreatitis shows deformity of the distal CBD, and numerous small radiolucent calculi are shown.

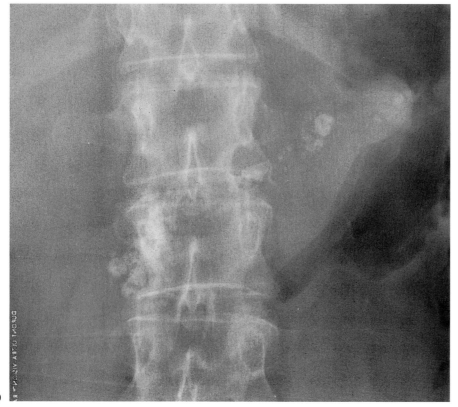

(a)

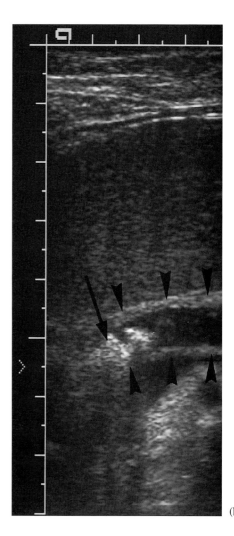

(b)

Fig. 9.28 Chronic pancreatitis. (a) The plain film of the epigastrium shows multiple foci of coarse calcification in the distribution of the pancreas. The appearance is characteristic of chronic pancreatitis and indicates severe ductal damage. (b) A transverse abdominal ultrasound scan in the same patient (5 MHz) shows marked thickening and dilatation of the pancreatic duct (arrowheads), which measured 7 mm in diameter. One of several intraduct calculi is indicated by the arrow.

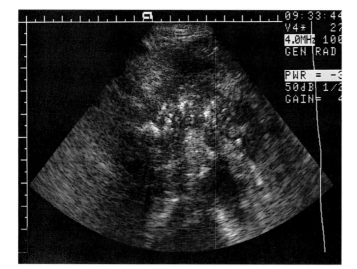

Fig. 9.29 Chronic pancreatitis. A transverse upper abdominal ultrasound scan shows widespread punctate calcification within the gland.

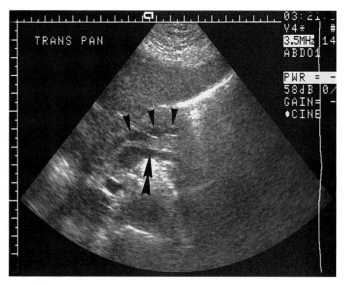

Fig. 9.30 Chronic pancreatitis. Transverse upper abdominal ultrasound shows 'chain-of-lakes' deformity of the pancreatic duct, resulting from multiple strictures and intervening dilated segments (arrowheads). The splenic vein is indicated (double arrowhead). (Courtesy of Dr Laura M. Wilkinson.)

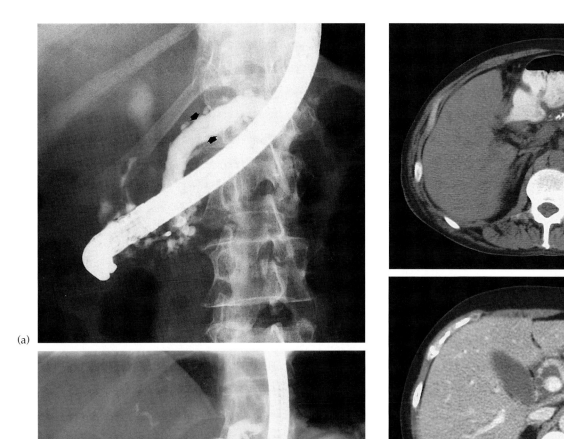

(a)

(b)

(a)

(b)

Fig. 9.31 Chronic pancreatitis. (a) An ERCP in a patient with alcoholic liver disease and clinical features of chronic pancreatitis shows massive dilatation of the main pancreatic duct, with a lack of filling of the tail of the gland. The duct measures 14 mm between the arrowheads. There is marked deformity and dilatation of multiple tributaries. (b) A second case shows similar features and includes marked dilatation of tributaries in the head.

Fig. 9.32 Chronic pancreatitis. (a) A 52-year-old male patient with a long history of alcohol abuse and recurrent epigastric pain is shown to have widespread pancreatic calcification on this unenhanced CT scan. Pancreatic calcification is rare in gallstone-induced chronic pancreatitis. (b) This spiral CECT shows an irregularly dilated pancreatic duct (arrow) associated with calculi and pancreatic atrophy.

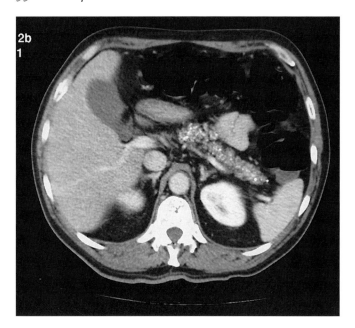

Fig. 9.33 Chronic pancreatitis. This spiral CECT in a diabetic patient shows very fine punctate calcification throughout the gland.

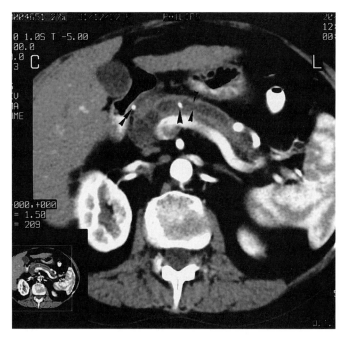

Fig. 9.34 Chronic pancreatitis. A spiral CECT shows marked irregular dilatation of the pancreatic duct (between small arrowheads) and a calculus is shown within the duct (large arrowhead). The splenic vein is densely opacified with contrast behind the pancreas and the gastroduodenal artery is also shown (double arrowhead).

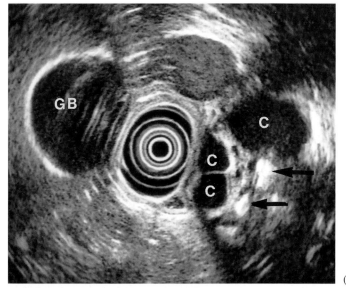

(a)

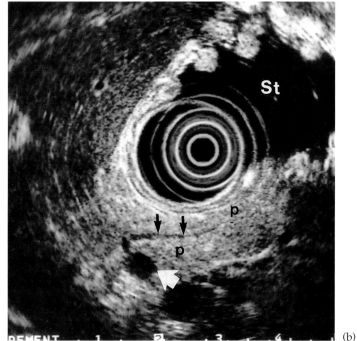

(b)

Fig. 9.35 Chronic pancreatitis, endoscopic ultrasound.
(a) The pancreatic head in patient with established chronic pancreatitis. The well-defined cysts (C) and echogenic foci of calcification (arrows) can be clearly seen. Endoscopic US may show early subtle changes of parenchymal heterogenicity and duct irregularities. GB, gallbladder. (b) The endoscopic US demonstrates small cysts with great sensitivity (white arrow). p, pancreas; St, stomach; black arrows, pancreatic duct. (Fig. 9.35b is reprinted from [24] with permission; courtesy of Dr Alison McLean.)

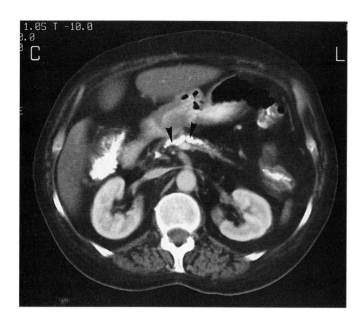

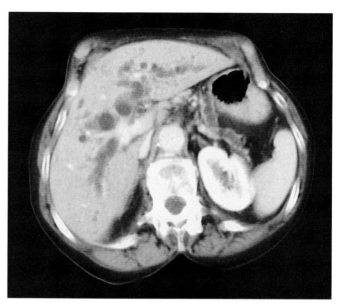

Fig. 9.36 Chronic pancreatitis leading to atrophy. This spiral CECT shows extensive pancreatic calcification (arrowheads), the volume of the gland parenchyma being severely reduced.

Fig. 9.38 Pancreatic-duct obstruction secondary to ampullary stenosis. A 74-year-old female patient with a major degree of biliary-tract obstruction was examined. The spiral CECT shows gross intrahepatic biliary-tract dilatation, which on lower sections was seen to extend to the distal end of the bile duct. There is gross dilatation of the pancreatic duct, associated with severe pancreatic atrophy. Pancreatic cancer or ampullary cancer could produce a similar appearance.

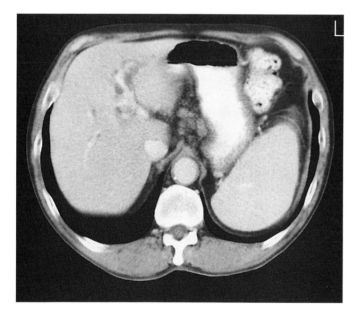

Fig. 9.37 Chronic pancreatitis complicated by biliary-tract obstruction. A spiral CECT in a 65-year-old male patient with chronic pancreatitis complicated by pseudocyst formation shows dilatation of the intrahepatic bile ducts. Left gastric varices are also shown, in association with portal hypertension. The pseudocyst is not visible on this section.

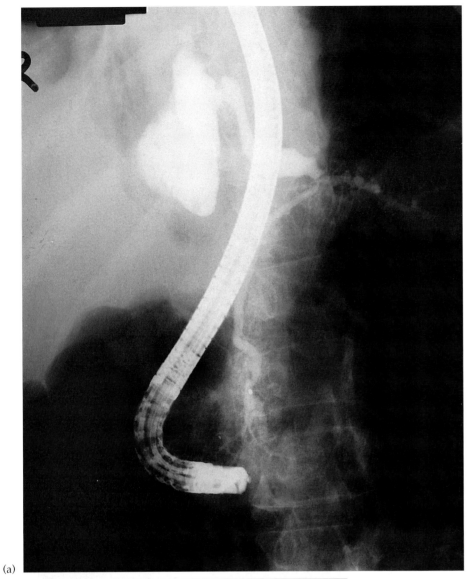

(a)

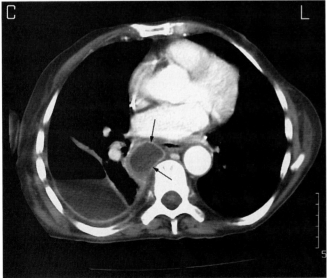

(b)

Fig. 9.39 Pancreaticopleural fistula. (a) An ERCP shows relatively normal filling of the downstream portion of the main pancreatic duct, but the contrast is seen to escape from the duct near its midpoint into an irregular fistula, which eventually drains into a loculated cavity in the right pleura. Upstream from the fistula, the pancreatic duct is markedly irregular, in keeping with chronic pancreatitis. (b) A spiral CT shows a posterior mediastinal pseudocyst (arrows), which on lower slices is seen to communicate with the pleural effusion. A pneumothorax is also present, following needle aspiration.

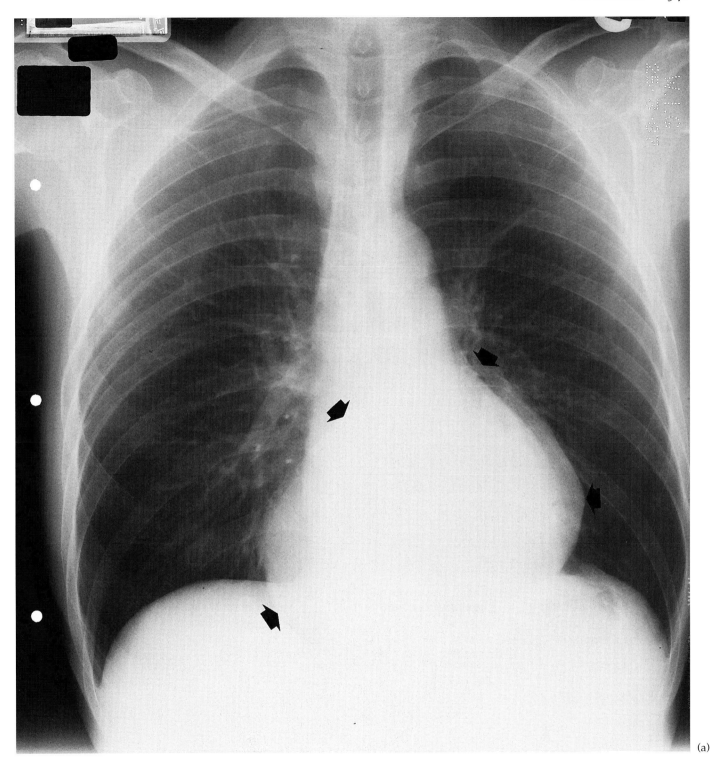

(a)

**Fig. 9.40 Mediastinal pseudocyst complicating chronic
pancreatitis.** (a) The patient presented with palpitation and
tachycardia. A posteroanterior chest X-ray showed an unusual
flask-shaped opacity (arrowheads) superimposed on the heart
shadow.

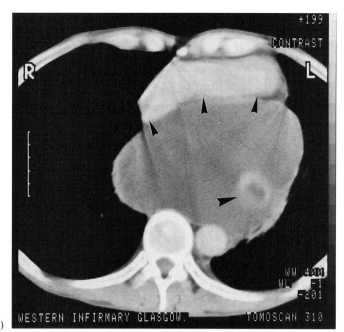

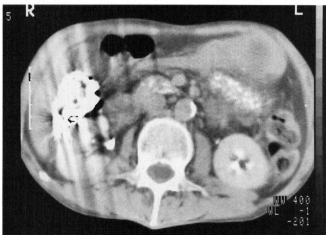

(b)

(c)

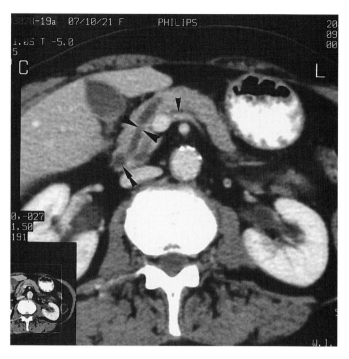

Fig. 9.41 Benign stricture of the pancreatic duct. The spiral CECT shows quite marked dilatation of the pancreatic duct (between large arrowheads). The small arrowhead indicates the fat plane between the splenic vein and the posterior surface of the pancreas and should not be confused with the pancreatic duct. The uncinate process tributary is also dilated. The CBD is normal (double arrowhead). The distinction between benign and malignant strictures may be impossible.

Fig. 9.40 *Continued.* (b) A CECT shows a well-defined cystic lesion within the mediastinum, causing gross anterior displacement of the heart (small arrowheads), and the cyst is seen to completely surround the oesophagus (large arrowhead). (c) The cyst was followed through the diaphragm and had its origin in the lesser sac. The body, tail and uncinate process of the pancreas are seen to be extensively calcified. (Reprinted from *Clinical Radiology*, 1992, **45**, 128–130 with permission.)

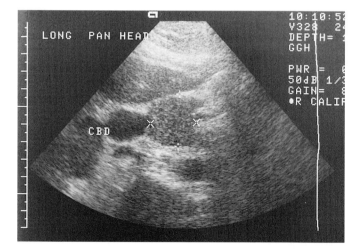

Fig. 9.42 Carcinoma of the head of the pancreas. A 51-year-old female patient presented with a short history of obstructive jaundice. This oblique US scan of the upper abdomen shows marked dilatation of the distal end of the bile duct immediately above a solid mass lesion in the head of the pancreas measuring 30 mm in diameter. CBD, common bile duct.

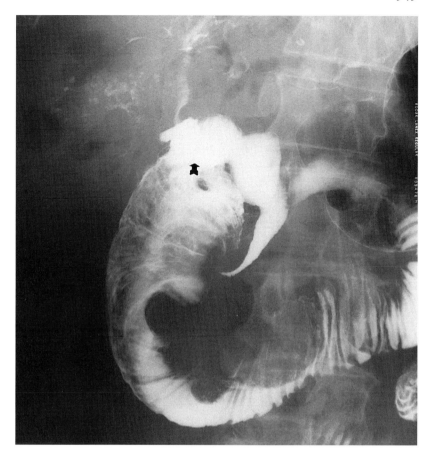

Fig. 9.43 Carcinoma of the head of the pancreas.
A double-contrast barium meal in a patient with
progressive weight loss, abdominal pain and
obstructive jaundice shows a very extensive
lobulated filling defect, causing gross deformity of
the concave aspect of the second and third parts
of the duodenum. Contrast entered the dilated
bile duct via a spontaneous fistula (arrow). The
duodenal deformity corresponds with Frostberg's
'reversed 3' sign [11] and is consistent with
advanced pancreatic malignancy, although the
appearance is not specific and is more frequently
seen in pancreatitis.

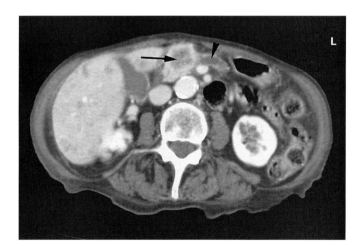

Fig. 9.44 Carcinoma of the head of the pancreas. A spiral CECT
in a patient with profound weight loss and recent jaundice shows
an irregular low attenuation lesion (arrow) within the head of the
pancreas associated with marked obstruction of the pancreatic
duct (arrowhead). Liver metastases are also visible.

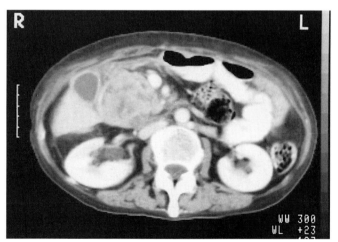

Fig. 9.45 Carcinoma of the head of the pancreas. This shows a
larger pancreatic tumour in a patient with obstructive jaundice.
Pancreatic-duct obstruction was also apparent on higher sections.

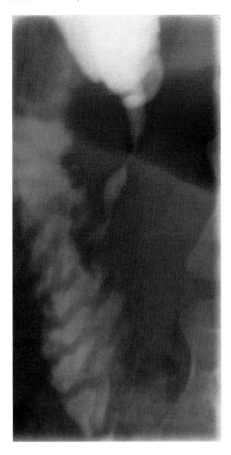

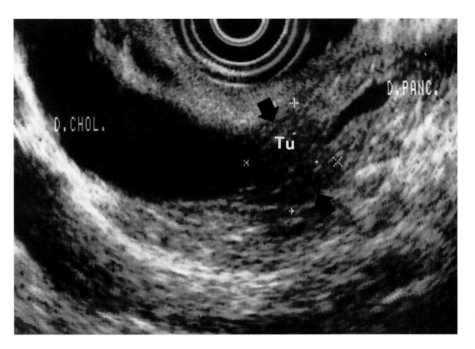

Fig. 9.47 Carcinoma of the head of the pancreas, endoscopic ultrasound. In small, potentially operable, pancreatic cancers, endoscopic US may contribute useful information. A small hypoechoic, rounded mass (Tu) (1.5 cm) is demonstrated obstructing both the CBD and, to a lesser extent, the pancreatic duct. The demonstration of portal and splenic vein involvement is well seen on endoscopic US, although arterial involvement is better demonstrated by spiral CECT. Some small pancreatic tumours may be occult on even high-quality CT and, in such patients, endoscopic US can demonstrate tumour with a high sensitivity (up to 93%). (Courtesy of Dr Alison McLean.)

Fig. 9.46 Carcinoma of the head of the pancreas. Percutaneous transhepatic cholangiography in a 29-year-old male patient with a 4-week history of obstructive jaundice shows an irregular stricture of the distal CBD associated with deformity of the medial wall of the duodenum. He quickly developed bone metastases and died within 4 months.

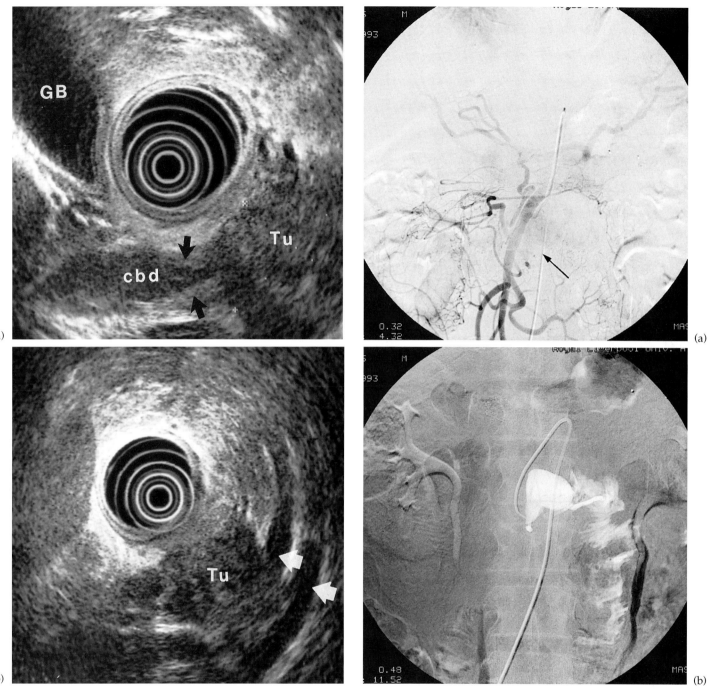

Fig. 9.48 Pancreatic carcinoma, endoscopic ultrasound. (a) A large, 4 cm, carcinoma (Tu) in the head of the pancreas is demonstrated as a mass of mid- to low-level echogenicity, obstructing the common bile duct (cbd) with thickening of the distal duct, consistent with infiltration (arrows). GB, gallbladder. (b) The tumour is extending inferiorly to involve both the superior mesenteric vein and the superior mesenteric artery (arrows). (Courtesy of Dr Alison McLean.)

Fig. 9.49 Jejunal artery pseudoaneurysm. (a) Selective mesenteric arteriogram shows a pseudoaneurysm (arrow) arising from the first jejunal artery. The patient had a major gastrointestinal haemorrhage 10 days after a Whipple's procedure for pancreatic carcinoma. (b) A selective jejunal arteriogram shows the pseudoaneurysm communicating with the distal pancreatic duct and small bowel. (Courtesy of Dr Richard D. Edwards.)

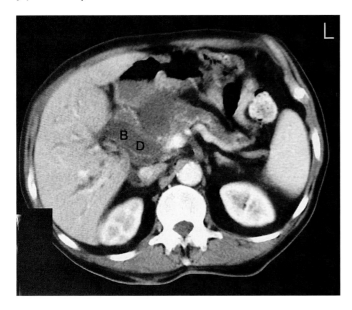

Fig. 9.50 Mucinous cystadenocarcinoma of the pancreas. A 77-year-old male patient had jaundice, but no history of pancreatitis. A cystic mass lesion is shown in the head of the pancreas and this is associated with gross dilatation of the bile duct and of the pancreatic duct.

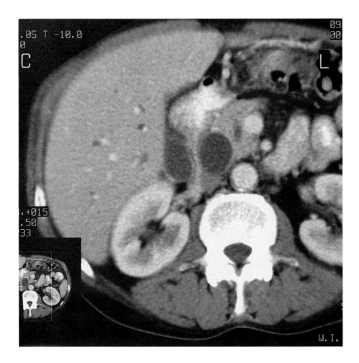

Fig. 9.51 Ampullary carcinoma. A spiral CECT of a patient with painless, obstructive jaundice shows marked dilatation of the CBD within the pancreas. The second part of the duodenum is compressed between the gallbladder and bile duct. There was positive histology for ampullary carcinoma.

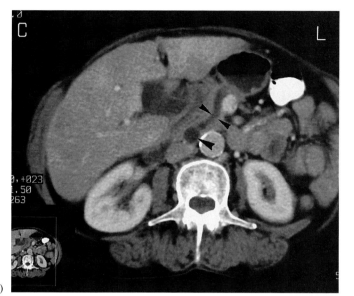

(a)

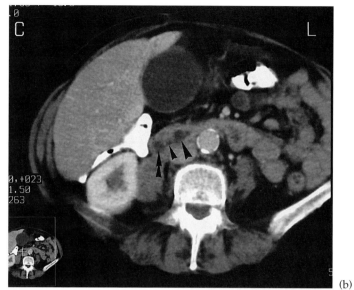

(b)

Fig. 9.52 Villous adenoma of the ampulla of Vater. (a) The CBD is seen to be dilated (large arrowhead), together with the pancreatic duct (small arrowheads). (b) At the level of the ampulla of Vater, the lumen of the duodenum is indicated by the double arrowhead and the bile duct by the large arrowhead, and a tiny lesion (small arrowhead) may represent a very small tumour. (c) ERCP shows marked dilatation of the biliary tree and the pancreatic duct. Endoscopic cytology was positive and the head of the pancreas was resected. Histology of the resection specimen revealed a tiny villous adenoma of the ampulla.

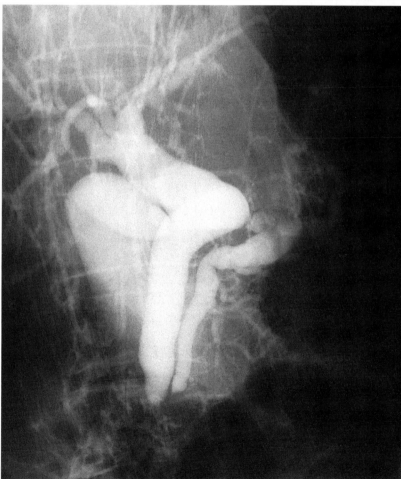

(c)

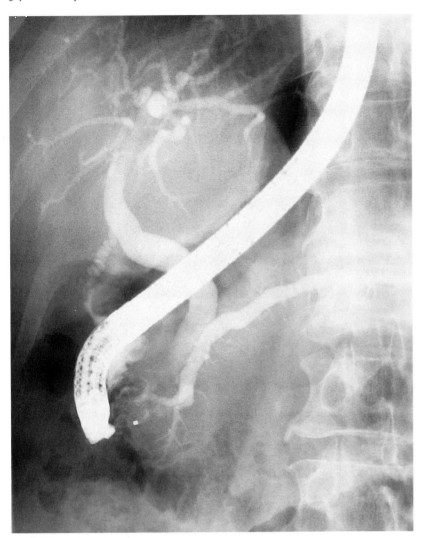

Fig. 9.53 Benign ampullary stenosis. An ERCP
in a patient with biliary-tract obstruction shows
dilatation of both the pancreatic duct and the bile
duct. The nature of the obstructing lesion has not
been demonstrated. Pancreatectomy was
performed, with no trace of neoplasm in the
resected specimen.

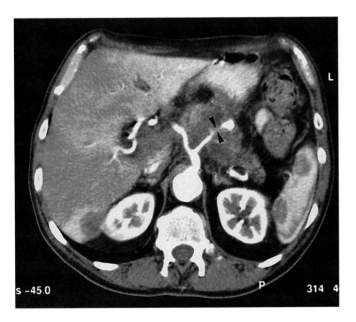

Fig. 9.54 Carcinoma of the body of the pancreas. This spiral
CECT shows irregular expansion of the body of the pancreas,
with uneven enhancement and evidence of encasement of the
splenic artery (arrowheads). There was positive histology. A liver
metastasis is also shown.

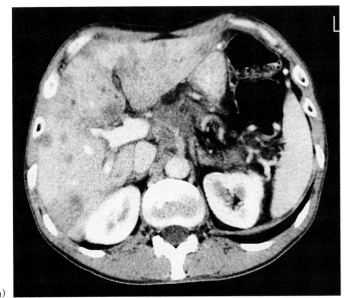

(a)

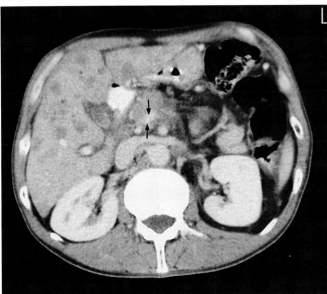

(b)

Fig. 9.55 Carcinoma of the neck and body of the pancreas.
(a) There is an extensive solid mass lesion involving the neck and body, with patency of the portal vein, but encasement of the hepatic artery. There are multiple liver metastases. (b) The SMV is seen to be encased in tumour (arrows).

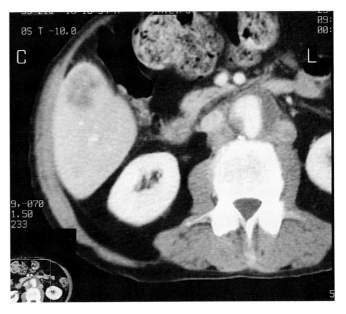

Fig. 9.56 Carcinoma of the pancreas with metastatic disease.
Enlarged lymph nodes are seen adjacent to a small aortic aneurysm. One of multiple liver metastases is also visible. Pancreatic cancer was proved.

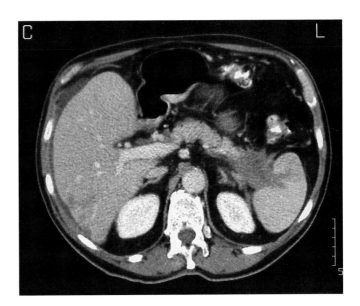

Fig. 9.57 Carcinoma of the tail of the pancreas with liver metastases. There is a solid, low-attenuation, mass lesion in the tail of the pancreas extending into the hilum of the spleen. Approximately 12% of all pancreatic cancers are in the tail, 25% in the body and 50–60% in the head.

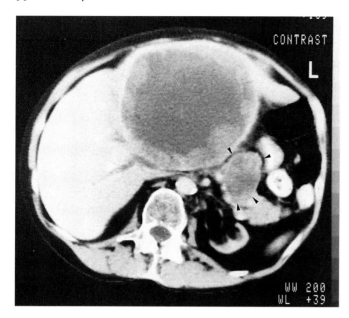

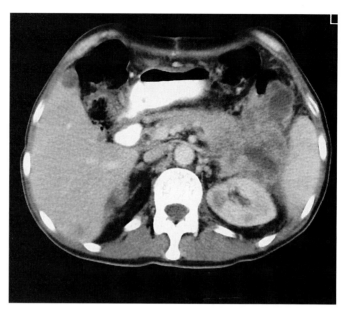

Fig. 9.58 Pancreatic cystadenocarcinoma with metastatic liver disease. A huge solitary liver metastasis is shown replacing the left lobe. The primary lesion is shown in the tail of the pancreas (arrowheads).

Fig. 9.59 Cystadenocarcinoma of the pancreas. Left upper quadrant pain and a palpable mass were present in a 63-year-old male. There is a large, complex, left upper quadrant, mass lesion contiguous with the body and tail of the pancreas invading the anterior surface of the left kidney.

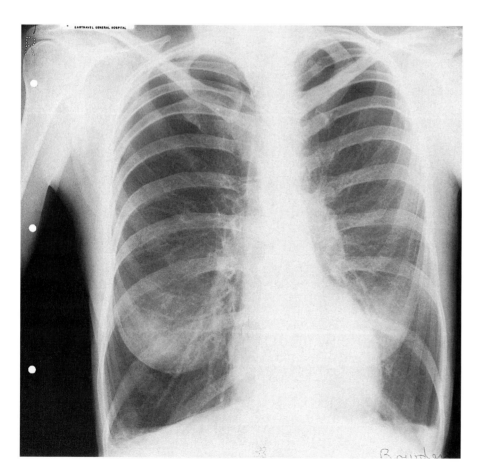

Fig. 9.60 Bilateral pneumothorax with pancreatic cancer. This patient developed bilateral pneumothorax during percutaneous coeliac ganglion block for intractable pain resulting from pancreatic cancer.

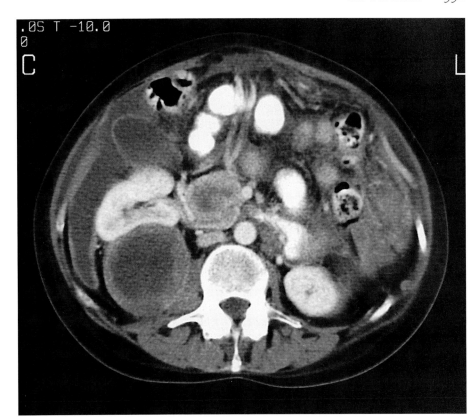

Fig. 9.61 Metastatic disease in the pancreas. A spiral CECT in a 45-year-old female patient with widespread metastatic malignant melanoma shows an irregular, low-attenuation, mass lesion expanding the head of the pancreas. A separate, large, retroperitoneal tumour deposit is seen to cause marked anterior displacement of the right kidney. Ascites is also present.

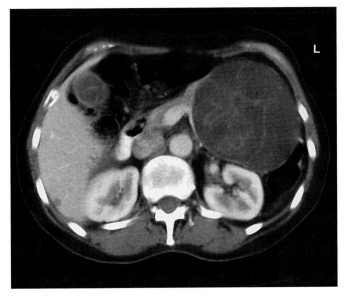

Fig. 9.62 Mucinous cystadenoma of the pancreas. A 57-year-old female patient with painless swelling in the left upper quadrant had no history of pancreatitis. The spiral CECT shows a very well-circumscribed, thin-walled, low-attenuation, mass lesion with delicate strands or septa within it. Diagnostic percutaneous aspiration produced obvious mucus. The lesion was completely excised surgically and pathology revealed no evidence of malignancy.

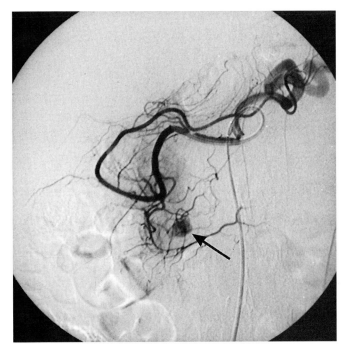

Fig. 9.63 Pancreatic insulinoma. This selective gastroduodenal arteriogram shows a round, enhancing lesion in the head of pancreas (arrow), supplied by the superior pancreaticoduodenal artery. The appearances are characteristic of a neuroendocrine tumour, in this case an insulinoma. (Courtesy of Dr Richard D. Edwards.)

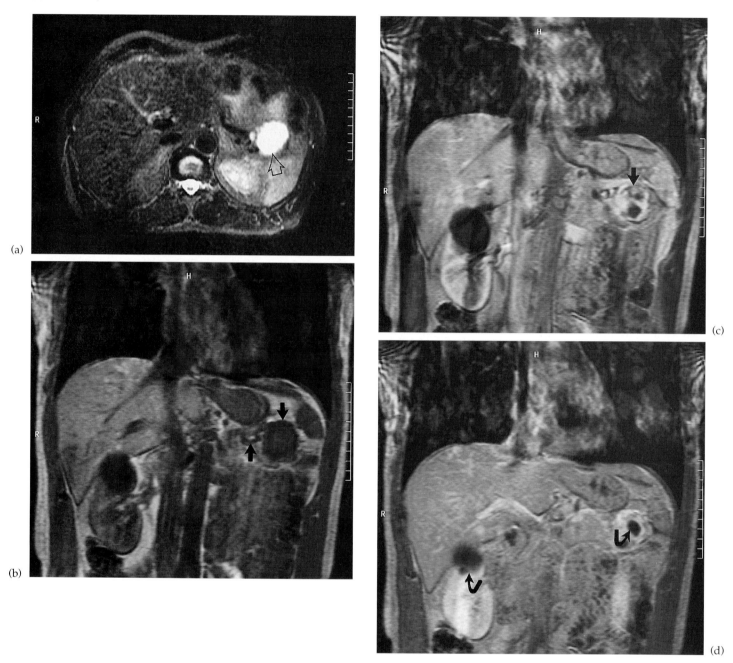

(a)

(b)

(c)

(d)

Fig. 9.64 Pancreatic insulinoma. This patient is a 63-year-old male with a 6-year history of recurrent hypoglycaemic attacks. (a) An axial STIR of the liver shows a 3.5 cm high-signal mass on the anterior aspect of the tail of the pancreas (open arrow). (b) A coronal T_1 GRE pre gadolinium enhancement shows a low-signal mass with associated vessel (arrows). (c) At 30 s and (d) 5 min after gadolinium enhancement (0.1 mmol/kg), there is early (straight arrow) and maintained peripheral enhancement of the lesion. There remains central non-enhancement, in keeping with cystic change (curved arrow). Surgical pathological confirmation. Curved arrow (right), incidental right simple cyst. (Courtesy of Dr Graeme Houston.)

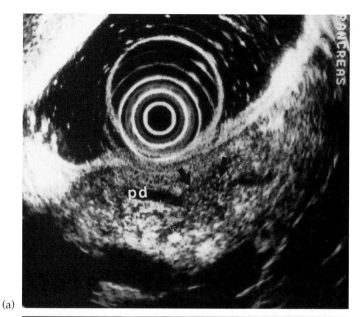

(a)

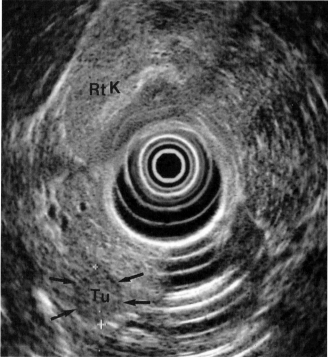

(b)

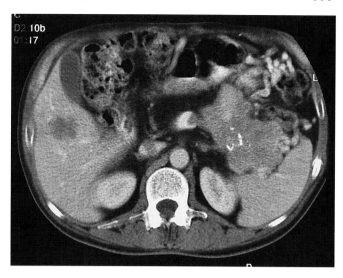

Fig. 9.66 Recurrent pancreatic glucagonoma. A 48-year-old male patient with previous pancreatic resection for glucagonoma had a follow-up spiral CECT, which showed a lobulated, irregular, solid, mass lesion in the region of the tail of the pancreas, with extension into the superior mesenteric vein. Gastrosplenic varices are shown as a result of previous splenic vein thrombosis. A metastasis is shown in the right lobe of the liver.

Fig. 9.65 Pancreatic islet-cell tumour, endoscopic ultrasound. In expert hands, the sensitivity of endoscopic US for the detection of small pancreatic islet-cell tumours is high—up to 82%. These small tumours may be difficult to locate on CT or MRI. On endoscopic US, they are characteristically seen as small, relatively well-defined hypoechoic lesions. (a) This demonstrates a 1.3 cm, slightly irregular, hypoechoic lesion (arrows) in relation to the pancreatic duct (pd) in a patient with multiple endocrine neoplasia. (b) This demonstrates a 1.3 cm, slightly hypoechoic mass (Tu) within the uncinate process, subsequently verified as a small insulinoma. RtK, right kidney. (Courtesy of Dr Alison McLean.)

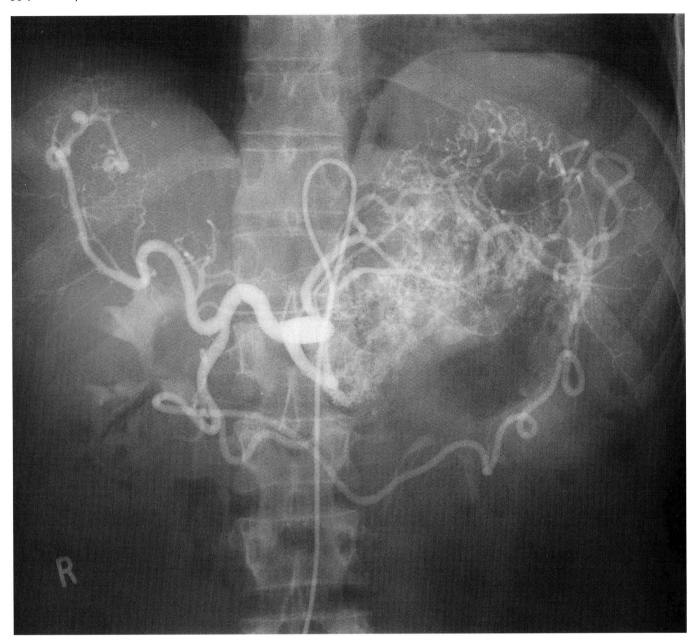

Fig. 9.67 Non-functioning islet-cell tumour of the pancreas. A selective coeliac arteriogram shows extensive tumour circulation in the region of the pancreatic bed. This patient had a large, non-functioning, neuroendocrine tumour of the pancreas, supplied by the splenic and left gastric arteries. A parasitic blood supply was also derived from the superior and inferior mesenteric arteries (not shown). A solitary, vascular, hepatic metastasis is also noted. (Courtesy of Dr Richard D. Edwards.)

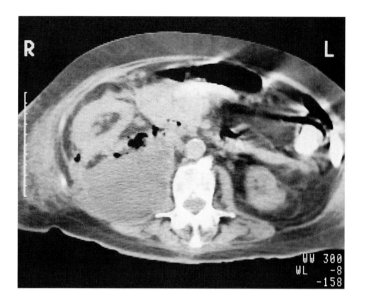

Fig. 9.68 ERCP sphincterotomy complicated by retroperitoneal abscess. The patient became septic soon after ERCP with sphincterotomy. The CT scan 4 weeks later shows a large fluid collection behind the head of the pancreas and right kidney, with pockets of gas within it. Pus was drained under ultrasound with a 12 F catheter.

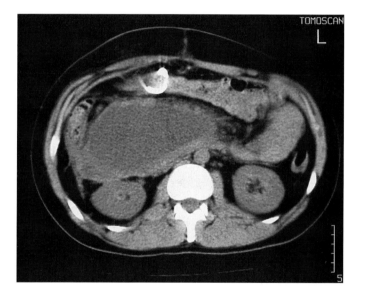

Fig. 9.69 Post-traumatic pancreatic pseudocyst. A public-house stabbing resulted in colonic perforation, which was surgically repaired. The patient subsequently developed a pancreatic pseudocyst. An unenhanced CT scan shows a relatively well-defined pseudocyst in the right upper quadrant. A drainage catheter was inadvertently placed in the transverse colon rather than in the pseudocyst.

10: The Anterior Abdominal Wall, Diaphragm, Peritoneal Cavity and Mesentery, Visceral Vessels and Lymph Nodes

Anterior abdominal wall

The layers of the anterior abdominal wall consist of skin, subcutaneous fascia, muscle layers, transversalis fascia, extraperitoneal fat and peritoneum. The lateral muscles of the anterior abdominal wall comprise three layers. The outermost consists of the external oblique muscle, which arises from the lower eight ribs; the fibres are directed downwards, forwards and medially. The lowermost fibres run vertically downwards and are inserted into the anterior two-thirds of the iliac crest. The remaining fibres become aponeurotic near the linea semilunaris and pass in front of the rectus abdominis muscle to reach the midline. The lower border of the aponeurosis of the external oblique forms the inguinal ligament, which extends from the anterior superior iliac spine to the pubic tubercle. The internal oblique lies under cover of the external oblique muscle. It arises from the thoracolumbar fascia, the iliac crest and the lateral two-thirds of the inguinal ligament. The fibres are directed upwards, forwards and medially. The intermediate fibres form an aponeurosis, which is inserted into the linea alba in the midline. The transversus abdominis is the deepest muscle layer of the lateral abdominal wall and the fibres are directed predominantly horizontally. The rectus abdominis arises from the pubic crest and widens as it passes upwards to be inserted in an almost horizontal line into the xiphoid process and the seventh, sixth and fifth costal cartilages. The medial border lies alongside the linea alba and the lateral border corresponds with the linear semilunaris. The rectus abdominis sheath is a strong, but incomplete, aponeurotic envelope, which is formed by the aponeuroses of the three lateral abdominal muscles. Above the horizontal arcuate line, the posterior layer of the internal oblique aponeurosis and the transversalis aponeurosis passes behind the rectus muscle. Below the arcuate line, the aponeurosis of all three muscles passes anterior to the rectus abdominis.

Diaphragm

The diaphragm is the principal muscle of respiration and is a dome-shaped musculotendinous partition separating the thoracic from the abdominal cavity. The tendinous part (central tendon) is completely surrounded by the peripheral muscular portion. There are three large openings, namely for the inferior vena cava (IVC) within the central tendon and two in the muscular part for the aorta and the oesophagus. The oesophageal opening is at the level of T12 and, in addition, its transmits the vagus nerves and the oesophageal branches of the left gastric artery and vein. This aperture lies in front and to the left of the aortic hiatus. The diaphragmatic crura are tendinous structures with origins on the anterolateral aspect of the upper lumbar spine. The right crus is larger and longer than the left and arises from L1, 2 and 3, whereas the left crus takes its origin only from the upper two lumbar vertebrae. On CT, the crura may have a nodular appearance [1], which should not be confused with enlarged retrocrural lymph nodes, which normally do not exceed 6 mm.

Peritoneal cavity and mesentery

The peritoneum is a highly absorptive serous membrane, which lines the abdominal and pelvic cavities. This parietal peritoneum is related to the viscera in the abdomen and pelvis, which are covered to a variable extent by visceral peritoneum (that is, a serous coat). In males, the peritoneum forms a completely closed sac. In the female, it communicates with the cavities of the uterus and vagina via the abdominal openings of the uterine tubes. There is therefore the potential for the spread of infection by this route. Above the umbilicus, there is a fold of peritoneum comprising the two layers of the falciform ligament, which pass upwards to the liver. The lower border of the falciform ligament is free and it contains the ligamentum teres. The peritoneum lining the anterior abdominal wall sweeps over the inferior surface of the diaphragm and is then reflected on to the stomach and liver. The lesser omentum is a broad peritoneal sheet attaching the lesser curve of stomach and proximal duodenum to the medial aspect of the liver. The greater omentum is a large peritoneal apron, which connects the transverse colon to the stomach. Developmentally, its upper part consisted of two layers and its lower part of four layers of peritoneum, but these usually become completely fused. The posterior two layers, having enclosed the transverse colon, pass backwards and upwards to the posterior abdominal wall as the transverse mesocolon, where they separate along the anterior border of the pancreas. The superior layer passes upwards over the posterior abdominal wall before being reflected on to the liver. The inferior layer passes downwards and forms a complete posterior abdominal-wall covering inferior to the pancreas. Along a line which passes obliquely downwards and to the right, the peritoneum is lifted from the posterior abdominal wall to form the mesentery, which is a broad, double, peritoneal layer containing mesenteric vessels and enclosing the jejunum and the ileum. Inferior to the root of the mesentery, the peritoneum continues downwards to cover the pelvic viscera, before being reflected upwards on to the anterior abdominal wall. The blind sac of peritoneum posterior to the stomach and anterior to the pancreas is the lesser sac (omental bursa). It is, in effect, a diverticulum or a recess of the greater sac, with which it communicates through a single opening, the foramen of Winslow (epiploic foramen). This lies behind the right free border of the lesser omentum.

The various peritoneal ligaments naturally divide the peritoneal cavity into other compartments, as well as the lesser sac. These can be very important with respect to the distribution of fluid and the spread of disease, especially infection. In effect, the peritoneal space is a complicated potential cavity, in which several compartments are anatomically interconnected. The main division is between superomesocolic and inframesocolic regions. The former is more complex and is further divided into right and left sides, and these are further subdivided by the upper abdominal viscera, peritoneal ligaments and mesenteries. The inframesocolic space is divided into right and left infracolic compartments, paracolic gutters, paravesical recesses and the pouch of Douglas. The lesser sac lies behind the lesser omentum, stomach, duodenum and gastrocolic ligament. It lies anterior to the body of the pancreas and spleen. The left gastric artery, coronary vein and lymph nodes lie between the layers of the gastrohepatic ligament. The middle colic vessels lie within the layers of the transverse mesocolon. The sigmoid mesocolon contains sigmoid and haemorrhoidal vessels. Free intraperitoneal fluid can be detected by CT in amounts of 50 ml or more [1]. Fluid in the peritoneal cavity can also be readily detected by ultrasound. Computerized tomography is superior to plain X-rays in detecting free peritoneal air, which collects anteriorly behind the abdominal wall. In the postoperative patient, small amounts of air may be visible on CT scans for up to 1 week.

Visceral arteries

The coeliac artery arises from the anterior aspect of the abdominal aorta immediately below the aortic hiatus in the diaphragm. It is usually 1–2 cm long and passes forwards above the pancreas before dividing into the left gastric, splenic and hepatic arteries. The superior mesenteric artery (SMA) arises from the aorta behind the pancreas and descends at an acute angle, at first anterior to the uncinate process of the pancreas and the third part of the duodenum, before entering the root of the mesentery. Close to its origin, the SMA gives rise to the inferior pancreaticoduodenal artery. The jejunal and ileal arteries form a series of 12–15 branches, which arise from the left side of the main trunk and which supply the jejunum and ileum. They break up into branches which divide and reunite to form a connected series of arcades. From the terminal arcades, smaller branches, the vasa recta, pass to the mesenteric border of the gut, where the vessels alternately pass to the opposite sides of the bowel and penetrate the wall obliquely. Within the wall, they form free anastomoses with each other.

The inferior mesenteric artery (IMA) arises from the front or from a left anterolateral aspect of the distal abdominal aorta approximately 3 cm above the bifurcation. It supplies the splenic flexure, the descending and pelvic colon and upper rectum. The IMA terminates in the right and left superior haemorrhoidal branches. Its highest branch is the left colic, branches of which anastomose with the branches of the middle colic branch of the SMA. The left colic artery is often absent. Other branches derived from the IMA supply the descending and sigmoid colon and proximal rectum. The marginal artery of Drummond [2–4] refers to a vascular arcade which runs along the mesenteric border of the large bowel. An enlarged marginal artery may provide a collateral pathway between the SMA and the IMA territories, but anatomically this vessel is not always complete. Griffiths' point refers to a zone of potentially poor anastomotic connection [5]. The arc of Riolan is a more centrally located collateral pathway within the large-bowel mesentery, between the IMA and SMA [2]. The development of collaterals connecting the superior rectal arteries and the middle and inferior rectal arteries can provide a vital circulation in occlusive lower-limb arterial disease.

Lymph nodes

In the abdomen and pelvis, lymph nodes are vitally important in the control of the spread of disease, especially malignant disease, and the distinction between normal and abnormal lymph nodes is a major challenge to the diagnostic radiologist. Cross-sectional imaging by ultrasound, CT and MRI have completely replaced lymphangiography in the detection of lymphadenopathy. To this end, the principal modality at the present time is CT scanning, with its remarkably good resolution and speed of operation. However, the detection of lymph-node pathology by CT is entirely dependent on demonstrating enlarged lymph nodes. Criteria for the enlargement of different lymph-node groups in the abdomen and pelvis have been proposed by Dahnert [6]. Lymph nodes larger than 6 mm in the retrocrural area, greater than 8 mm in the gastrohepatic ligament and greater than 6 mm in the porta hepatis are considered abnormal. Lymph nodes larger than 10 mm in the retroperitoneal, coeliac, SMA, pancreaticoduodenal and perisplenic groups are considered abnormal. In the pelvis, the upper normal limit is said to be 15 mm.

Normal-sized lymph nodes are seen in most CT examinations in many intra-abdominal locations. Endoscopic ultrasound may demonstrate lymph nodes as small as 2 mm. Husband and others [7–9] consider that, in the pelvis, 8 mm should be the maximum short-axis diameter and, in the upper para-aortic area lymph nodes larger than 8 mm are considered abnormal. At the aortic bifurcation, 10 mm is the upper limit of normal.

References

1 Burgener F.A. & Kormano M. (1996) *Differential Diagnosis in Computed Tomography*. Stuttgart: Thieme Medical Publishers, 211.
2 Reuter S.R., Redman H.C. & Cho K.J. (1986) *Gastro-intestinal Angiography*, 3rd edn. Philadelphia: W.B. Saunders.
3 Kadir S., Lundell C. & Saeed M. (1991) Coeliac, inferior and superior mesenteric arteries. In: Kadir S. (ed.) *Atlas of Normal and Variant Angiographic Anatomy*. Philadelphia: W.B. Saunders, 297–364.
4 Ruzika F.F., Jr & Rossi P. (1970) Normal vascular anatomy of the abdominal viscera. *Radiological Clinics of North America* **8**, 3–29.
5 Meyers M.A. (1976) Griffiths' point: critical anastomosis at the splenic flexure. Significance in ischaemia of the colon. *American Journal of Roentgenology* **126**, 77–94.
6 Dahnert W. (1996) *Radiology Review Manual*, 3rd edn. Baltimore: Williams & Wilkins, 566.
7 Husband J. (1996) Nodal lymphoma—the abdomen and pelvis. In: *Proceedings of the London CT/MRI Course*. Gleneagles, Scotland, 82–86.
8 Dorfman R.E., Alpern M.B., Goss B.H. *et al.* (1991) Upper abdominal lymph nodes: criteria for normal size determined with CT. *Radiology* **180**, 319–322.
9 Vinnicombe S.J., Norman A.R., Nicolson V. & Husband J.E. (1995) Normal pelvic lymph nodes, evaluation with CT after bi-pedal lymphangiography. *Radiology* **194** (2), 349–355.

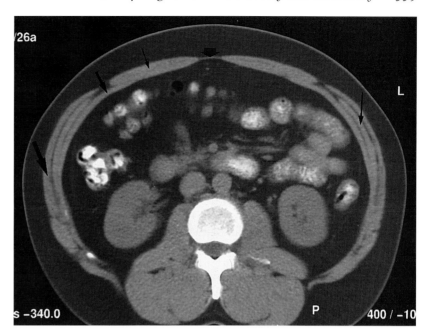

Fig. 10.1 Normal anterior abdominal wall. Spiral CT at the level of the third part of the duodenum. The three muscular layers of the abdominal wall are clearly visible, contrasting with the subcutaneous fat and intra-abdominal fat. Arrowhead, linea alba; short thin arrow, rectus abdominis; short thick arrow, transversus abdominis; long thin arrow, internal oblique; long thick arrow, external oblique.

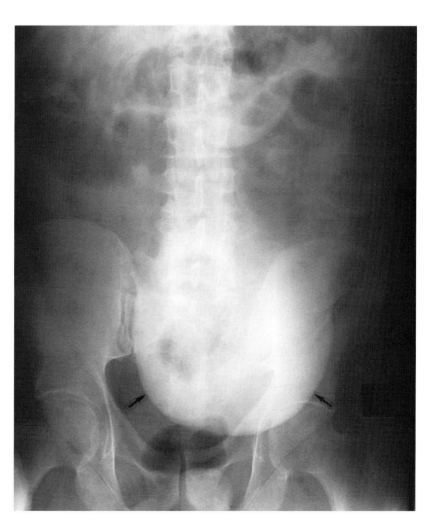

Fig. 10.2 Incisional hernia. A plain abdominal X-ray shows a large homogeneous opacity projected in the lower abdomen and pelvis with a very well-circumscribed inferior margin (arrows). This was caused by a large incisional hernia of the anterior abdominal wall.

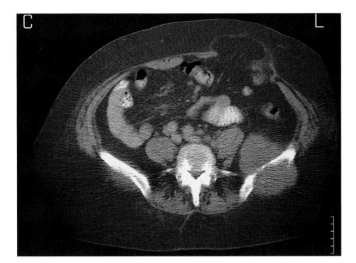

Fig. 10.3 Incisional hernia. A spiral CT through the lower abdomen of a female patient shows an extensive defect in the anterior abdominal wall on the left side containing fat. The patient also has extensive destruction of the blade of the ilium on the left side, associated with soft-tissue swelling both inside and outside the pelvis, displacing the left psoas muscle, caused by lymphoma.

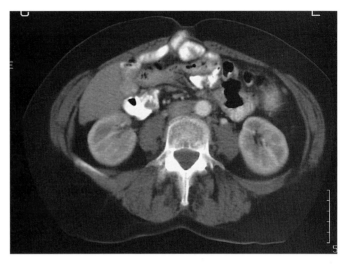

Fig. 10.5 Paraumbilical hernia. A spiral contrast-enhanced CT (CECT) in a patient with metastatic liver disease (not shown) shows a defect in the linea alba adjacent to the umbilicus containing a loop of contrast-filled bowel.

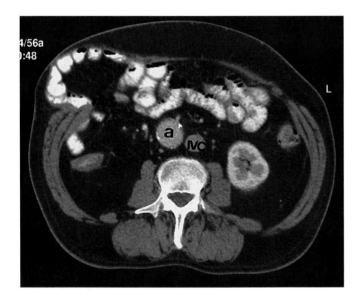

Fig. 10.4 Incisional hernia containing small bowel. A spiral CT scan shows a fairly extensive, right-sided, anterior, abdominal-wall defect, with a wide hernia sac containing contrast-filled small bowel. In addition, the patient is noted to have a left-sided inferior vena cava (IVC)—that is, a persisting left supracardinal vein. The incidence is 1/200. a, aorta.

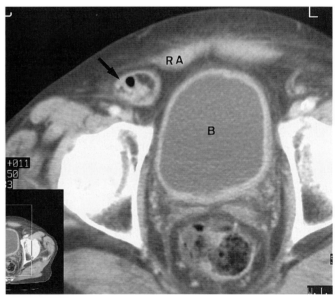

Fig. 10.6 Inguinal hernia. A spiral CECT shows a small hernia sac in the right groin (arrow), lying anterior to the common femoral artery and vein and posterolateral to the rectus muscle (RA). B, bladder.

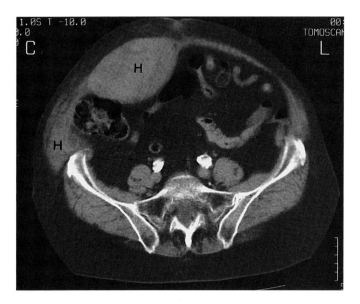

Fig. 10.7 Rectus-sheath haematoma. A 71-year-old female patient on warfarin developed painful, tender swelling in the right side of her abdomen and flank. The spiral CT shows a lens-shaped haematoma (H) within the anterior abdominal wall on the right side in the distribution of the rectus sheath, limited in the midline by the linea alba. The left rectus muscle is markedly atrophic. The haematoma is seen to extend within the oblique muscles on the right side as far as the iliac crest. (Courtesy of Dr George Stenhouse.)

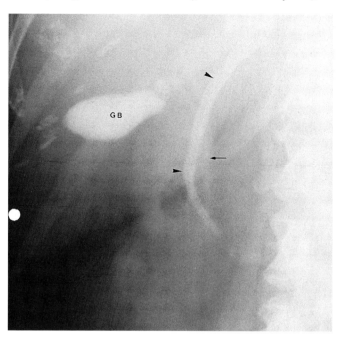

Fig. 10.9 Ossification in a laparotomy scar. A normal oral cholecystogram shows contrast in the gallbladder (GB) and common bile duct (arrow). In addition, however, there is a scimitar-shaped calcified or ossified opacity projected over the right upper quadrant (arrowheads). This was the result of scar tissue following previous gastroduodenal surgery.

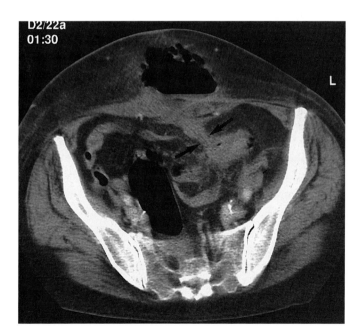

Fig. 10.8 Abscess of the anterior abdominal wall. A 54-year-old female patient had a 2-week history of increasing abdominal pain. Clinically there was diffuse swelling of the anterior abdominal wall, which was red, hot and exquisitely tender. Spiral CECT shows an irregular gas-filled cavity with a small amount of fluid within the subcutaneous fat of the anterior abdominal wall, together with diffuse swelling of the muscle layer deep to it. In addition, there is a thick strand of soft tissue (arrows), apparently in continuity with the sigmoid colon, which shows evidence of

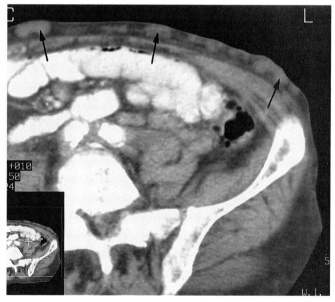

Fig. 10.10 Collateral veins in the anterior abdominal wall. Multiple subcutaneous opacities (arrows) are seen in this 83-year-old male patient with thrombosis of the inferior vena cava.

diverticular disease. The abscess was decompressed with a percutaneous drain, but, within 24 h, the patient had a faecal fistula. After a short interval, diverticular disease was confirmed by double-contrast barium enema (DCBE) and colonic resection performed.

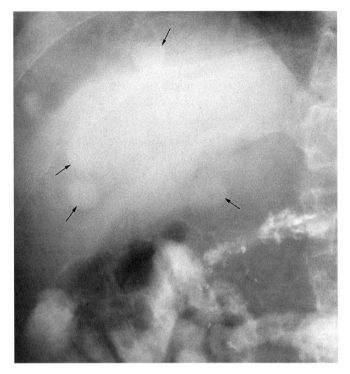

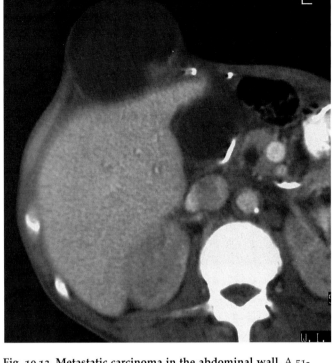

Fig. 10.11 Subcutaneous neurofibromatosis (von Recklinghausen's disease). Part of a barium follow-through study shows multiple, well-circumscribed opacities of soft-tissue density superimposed on the liver shadow (arrows). These corresponded with visible subcutaneous neurofibromata. Lesions of soft-tissue density within the liver cannot be visualized on plain films because of a lack of inherent contrast.

Fig. 10.13 Metastatic carcinoma in the abdominal wall. A 51-year-old male patient had a previous oesophagogastrectomy for carcinoma, but recently developed soft-tissue swelling within the anterior abdominal wall. There is a well-circumscribed, very low-attenuation, mass lesion within the abdominal wall, in keeping with a metastatic deposit. Histological confirmation.

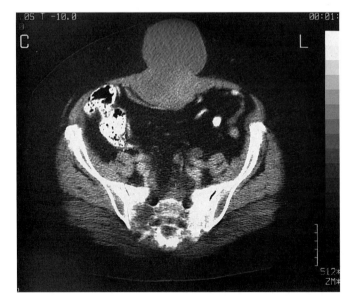

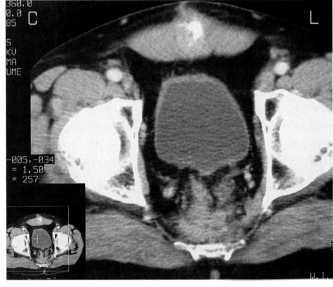

Fig. 10.12 Metastatic carcinoma in the anterior abdominal wall. A spiral CT in an obese patient with a palpable anterior abdominal-wall mass lesion shows a very well-circumscribed solid mass. This is largely within the subcutaneous fat, but is seen to be contiguous with a mass infiltrating the muscle layer, which proved to be a recurrent carcinoma from an ovarian primary in the laparotomy scar.

Fig. 10.14 Calcified metastasis in the anterior abdominal wall. The patient had a previous AP resection of rectal adenocarcinoma resulting in local recurrence, as well as liver metastases. The spiral CECT shows an irregular calcified mass in the laparotomy scar. There is extensive presacral tumour recurrence, with early destruction of the left lateral border of the sacrum. Calcification is typical of mucin-secreting adenocarcinoma.

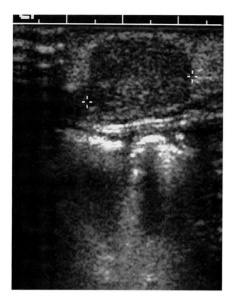

Fig. 10.15 Abdominal-wall metastasis. Ultrasound scan (7 MHz) in a patient who presented originally with a sigmoid stricture, which was found to be due to invasion by ovarian carcinoma. There is a well-circumscribed, solid, 19 mm, mass lesion within the anterior abdominal wall 2 years after surgery. The biopsy was positive.

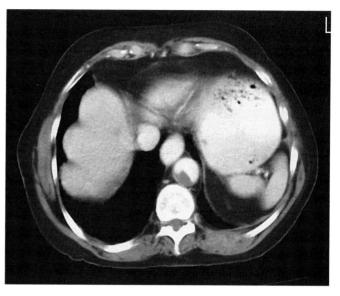

Fig. 10.17 Scalloping of the diaphragm. In elderly patients, the periphery of the liver may have a scalloped appearance, caused by diaphragmatic slings. This is a normal variant. It may be sufficient to produce an accessory fissure.

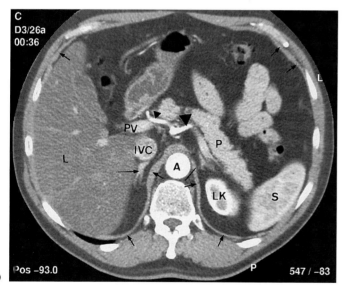

(a)

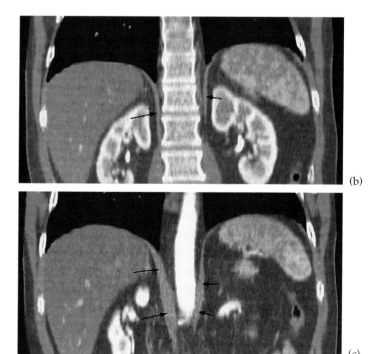

(b)

(c)

Fig. 10.16 Normal diaphragm. (a) A spiral CECT at the level of the right adrenal gland (long arrow). The diaphragm is shown with the aperture for the aorta (A). IVC, inferior vena cava; L, liver; LK, left kidney; P, pancreas; PV, portal vein; S, spleen; short arrows, diaphragm; small arrowhead, hepatic artery; large arrowhead, splenic artery. (b) A coronal reconstruction of the spiral CECT shows the right crus (long arrow) and left crus (short arrow) arising from the lumbar spine. (c) A further coronal section in the plane of the aorta again shows the right crus (long arrows) and left crus (short arrows).

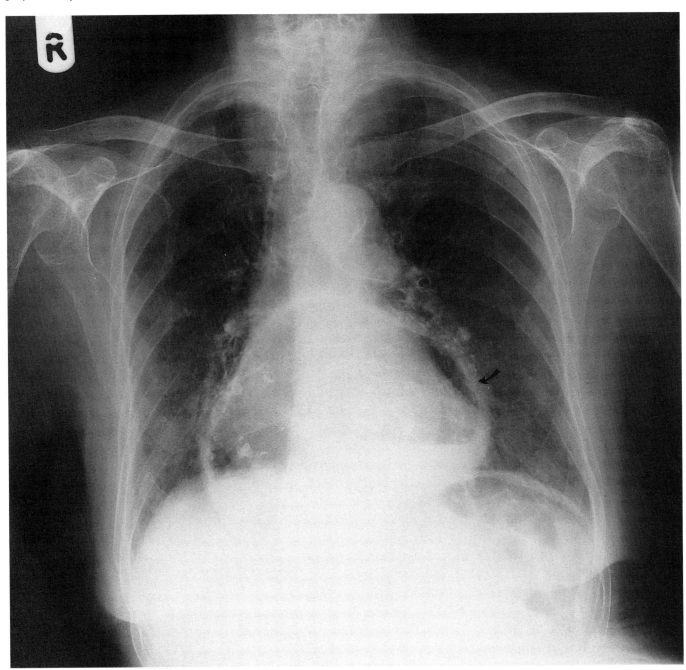

Fig. 10.18 Hiatus hernia of the diaphragm. A PA chest X-ray in
an elderly female patient shows a large, well-circumscribed
shadow (arrow) containing air and two fluid levels, caused by
fixed herniation of the stomach through the diaphragm.

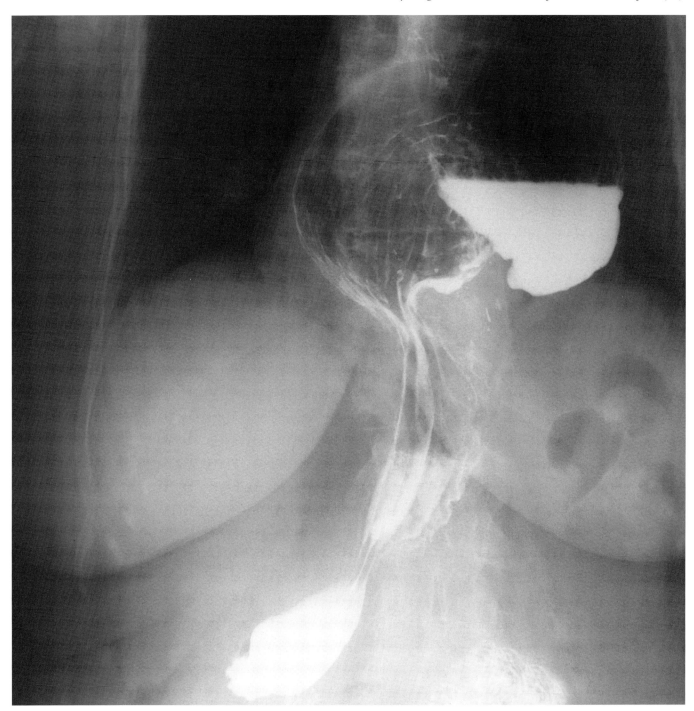

Fig. 10.19 Fixed, mixed sliding and paraoesophageal hernia. An erect double-contrast barium meal (DCBM) shows a substantial portion of the stomach distended with CO_2 within the mediastinum. The oesophagogastric junction is above the diaphragm, indicating the sliding mechanism and, in addition, part of the body of the stomach has rolled into the mediastinum alongside the oesophagus, resulting in an unobstructed partial volvulus.

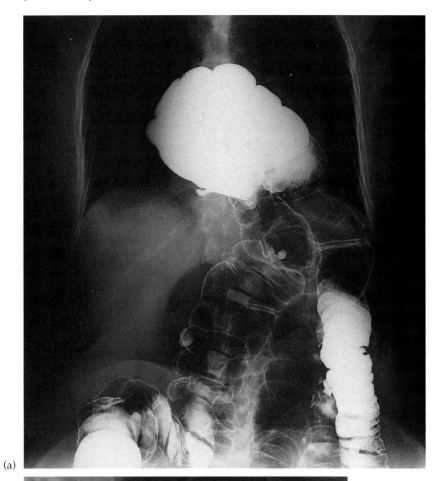

(a)

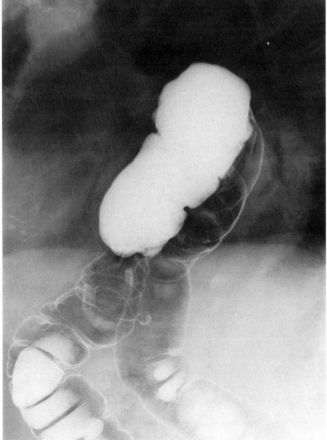

(b)

Fig. 10.20 Paraoesophageal colonic hernia. (a) A DCBE shows a large loop of splenic flexure extending through a wide orifice into the mediastinum. On this frontal projection, it is impossible to determine whether the hernia is anterior (Morgagni), posterior (Boschdalek) or central. (b) The lateral projection shows that the hernia is in a central position.

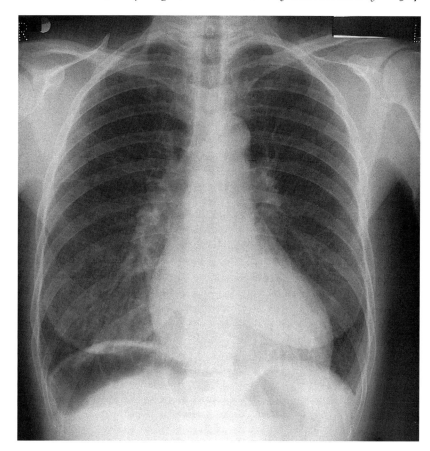

Fig. 10.21 Interposition of bowel between the right hemidiaphragm and the liver. A PA chest X-ray in a patient with no relevant symptoms. A loop of small bowel is seen to be interposed between the right hemidiaphragm and the liver. This needs to be distinguished from a pneumoperitoneum. In this case, the circular fold pattern of the small bowel is apparent. On a previous chest X-ray taken 3 days previously, this phenomenon, which is sometimes known as Chilaiditis' syndrome, was not present.

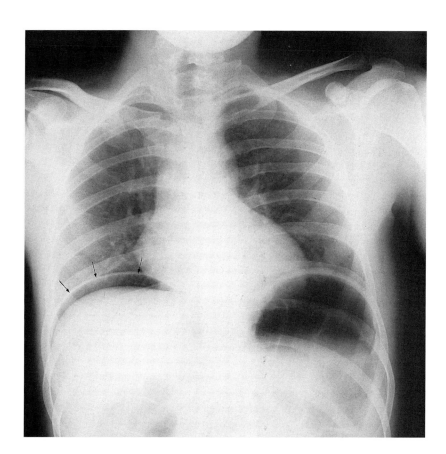

Fig. 10.22 Air under the diaphragm, pneumoperitoneum. An erect chest X-ray in a patient with a duodenal ulcer perforation shows the diaphragm (arrows) profiled by air. Anatomically, the line depicting 'the diaphragm' consists of parietal peritoneum, diaphragm, parietal pleural and visceral pleura.

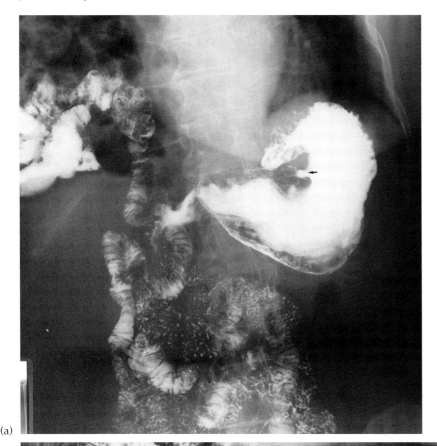

(a)

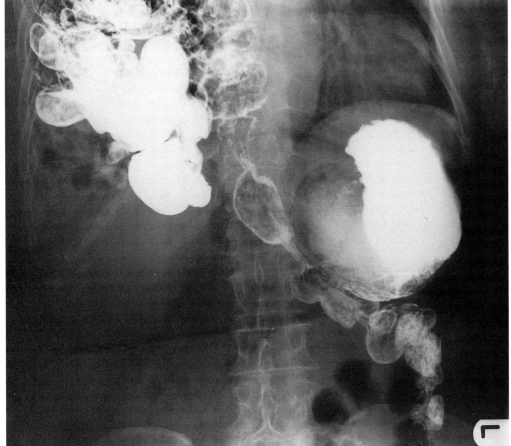

(b)

Fig. 10.23 Eventration of the right hemidiaphragm. The patient had a history of abdominal pain and some weight loss. A recent chest X-ray showed marked elevation of the right hemidiaphragm, with evidence of bowel interposed between the diaphragm and liver. (a) The barium-meal follow-through shows a penetrating ulcer crater on the lesser-curve aspect of the stomach (arrow). There is extensive contrast filling of the small bowel abnormally located between the diaphragm and liver. (b) A further film 30 min later shows extensive filling of the right side of the large bowel, which is also seen to be located in a suprahepatic position.

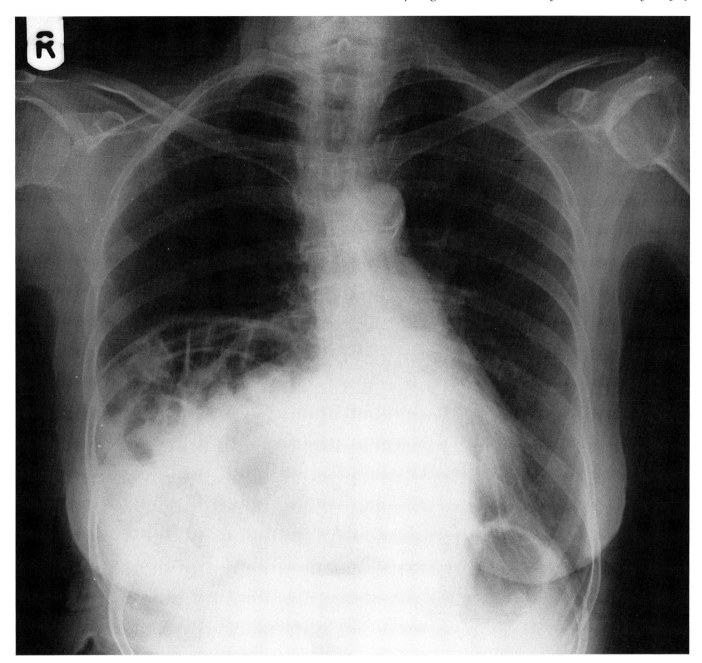

Fig. 10.24 Eventration of the right hemidiaphragm. The chest X-ray in a case similar to that in Fig. 10.23 shows marked elevation of the right hemidiaphragm, with multiple bowel loops interposed between the diaphragm and the liver.

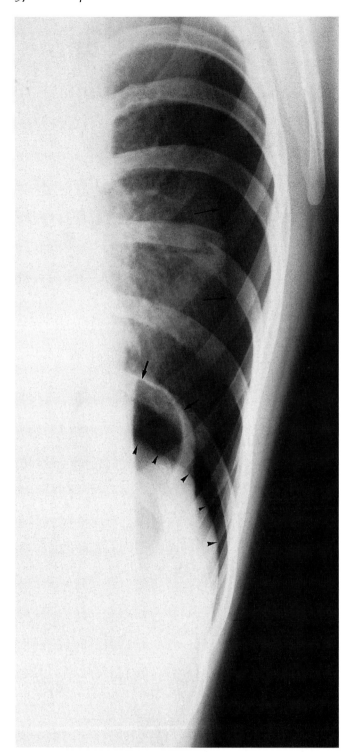

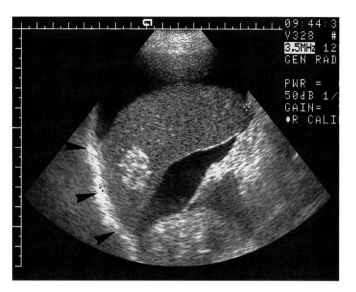

Fig. 10.26 Free fluid in the peritoneal cavity, ascites. A longitudinal US scan in the left upper quadrant shows free fluid anterior and posterior to the spleen. An incidental finding is an echogenic focal lesion within the spleen, in keeping with a haemangioma. Arrowheads, left hemidiaphragm.

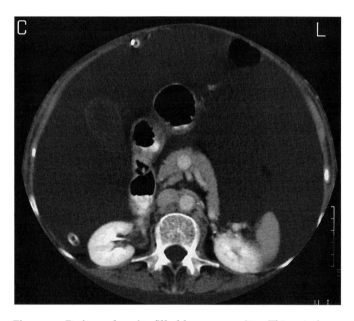

Fig. 10.27 Peritoneal cavity filled by gross ascites. This spiral CECT shows marked abdominal distension by a large volume of ascitic fluid. This includes the lesser sac, which contrasts sharply with the stomach anteriorly and the pancreas posteriorly. A Leveen shunt is shown.

Fig. 10.25 Rupture of the left hemidiaphragm. A young adult female patient presented with a severe crush injury to the chest. The right lateral decubitus film of the chest (left side raised) shows a pneumothorax (long thin arrows). The left hemidiaphragm is indicated by the arrowheads and the stomach (short arrows) is seen to have herniated into the chest as a result of traumatic rupture of the diaphragm. A displaced rib fracture is also shown. These changes were confirmed surgically. (Courtesy of Dr Richard D. Edwards.)

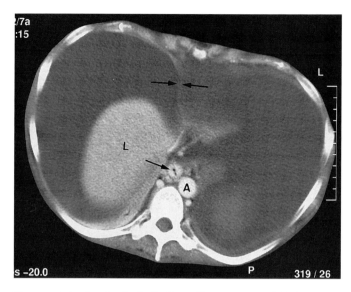

Fig. 10.28 Ascites in alcoholic liver disease. A spiral CECT through the upper abdomen shows a large volume of ascites, the right and left sides of the peritoneal cavity being divided by the double layer of peritoneum comprising the falciform ligament (double arrows). Varices are shown in relation to the distal oesophagus (single arrow). A, aorta; L, liver.

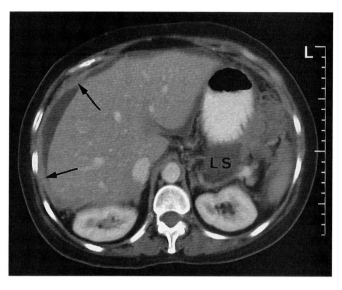

Fig. 10.30 Ascites with serosal metastases. A 53-year-old female patient had a history of ovarian carcinoma. A relatively small amount of ascites is shown, including fluid in the lesser sac (LS). The parietal peritoneum is irregularly thickened, in keeping with serosal tumour (arrows).

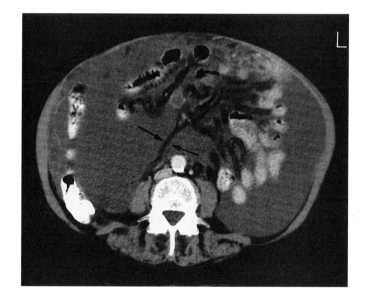

Fig. 10.29 Right and left inframesocolic compartments of the peritoneal cavity. Spiral CECT in a patient with ascites in whom the small-bowel mesentery is clearly shown (arrows). The peritoneal cavity below the transverse mesocolon is divided into right and left compartments by the small-bowel mesentery.

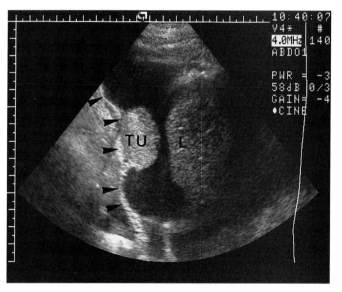

Fig. 10.31 Serosal metastasis, diaphragmatic peritoneum. Longitudinal US scan of upper abdomen showing a large deposit of metastatic tumour (TU), measuring almost 3 cm in diameter, arising from the peritoneum covering the right hemidiaphragm (arrowheads). Ascites is present. The primary tumour was a colonic adenocarcinoma. L, liver.

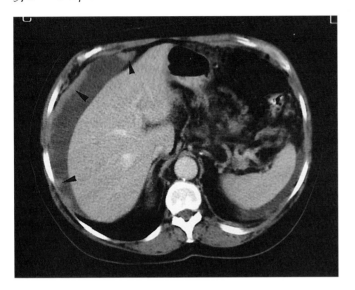

Fig. 10.32 Serosal metastases and ascites. A spiral CECT in a 64-year-old female patient with a pelvic mass. Ascites is present and the parietal peritoneum is irregularly thickened (arrowheads) by deposits of tumour. Ovarian primary carcinoma was proved.

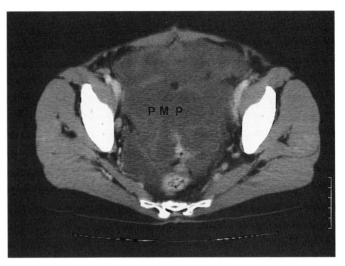

Fig. 10.34 Pseudomyxoma peritonei. A 55-year-old female patient with progressive abdominal distension had a spiral CECT which showed a complex loculation of low-attenuation material throughout the abdomen and pelvis. The patient was found to have an ovarian carcinoma and the loculated material consisted of gelatinous mucin, which is produced by metastatic visceral and parietal peritoneal deposits. Typically these are seeded after the rupture of benign or malignant mucin-secreting tumours of the ovary or appendix. Neoplasms of the stomach, pancreas and large bowel are less common causes. PMP, pseudomyxoma peritonei.

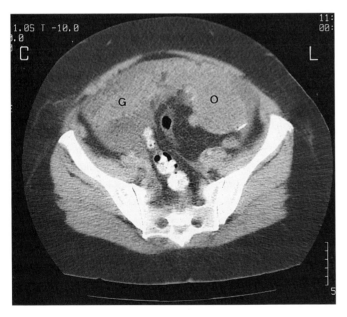

Fig. 10.33 Metastatic tumour in the greater omentum. A spiral CECT in 52-year-old female patient with abdominal swelling showing, as well as ascites, massive thickening of the greater omentum (GO). This was caused by metastatic involvement (omental cake) resulting from carcinoma of the ovary.

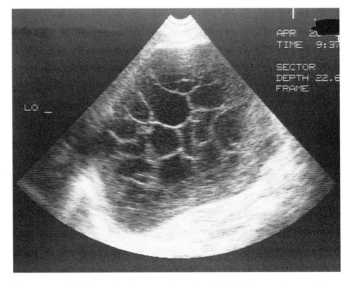

Fig. 10.35 Subphrenic abscess. Longitudinal US scan through the right upper quadrant 10 days after abdominal surgery. Malaise, right upper quadrant pain, pyrexia and a white-cell count of 17 000 were found. There is a very large, septated, largely transonic, mass lesion between the diaphragm and right lobe of liver. Pus was drained percutaneously.

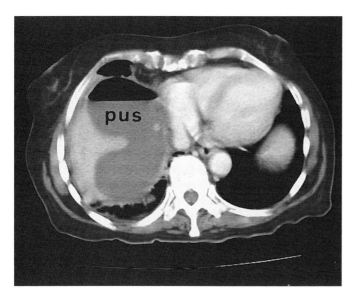

Fig. 10.36 Subphrenic abscess. A spiral CT scan following abdominal surgery for radiation damage to the bowel. A large abscess cavity containing fluid (pus) and gas is interposed between the right hemidiaphragm and right lobe of liver.

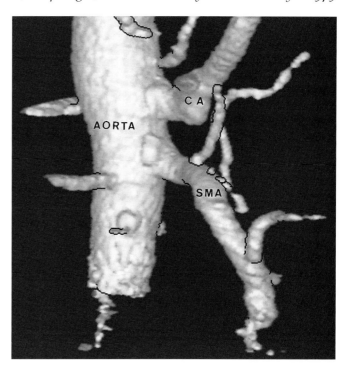

Fig. 10.38 Normal visceral arteries. A 3-D reconstruction of a spiral CECT using the shaded-surface technique shows a lateral projection of the abdominal aorta, the coeliac artery (CA) and the proximal superior mesenteric artery (SMA). (Courtesy of Dr Andrew Watt.)

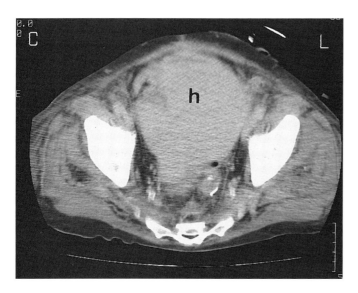

Fig. 10.37 Haematoma in the peritoneal cavity. At 7 days post colonic resection there was a fall in haemoglobin in this patient. A spiral CECT scan through the pelvis shows a large fairly homogeneous mass (h) filling a large part of the pelvis. Percutaneous aspiration confirmed haematoma.

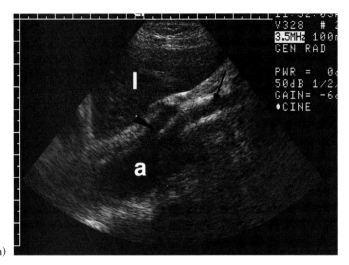

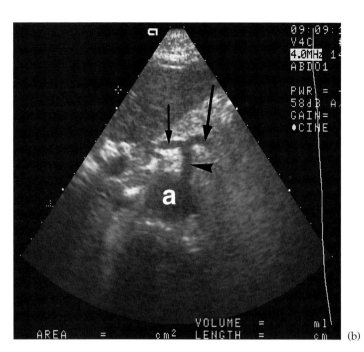

(a)

(b)

Fig. 10.39 Normal visceral arteries, ultrasound. (a) A sagittal midline section shows the upper abdominal aorta (a), coeliac axis (arrowhead) and SMA (arrow). l, left lobe of liver. (b) A transverse US section through the upper abdomen shows the abdominal aorta (a), coeliac axis (arrowhead), hepatic artery (small arrow) and splenic artery (long arrow). This method has the advantages of speed and low cost.

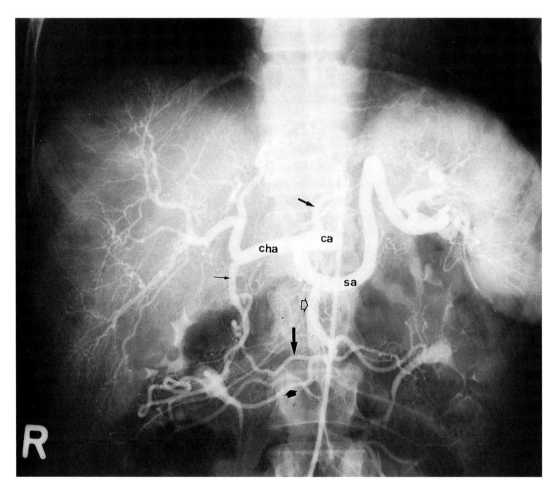

Fig. 10.40 Normal coeliac arteriogram. An AP projection of a selective coeliac arteriogram shows contrast filling of the coeliac artery (ca), common hepatic artery (cha), splenic artery (sa) and left gastric artery (short thick arrow). The gastroduodenal artery is also shown (short thin arrow) and there is retrograde filling of the SMA (open arrowhead) via the inferior pancreaticoduodenal artery (black arrowhead). Large arrow, right gastroepiploic artery.

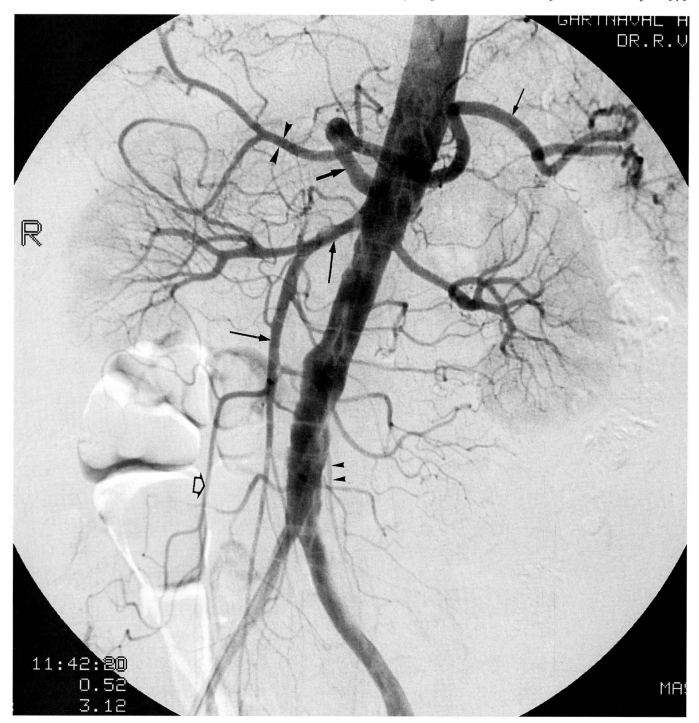

Fig. 10.41 Normal visceral arteries. A digital-subtraction angiogram (DSA) with abdominal aortic injection of contrast via a right, femoral catheter. Short thick arrow, coeliac artery; small thin arrow, splenic artery; large arrowheads, common hepatic artery; large thin arrows, SMA; open arrowhead, ileocolic artery; small arrowheads, IMA.

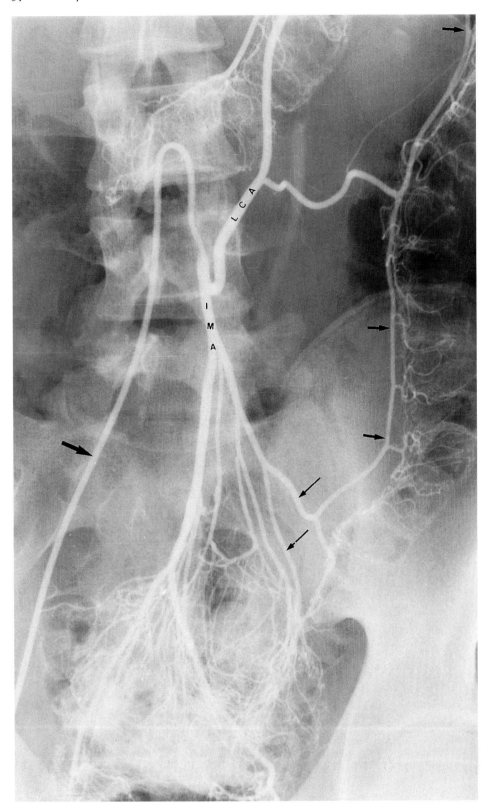

Fig. 10.42 Normal inferior mesenteric angiogram. Selective injection into the inferior mesenteric artery (IMA) shows the left colic artery (LCA), sigmoid arteries, two of which are indicated by the thin arrows, and the marginal artery of Drummond adjacent to the mesenteric border of the colon (short thick arrows). Normal filling of the vasa recta within the bowel wall is also shown. Large arrow, selective catheter.

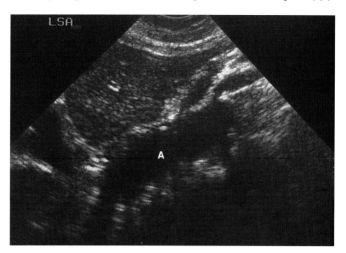

Fig. 10.43 Stenosis of the coeliac and superior mesenteric arteries. A 67-year-old female patient presented with abdominal pain after food and weight loss. This longitudinal US scan in the plane of the aorta shows stenoses of the origins of both the coeliac artery and the SMA. A, aorta.

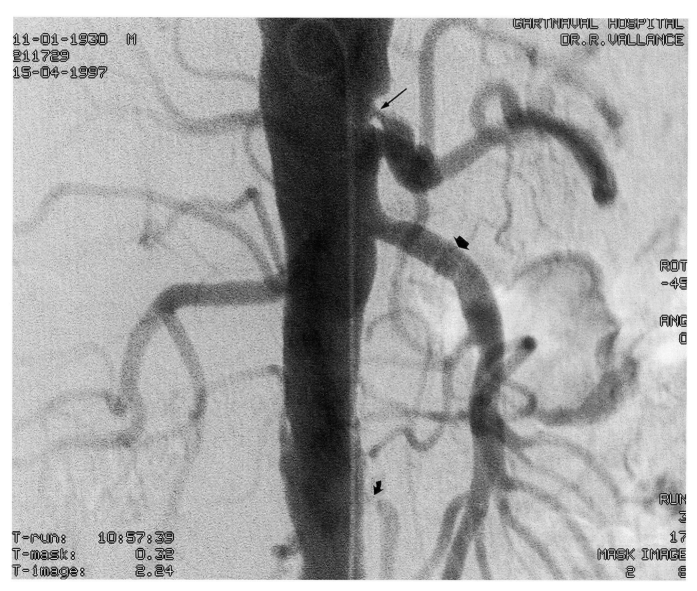

Fig. 10.44 Stenosis of the coeliac and inferior mesenteric arteries. The diabetic patient has peripheral vascular disease and a non-functioning left kidney. The DSA (lateral projection) shows tight stenoses of the coeliac artery origin (long arrow) and of the IMA (short curved arrow). The SMA is virtually normal (arrowhead).

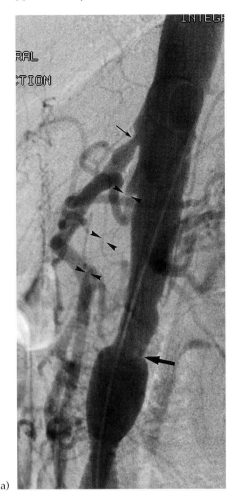

(a)

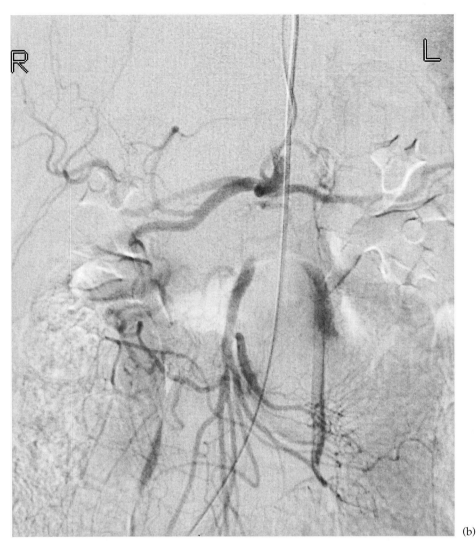

(b)

Fig. 10.45 Stenosis of the coeliac artery and occlusion of the SMA. A 59-year-old patient developed left-sided ischaemic colitis following an aortic-bifurcation graft (ABG). (a) The lateral aortogram shows stenosis of the origin of the coeliac artery (small arrow). The SMA is seen to be occluded for approximately 4 cm (arrowheads). Large arrow, proximal end of the ABG. (b) An AP projection in the same patient with selective injection into the coeliac artery shows collateral filling of the SMA beyond the occlusion via the pancreaticoduodenal circulation. The inferior mesenteric artery in this case was occluded.

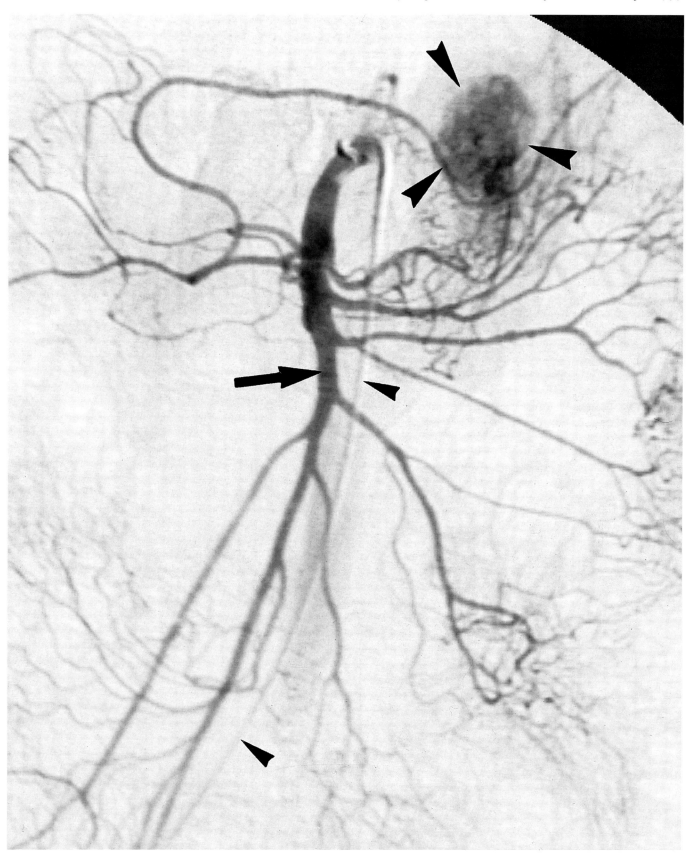

Fig. 10.46 Jejunal leiomyoma, superior mesenteric angiography.
A 69-year-old female patient presented with massive melaena,
resulting in shock requiring a major blood transfusion. Upper
gastrointestinal endoscopy revealed no proximal source of
bleeding. Selective superior mesenteric angiography using DSA
shows a highly vascular lesion in the left upper quadrant (large

arrowheads). The bleeding was controlled by placing
embolization coils in the first jejunal branch of the SMA. Four
days later a tumour was surgically excised from the proximal
jejunum and the histology indicated leiomyoma. Arrow, SMA;
small arrowheads, selective catheter. (Courtesy of Dr Richard D.
Edwards.)

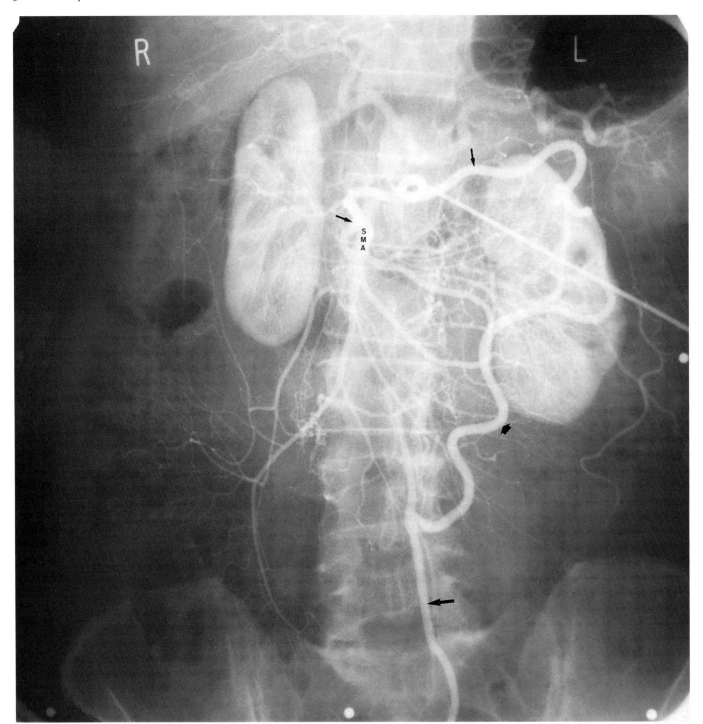

Fig. 10.47 Collateral filling of the occluded IMA from the SMA.
This translumbar aortogram shows an enlarged middle colic
artery (small arrows) filling from the superior mesenteric artery
(SMA), resulting in retrograde filling of the left colic artery
(arrowhead), resulting in opacification of an enlarged inferior
mesenteric artery (large arrow), which contributes blood to the
lower limbs in a patient with bilateral iliac artery occlusions.

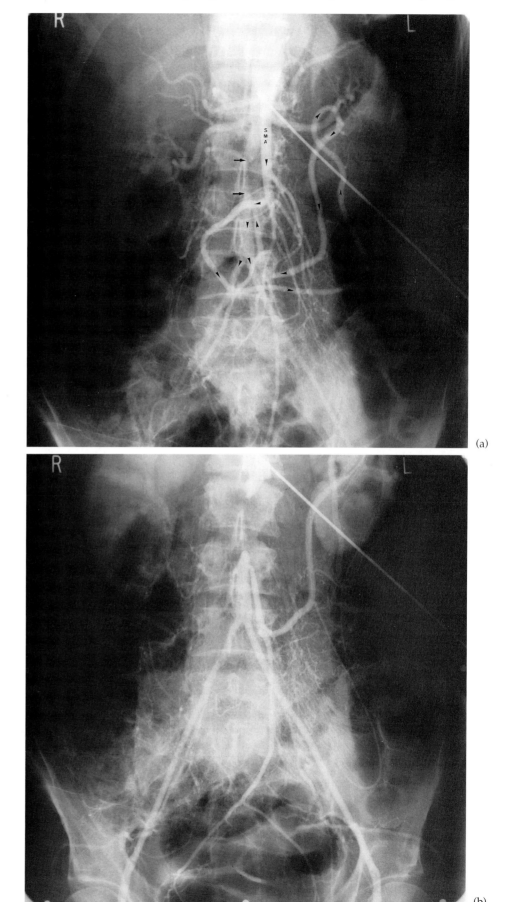

(a)

(b)

Fig. 10.48 Occlusion of the abdominal aorta between the SMA and IMA. (a) A translumbar aortogram shows a 5 cm occlusion of the abdominal aorta distal to the origin of the superior mesenteric artery (SMA) and proximal to the origin of the IMA. Arrows, aortic occlusion; arrowheads, direction of blood flow. (b) There is a well-developed collateral circulation provided by these two visceral arteries.

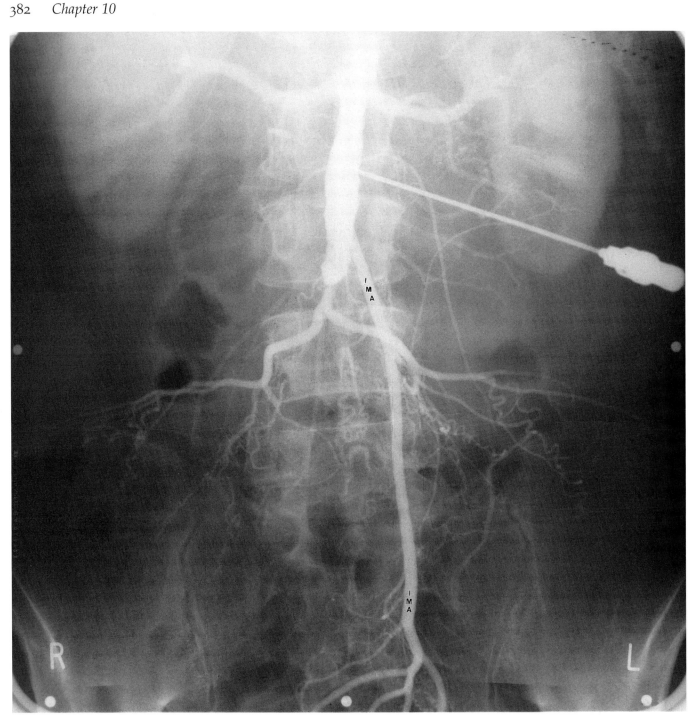

Fig. 10.49 Hypertrophy of the IMA associated with aortoiliac occlusion. A translumbar aortogram in a patient with bilateral buttock claudication (Leriche syndrome). The abdominal aorta is seen to be occluded and collateral flow is provided by a much enlarged inferior mesenteric artery (IMA) and enlarged lumbar arteries.

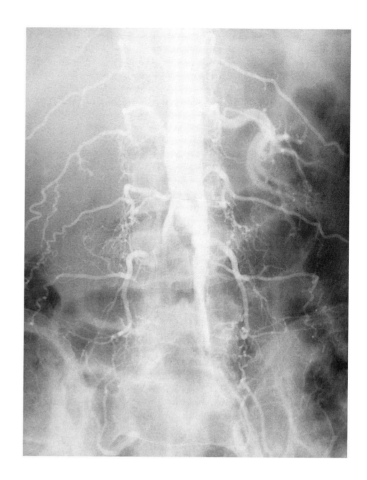

Fig. 10.50 Acute embolic occlusion of the abdominal aorta and visceral arteries. A 78-year-old male patient 7 days post myocardial infarction developed dramatically sudden bilateral lower-limb ischaemia and some abdominal distension. This abdominal arteriography via the left brachial artery access shows irregular occlusion of the distal abdominal aorta, with no filling of visceral arteries except the left renal. This was the result of a 'saddle embolus' resulting from mural thrombus in the left ventricle.

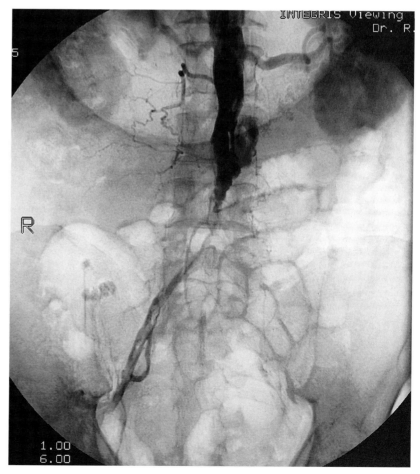

Fig. 10.51 Acute infarction of the bowel associated with aortic thrombosis in severe aortoiliac disease. A 68-year-old male patient with known peripheral vascular disease developed sudden-onset abdominal pain and distension associated with pulseless lower limbs. A DSA via the left brachial approach shows occlusion of the distal abdominal aorta, with irregular filling of the lumen of an aortic aneurysm. There is slight collateral filling of the iliac system on the right side containing thrombus. Some filling of the hepatic artery is shown, but no SMA or IMA patency is apparent and there is generalized gaseous distension of the small bowel. At emergency laparotomy, there was very extensive infarction of the small and large bowel.

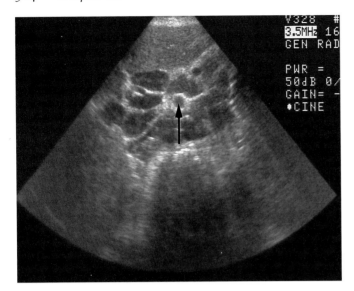

Fig. 10.52 Retroperitoneal para-aortic lymphadenopathy. A 74-year-old female patient with abdominal swelling, pain and weight loss developed a palpable left-sided abdominal mass. A transverse US scan of the upper abdomen shows a major degree of lymphadenopathy completely surrounding the abdominal aorta. The spleen was also found to be enlarged to 19 cm. Non-Hodgkin's lymphoma was diagnosed. Arrow, aorta.

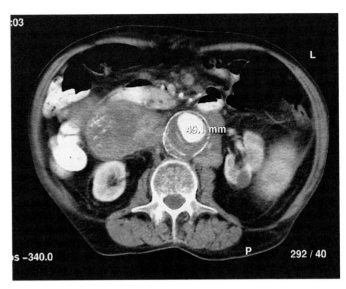

Fig. 10.54 Calcified lymphadenopathy in non-Hodgkin's lymphoma. A 72-year-old male patient with clinical relapse of known high-grade non-Hodgkin's lymphoma was previously treated by chemotherapy. A stippled calcification is shown within the right-sided retroperitoneal mass, which is seen to displace the duodenum forwards. The patient also has a moderate-sized abdominal aortic aneurysm measuring 49 mm transversely, the wall of which is calcified. (Courtesy of Dr Richard D. Edwards.)

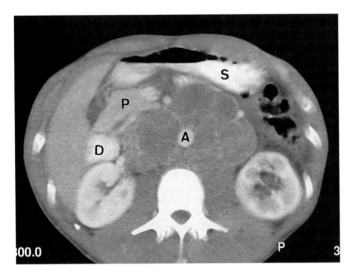

Fig. 10.53 Retroperitoneal metastatic carcinoma. A lymph-node biopsy from the neck of a 35-year-old male patient with abdominal pain and swelling indicated adenocarcinoma. A spiral CECT shows a major degree of low-attenuation lymphadenopathy completely surrounding the abdominal aorta (A). The stomach (S), head of pancreas (P) and mesenteric vessels are displaced forwards. No primary lesion was identified. D, duodenum.

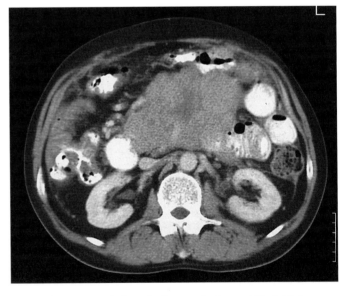

Fig. 10.55 Mesenteric lymphadenopathy in non-Hodgkin's lymphoma. A 50-year-old male patient with a central abdominal solid mass associated with infiltration of the wall of an adjacent small bowel loop underwent a spiral CECT. The great majority of small-bowel lymphomata are secondary to mesenteric nodal primary lymphoma.

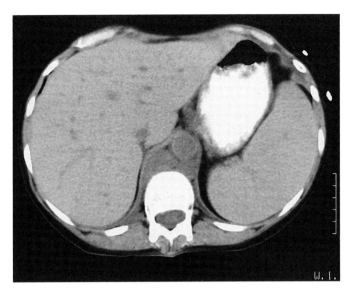

Fig. 10.56 Retrocrural lymphadenopathy. This 62-year-old female patient had known non-Hodgkin's lymphoma. The retrocrural nodes are seen to be enlarged (upper normal limit = 6 mm). The patient also had widespread retroperitoneal disease and splenomegaly.

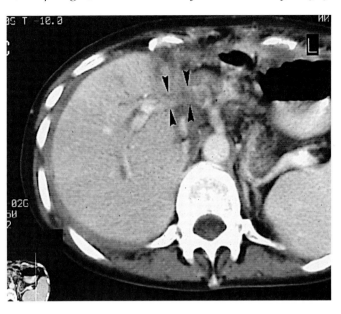

Fig. 10.58 Coeliac lymphadenopathy associated with cholangiocarcinoma encasing the portal vein. The spiral CECT shows enlarged lymph nodes on both sides of the coeliac axis and the portal vein is seen to be encased in tumour (arrowheads).

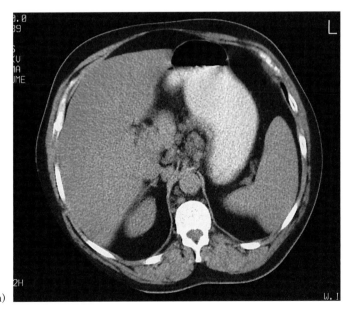

(a)

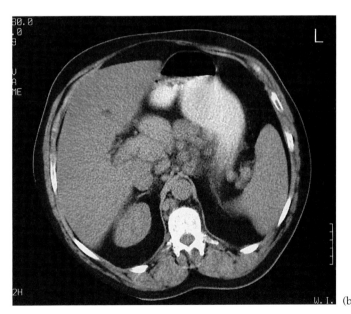

(b)

Fig. 10.57 Coeliac, liver hilar and left gastric lymphadenopathy. (a) A spiral CT in a patient with known lymphoma shows left gastric nodal enlargement, causing extrinsic compression of the lesser curve of the stomach. (b) Coeliac and gastrohepatic lymph nodes are also seen to be enlarged, as well as retrocrural nodes.

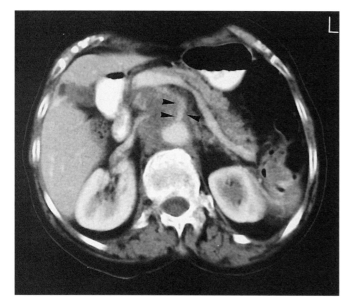

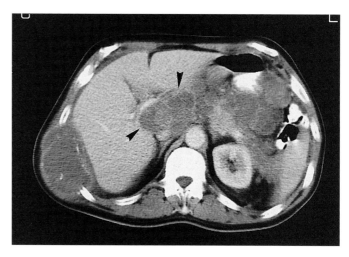

Fig. 10.61 Lymphadenopathy in the porta hepatis. A spiral CECT in a 62-year-old male patient with widespread metastatic malignant melanoma shows a solid mass lesion in the porta hepatis (arrowheads), together with multiple deposits in the left upper quadrant and also in the abdominal wall on the right side.

Fig. 10.59 Lymphadenopathy encasing the SMA. The spiral CECT shows loss of definition of the margins of the SMA, which is seen to be surrounded by lymphadenopathy in a patient with metastatic ovarian carcinoma. The splenic vein and pancreas are seen to be displaced forwards. Arrowheads, SMA.

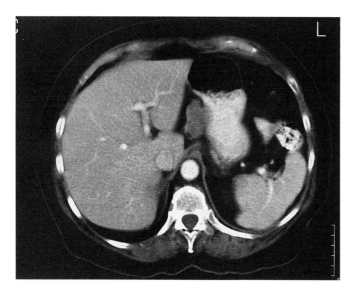

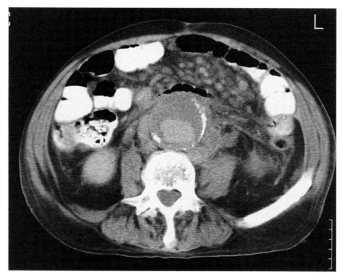

Fig. 10.60 Left gastric lymphadenopathy, malignant melanoma. The spiral CECT in a patient with widespread metastatic malignant melanoma shows a 3 cm mass lesion involving left gastric nodes contiguous with the lesser curve of the stomach.

Fig. 10.62 Mesenteric lymphadenopathy. A spiral CECT in a male patient with prostatic carcinoma shows multiple enlarged mesenteric nodes, together with para-aortic lymphadenopathy, related to a moderate-sized abdominal aortic aneurysm.

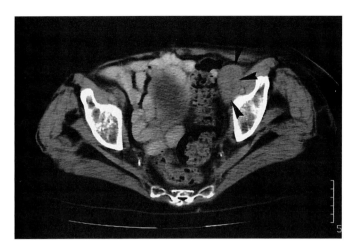

Fig. 10.63 Left iliac lymphadenopathy. A spiral CT scan was taken in a 70-year-old female patient with non-Hodgkin's lymphoma which had been previously treated with chemotherapy with a good response. There was recent swelling of the left lower limb, and a normal venogram. There is a discrete lymph-node mass in the left iliac fossa, almost 5 cm in diameter (arrowheads), displacing the sigmoid colon medially.

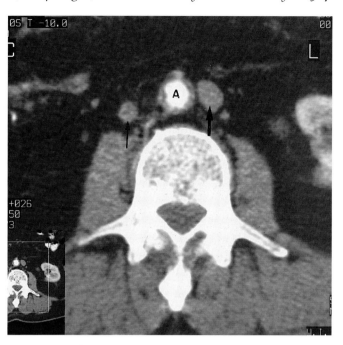

Fig. 10.65 Duplication of the IVC. This spiral CECT in a male patient with no relevant symptoms shows a well-circumscribed structure adjacent to the abdominal aorta (A) on the left side (thick arrow). On other sections, the tubular nature of the structure was apparent, becoming continuous with the left renal vein. It should not be confused with lymphadenopathy. The right-sided IVC (thin arrow) is of smaller calibre than usual.

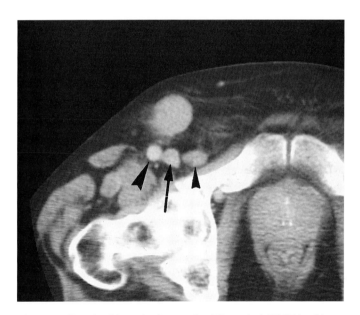

Fig. 10.64 Inguinal lymphadenopathy. The spiral CECT in this 71-year-old male patient with carcinoma of anus and mass in right groin shows a 2.5 cm mass lesion in the right groin lying anterior to the femoral artery (large arrowhead) and femoral vein (arrow). A second enlarged lymph node is shown in the femoral canal (small arrowhead).

Index